Practical Periodontal Diagnosis and Treatment Planning

# Practical Periodontal Diagnosis and Treatment Planning

*Edited by Serge Dibart and Thomas Dietrich*

Second Edition

**WILEY** Blackwell

*Edition History*
Blackwell Publishing (1e, 2010)

*Registered Office*
John Wiley & Sons, Inc., 111 River Street, Hoboken, NJ 07030, USA

For details of our global editorial offices, customer services, and more information about Wiley products visit us at www.wiley.com.

Wiley also publishes its books in a variety of electronic formats and by print-on-demand. Some content that appears in standard print versions of this book may not be available in other formats.

*Limit of Liability/Disclaimer of Warranty*
The contents of this work are intended to further general scientific research, understanding, and discussion only and are not intended and should not be relied upon as recommending or promoting scientific method, diagnosis, or treatment by physicians for any particular patient. In view of ongoing research, equipment modifications, changes in governmental regulations, and the constant flow of information relating to the use of medicines, equipment, and devices, the reader is urged to review and evaluate the information provided in the package insert or instructions for each medicine, equipment, or device for, among other things, any changes in the instructions or indication of usage and for added warnings and precautions. While the publisher and authors have used their best efforts in preparing this work, they make no representations or warranties with respect to the accuracy or completeness of the contents of this work and specifically disclaim all warranties, including without limitation any implied warranties of merchantability or fitness for a particular purpose. No warranty may be created or extended by sales representatives, written sales materials or promotional statements for this work. This work is sold with the understanding that the publisher is not engaged in rendering professional services. The advice and strategies contained herein may not be suitable for your situation. You should consult with a specialist where appropriate. The fact that an organization, website, or product is referred to in this work as a citation and/or potential source of further information does not mean that the publisher and authors endorse the information or services the organization, website, or product may provide or recommendations it may make. Further, readers should be aware that websites listed in this work may have changed or disappeared between when this work was written and when it is read. Neither the publisher nor authors shall be liable for any loss of profit or any other commercial damages, including but not limited to special, incidental, consequential, or other damages.

*Library of Congress Cataloging-in-Publication Data*
Names: Dibart, Serge, editor. | Dietrich, Thomas, 1969- editor.
Title: Practical periodontal diagnosis and treatment planning / edited by Serge Dibart, Thomas Dietrich.
Description: Second edition. | Hoboken, NJ : Wiley-Blackwell, 2024. | Includes bibliographical references and index.
Identifiers: LCCN 2023041028 (print) | LCCN 2023041029 (ebook) | ISBN 9781119830313 (hardback) |
    ISBN 9781119830320 (pdf) | ISBN 9781119830337 (epub) | ISBN 9781119830344 (ebook)
Subjects: MESH: Periodontal Diseases--diagnosis | Periodontal Diseases--therapy | Patient Care Planning |
    Evidence-Based Dentistry--methods
Classification: LCC RK450.P4 (print) | LCC RK450.P4 (ebook) | NLM WU 241 | DDC 617.6/32--dc23/eng/20231023
LC record available at https://lccn.loc.gov/2023041028
LC ebook record available at https://lccn.loc.gov/2023041029

Cover Image: © Serge Dibart
Cover Design: Wiley

Set in 9.5/12.5pt STIXTwoText by Integra Software Services Pvt. Ltd, Pondicherry, India

SKY10060715_112423

# Contents

# List of Contributors

## Editors:

**Serge Dibart, DMD**
Professor of Periodontology and Oral Biology Director,
Post-Graduate Program and 2nd Floor Specialty Clinics
Boston University School of Dental Medicine
100 East Newton Street Boston, MA

**Thomas Dietrich, MD, DMD, MPH**
Professor and Head of Oral Surgery The School of
Dentistry University of Birmingham 5 Mill Pool Way,
Birmingham B5 7EG United Kingdom

## Contributors:

**Massimo Di Battista, DMD, MSD**
Private Practice Limited to Periodontology and
Implant Dentistry,
Montréal, Québec, Canada

**Iain L.C. Chapple, DDS, PhD**
Professor, Director of Research Institute of Clinical
Sciences
Institute of Clinical Sciences
College of Medical & Dental Sciences
The University of Birmingham

**Sheilesh Dave, DDS, MSD, CAGS, deceased**
Practice limited to Periodontology and
Implant Dentistry 1333 8th Street SW Calgary,
Alberta, Canada

**Thomas Van Dyke, DDS, PhD**
Professor, Department of Periodontology and
Oral Biology Director, Clinical Research Center Boston
University School of Dental Medicine 100 East Newton
Street Boston, MA

**Paul S. Farsai, DMD, MPH, FACD**
Associate Professor, Director of Evidence-based Dentistry
and Behavioral Sciences Department of General Dentistry
Boston University School of Dental Medicine 72 East
Concord Street—Robinson Room 334, Boston, MA

**Jeremy Kernitsky-Barnatan, DDS, MSD**
Clinical Director and Clinical Assistant Professor
Advanced Education Program, Department of
Periodontology
Henry M. Goldman School of Dental Medicine
635 Albany Street, Suite G-200, Boston, MA

**Raman Kohli, DDS, MSc, FRCD(c)**
Practice limited to Periodontology and Implant Dentistry
3155 Harvester Rd., Suite 401 Burlington, Ontario, Canada

**Annika Kroeger Dr. med. dent.**
School of Dentistry, University of Birmingham, UK

**Cataldo W. Leone, DMD, DMSc**
Professor of Periodontology and Oral Biology Associate
Dean for Academic Affairs
Diplomate, American Board of Periodontology Boston
University Goldman School of Dental
Medicine 100 East Newton Street Boston, MA

**Luca Landi, MD, DDS**
Practice limited to Periodontology and Implant Dentistry
Via della Balduina 114 Roma, Italy

**Gail McCausland, DMD, M.Dent.Sci., FICD**
Clinical Professor and Assistant Dean for Academic
Affairs, Boston University Henry M. Goldman
School of Dental Medicine, 72 East Concord Street;
Robinson Suite B309
Boston, MA

**Lorenzo Montesani, DDS**
Implant Fellow, Department of Periodontology
Henry M. Goldman School of Dental Medicine
635 Albany Street, Suite G-200, Boston, MA

**Steven M. Morgano, DMD**
Professor and Director, Division of Postdoctoral
Prosthodontics Department of Restorative Sciences and
Biomaterials Boston University School of Dental Medicine
100 East Newton Street Boston, MA

**Christoph A. Ramseier, MAS**
Privatdozent, Scientific Associate, Periodontist SSO,
EFPMaster of Advanced Studies (MAS) in Periodontology
University of Bernzmk bernSchool of Dental
Medicine Department of Periodontology Freiburgstrasse
7CH-3010 Bern Switzerland

**Dimitra Sakellari, DDS, PhD**
Assistant Professor Department of Preventive Dentistry,
Periodontology, and Implant Dentistry Aristotle
University of Thessaloniki Dental School 212 A. Vas.
Olgas Avenue Thessaloniki, Greece

**Carolina Miller Mattos de Santana, DDS, MScD, PhD**
Associate Professor
Universidade Federal Fluminense, Department of
Periodontology
Rio de Janeiro, Brazil

**Ronaldo Barcellos de Santana, DDS, MScD, DSc**
Professor, Deputy Chair of Periodontology
Director of MSc program and Research in Periodontology
Temple University, Maurice H. Kornberg School of
Dentistry, Department of Periodontology and Oral
Biology, Philadelphia, USA

**Praveen Sharma BDS, MFDS (RCS Edin.), FHEA, FDS
(Restorative Dentistry) (RCS Edin.), PhD**
Associate Professor & Honorary Consultant in Restorative
Dentistry University of Birmingham School of Dentistry
Birmingham, UK

**Bradford Towne, DMD**
Retired, Oral and Maxillofacial Surgery, 3600 Golden
Cascade Ln, Indian Land, SC. USA

**Mehmet Ilhan Uzel, DMD, DSc**
Clinical Associate Professor, Department of Periodontics
Director, International Program in Periodontics and
Implant Dentistry University of Pennsylvania School of
Dental Medicine Robert Schattner Center, Evans Building
240 S. 40th Street Philadelphia, PA

**Clemens Walter Prof. Dr. med. dent**
Charité – Berlin University of Medicine, Department of
Periodontology, Oral Medicine and Oral Surgery
Berlin, Germany

# Preface

Welcome to the second edition of *Practical Periodontal Diagnosis and Treatment Planning*, skillfully edited by Serge Dibart and Thomas Dietrich. This edition delves into the foundational principles of periodontal and dental implant therapy, with a focus on processes that culminate in accurate diagnoses and well-rounded, pragmatic treatment planning. The methodology embraced is evidence-based, retaining the integrity of the first edition, while also offering a refreshingly practical approach. The reader is guided systematically from risk assessment through minimally invasive therapies to rehabilitation, whether through surgical tissue regeneration or dental implant therapy.

This edition confronts the complexities of the 2017 International Workshop Classification of Periodontal and Peri-implant Diseases and Conditions. It contrasts the new system with the 1999 classification, enlightening readers on the rationale and evolution that led to what is now known as the 2018 Classification. The reader is provided with a hands-on guide to implementation in day-to-day practice, along with comprehensive explanations of the radical changes in thinking that shaped the 2018 classification.

The book features three new and very engaging chapters. The first explores the classification topic mentioned above; the second delves into the rapid emergence of digital systems within dental practice. These systems now form the crux of three-dimensional planning in dento-facial aesthetics, extending beyond mere "in-silico" modeling by interfacing with contemporary recording techniques for dento-facial parameters, and transitioning through to innovative methods of implementation such as dynamic surgery with navigation and robotic placement systems. The final chapter on prosthetic rehabilitation, employing digitized systems, actualizes the initial planning and fulfills the patient care circle.

The third fresh chapter examines a subject of great contemporary relevance: the human pursuit of beauty and the harmonization of facial features. These considerations have increasingly become essential to the well-being and self-confidence of many individuals in the twenty-first century. The chapter delves into the meticulous knowledge and appreciation of applied facial anatomy, risk–benefit assessment, and the critically important concept of informed consent, required for the successful implementation of various facial tissue management strategies. Although the impact of such interventions can be transformative, a clear understanding of the risks, side effects, and psychological effects of facial remodeling is emphasized.

Doctors Dibart and Dietrich have once again orchestrated a harmonious collaboration of experts in their respective fields, updating the first edition of this vital textbook to resonate with the pulse of this rapidly changing and dynamic discipline. The book's relevance extends to periodontists, periodontal residents, general dentists with a special interest in this rapidly evolving field, oral surgeons, dental hygienists, and dental students alike. With something to offer the entire periodontal team, the evidence-based approach reassures readers that the content is delivered in a manner that is both balanced, state-of-the-art, and eminently practical.

*Iain L. C. Chapple*

# 1

## The Necessity of an Evidence-based Approach to Diagnosis and Treatment

*Paul Farsai and Thomas Van Dyke*

Today, the concept of evidence-based healthcare surrounding our clinical practice of dentistry is discussed more than ever. However, many times this term is used to define anything *but* "evidence-based dentistry" (EBD).

The term "evidence-based" has evolved through certain iterations through the years. Archie Cochrane initiated the discussion of putting into action the concept of science-based medicine when in 1971 he published *Effectiveness and Efficiency: Random Reflections of Health Services* (Cochrane 1972). In 1992 a clinical epidemiology group at McMaster University in Canada (Evidence Based Medicine Working Group 1992) published a paper on evidence-based healthcare (EBM Working Group 1992). Their article described their challenge to adopt an "evidence-based practice" (EBP) approach since it "de-emphasizes intuition, unsystematic clinical experience and pathophysiological rationale as sufficient grounds for clinical decision making." The paper was written with the clear intent of placing a greater emphasis on a systematic appraisal of the evidence.

The first well-defined use of the term "evidence-based" in the UK was in a 1996 *British Medical Journal* article by David Sackett et al. (Sackett et al. 1996) and was defined as the "... conscientious, explicit and judicious use of current best evidence in making decisions about the care of individual patients."

The term "current best evidence" is the operative word here, because it implies that our best available evidence should by definition change as we progress through more research findings, to the point that what was true as the best available evidence even as recently as ten years ago in dentistry in some respects is not even true today. Many examples come to mind, such as digital technologies in scanning, designing, milling, or printing restorations and appliances; the newer adhesive systems; newer generations of composites; more nonsurgical and adjunctive periodontal therapies; different dental implant systems, shapes, sizes, components or engineered surfaces; and more procedure-specific use of biomaterials as well as therapies, all due to better applied research results, and so on.

The American Dental Association (ADA) has defined the concept of EBD as:

> An approach to oral health care that requires the judicious integration of systematic assessments of clinically relevant scientific evidence, relating to the patient's oral and medical condition and history, with the dentist's clinical expertise and the patient's treatment needs and preferences.
>
> *(Sackett et al. 1996)*

EBD has five components. This premise is simply based on the notion that to perform a scientific search for the current best evidence, one must be able to interpret the clinical scenario, translate it into searchable terminology, and then find the best evidence by critically assessing the quality and the appropriateness of the published evidence to address the identified clinical scenario. The five components are:

1) **Translate a clinical problem into a question.** For example: A new patient who is pregnant comes to see you with a chief complaint that she wants a second opinion on her need for periodontal surgery. She has heard periodontal disease may cause low-birth-weight babies and asks, "Do I really need surgery, or could I just have dental cleanings (scaling and root planing) to prevent a low-birth-weight baby?" An easy method to translate a clinical scenario into a searchable format is by using the PICO structure. PICO is an acronym for **P**roblem, **I**ntervention (or Index, i.e., a category or condition), **C**omparison, and **O**utcome. So, by using PICO, one would devise the following structured format for the example described above:

How would I describe the dental **P**roblem or population?

"In *pregnant patients* ..."

Which main **I**ntervention or index am I considering?

"With *periodontal disease* ..."

What is the main **C**omparison or alternative?

"Compared to *pregnant people (patients) without periodontal disease*."

What is the **O**utcome to be studied?

"Is there a greater risk of "*low-birth-weight babies?*""

2) **Effectively search for the best evidence.** For this component, one must determine which databases to search and then use the appropriate databases and search filters to find the best evidence. The most common database is Medline (accessible via many free Internet portals such as www.pubmed.gov); however, there are many highly specialized databases such as Psychlit for behavioral research, Cancerlit for cancer literature, and NHSEED for economic evaluation research (UK) (see Chapter 4) As a source of high-level study designs, the Cochrane Oral Health Group (OHG), which originated in New England in 1994 and moved to Manchester (UK) in 1996, now has a registry (at the time of print) of 174 reviews, 28 protocols, and 214 subtopics in dentistry (https://oralhealth.cochrane.org). Summaries of the reviews are listed on the OHG website.

The term "filter" refers to the strategy for condensing thousands of articles into a more refined or limited set of relevant data. Filtration could be based on "human" topics, "English" language articles, a certain period of time (certain decade of research and beyond), and so on (many more filtration strategies are available). For the abovementioned example, a search of the best evidence yielded the following number of articles (at the time of print):

- 199,124 articles that include the word "pregnant"
- 100,793 articles that include the words "periodontal disease"
- 716 articles that include the words "pregnant" and "no periodontal disease"
- 59,888 articles that include the words "low-birth-weight": Clearly, reading more than 360,000 articles to address our clinical scenario is neither indicated nor necessary. By using just "human" subjects and "English" language as our limits for our filtration strategy, we came up with 198 articles that describe the association (or lack thereof) between periodontal disease in pregnant patients and low-birth-weight babies. A further review of the articles and additional filtration (specificity and sensitivity) yielded 37 articles that describe the potential link between pregnant patients with periodontal disease and the risk for preterm and low-birth-weight babies.

3) **Critically appraise the evidence.** One must critically read and evaluate the basis of the articles at hand (all 37 of the articles). This means that for this component level, one must assess at some foundational level the quality of the research methodology, the study design, the statistical analyses, and the conclusions that are published in each research article. It should be noted that the mere fact that an article is published (in a reputable journal or otherwise) does *not* mean that the study design, the research methods, the statistical analyses, or the conclusions were/are appropriate. Certain clinical or patient-centered questions can be best answered and more scientifically based if they are investigated through specific research designs or methods. For example, randomized control trials are suitable and indicated for the majority of therapeutic interventions, whereas cohort studies are suitable in design to answer questions on prognosis. Critical appraisal skills are evaluative skills that are taught and developed over time with appropriate supervision from knowledgeable and skilled individuals.

For our example, there are 37 studies that show some level of association between low-birth-weight and periodontal disease. The discrepancies come from the use of methods used in conducting the research, the appropriateness of the statistical analyses in interpreting the data, the various study designs compared in the studies, the process by which the data were collected, the criteria used for inclusion or exclusion of risk factors, or the lack of such parameters, and so on. However, care must be taken not to introduce bias, conscious or unconscious, at this step. Filters cannot be arbitrary or be used to eliminate studies that do not seem to support the beliefs of the evaluator of the studies. While the critical review of pertinent studies is intended to eliminate bias, there is that potential every time a decision is made on which studies to include. As a hypothetical example, a filter of studies of at least 9 months duration might be imposed, but the majority of studies are of 6 months duration. It is possible that the majority of studies of 6 months contradict one or two 9-month studies. Eliminating the shorter studies is eliminating valuable information and if only 9-month studies are reported, the outcome is biased.

4) **Apply appraisal results to clinical practice.** At this time, if one critically appraises and assesses the quality of the research findings for our abovementioned clinical scenario, the evidence is mounting and suggests a new risk factor—periodontal disease. Pregnant women who have periodontal disease may be seven times more likely to have a baby that is born too early and too small.

More research is certainly needed to confirm how periodontal disease may affect pregnancy outcomes. It appears that periodontal disease triggers increased levels of biological mediators that induce labor. Furthermore, data suggest that women whose periodontal condition worsens during pregnancy have an even higher risk of having a premature baby.

Therefore, by using the most current published clinical evidence available, clinicians in private practice can make the judicious recommendation to their patients that periodontal disease may in fact be a significant risk for a preterm, low-birth-weight baby.

We ask you, the reader, a rhetorical question now: Is this in fact what we are currently telling our patients? If not, then why? More importantly, what is the level of appropriate scientific evidence that supports these communications or recommendations with our patients? Certainly, then, an understanding of the levels of evidence in scientific research becomes necessary for any clinician to judiciously take the research recommendations and translate them to clinical practice (see Chapter 4).

5) **Evaluate application step and outcomes.** As with any treatment modality, good science and good patient care must be evaluated once it is rendered. Some therapy or treatment (or preventive care) can be assessed shortly after it has been rendered, and for other occasions, the evaluation of the applied care must be assessed within a much wider time span. Nevertheless, evaluation of outcomes is a necessary component of responsible and appropriate evidence-based healthcare.

From a study design standpoint, identifying whether periodontal disease actually causes preterm, low-birth-weight babies is very difficult to measure with the presence of other variables.

Ethical issues also arise in a clinical trial if periodontal treatment is withheld for an indefinite period from half of the subjects, so technically this question cannot be measured well.

Regardless of whether this association is proven or not, dentists have nothing to lose by encouraging their patients to take care of their teeth.

Other salient topics with respect to periodontal disease and systemic disease include the suggested link between cardiovascular disease and periodontal inflammation. There is a wealth of cross-sectional studies (which yield limited assessment opportunities) that suggest the association is not random, but longitudinal studies that evaluate outcomes (and allow for multiple assessments) that predict cardiovascular events in people with periodontitis have been lacking. New evidence has been recently reported that independently associates major adverse cardiovascular events (MACE) with periodontal disease activity. Periodontal disease activity is defined as active inflammation of the periodontium, as opposed to a history of periodontal disease that is most often defined by radiographic bone loss. In this study, periodontal inflammation was a significant predictor of MACE. Interestingly, investigation of the mechanism for this observation is consistent with increased periodontal inflammation causing increased arterial inflammation (Van Dyke et al. 2021). While the study and the proposed mechanism seem plausible, it is a single study that has to be repeated in other settings. Thus, advising patients that the association has been proven is still premature. However, advising patients that periodontitis is associated with increased *risk* for developing cardiovascular disease is supported by literature using evidence-based evaluations (Sanz et al. 2020; Tonetti and Van Dyke 2013).

## Problems with Introducing EBD

In the past 20 years, dentists have become more aware of the existence of EBD and generally, the progress from initial skepticism to a more positive attitude of the use of EBD is palpable among the members of the profession. This observation is reflected by the formation of the ADA's Center for Evidence Based Dentistry, the implementation of EBD concepts in dental school curricula dictated by new ADA Commission on Dental Accreditation (CODA) standards for teaching dental students, and by journals and meetings/conferences all over the world emphasizing EBD concepts.

However, the main barriers to the implementation of EBD into practice have also been identified in many studies (Iqbal and Glenny 2002; Sbaraini et al. 2012; Straub-Morarend et al. 2013). So why are dentists not putting EBD into practice?

### Amount of Evidence

There are currently about 500 journals related to dentistry and not all are relevant to all areas of dental practice, nor can a busy practitioner read any more than a small handful of articles routinely.

### Quality of Evidence

Because enhancing career prospects in academia is partially tied to the number of publications someone authors, much of the ever-increasing volume of evidence produced is not necessarily to increase the knowledge base, which in essence compromises quality. In addition, a number of publications that are widely read are not subject to peer review, and even when peer review exists, there is always the unfortunate reality of publication bias (defined as the tendency by both researchers and editors to publish positive reviews or results).

### Dissemination of Evidence

History has shown that even in the presence of good evidence, the application phase of EBD can take many years to become the norm or standard in practice. Unless good methods of dissemination are available, good evidence can go to waste. Conversely, even with scant or insignificant differences in evidence from the *status quo*, many new products and procedures have been introduced to the marketplace simply because interest and desire exists to integrate a change in practice.

### Practice Based on Authority Rather than on Evidence

Common practice in professional development and continuing education demonstrates that the dental school model, which uses techniques or therapies based on views of authority rather than evidence, may lead to the wrong or outdated treatment being performed.

## Advantages of EBD

### What Constitutes Evidence?

Personal clinical examination, including specific findings from history and results from tests, constitutes evidence. Research evidence is a manifestation of a much larger scale of interventions and, therefore, becomes a stronger tool for clinical decision making because it extends beyond individual experience. This should not, however, replace individual experience but rather anchor our clinical experience from years of practice. Sound reproducible research outcomes should enable clinicians to recognize gaps and uncertainties in their knowledge rather than wait for the next patient to expose our inadequacies. This implies a marriage between the research process and the clinical application of that process, hence the need for a continuous process of reading, learning, and applying a dynamic field of information.

### What Is Good Evidence?

The randomized controlled trial (RCT) study design is the gold standard for evidence for treatment-related questions. An even better level of evidence is a systematic review or a meta-analysis of a series of RCTs. However, this is only true for the clinical question regarding therapeutics. For other clinical questions, a study design hierarchy exists to determine the levels of evidence (see Chapter 4). This means that in the EBD process, no evidence is considered to be bad evidence; there are just levels of applicable good, better, and best evidence.

### Finding and Making Sense of Evidence

After finding the evidence, one needs to make sense of it. This appraisal should be critical; after all, no research design is perfect, and the health status of a person is at stake. The Critical Appraisal Skills Program (CASP) at Oxford University has developed a worksheet that can be used while reading and interpreting published articles to make sense of the evidence (https://www.cebm.ox.ac.uk/resources/ebm-tools/critical-appraisal-tools). The aim of the critical appraisal is to systematically consider the validity, results, and relevance to our own clinical practice.

EBD improves the effective use of research evidence in clinical practice. If used judiciously, it favors the early uptake of new and better treatments or results in the early rejection of ineffective treatments. It uses resources more effectively. For example, a systematic review of materials may lead to the earlier adoption of the most effective ones and the subsequent reduction in replacement levels, thereby saving resources.

EBD relies on evidence rather than authority for clinical decision-making. Regular reviewing of currently available literature should develop us as practitioners, so we attain the skills to evaluate evidence for ourselves based on our own experiences rather than have someone interpret the data for us.

To use this approach, we need to develop new interpretive skills for identifying clinical problems, searching literature by using conventional and electronic means, and improving our critical appraisal skills. In the same spirit, this book encompasses practical evidence-based developments in diagnosis and treatment planning for a periodontal patient.

## References

Evidence-Based Databases as part of the ADA Library. About EBD. https://www.ada.org/en/resources/ada-library/evidence-based-databases (accessed June 2021).

Cochrane, A.L. (1972). *Effectiveness and Efficiency: Random Reflections on Health Services*. London: Nuffield Provincial Hospitals Trust. https://www.nuffieldtrust.org.uk/research/efectiveness-and-efficiency-random-refections-on-health-services (accessed June 2021).

EBM Working Group (1992). Evidence based medicine. *JAMA* 268: 2420–2425.

Iqbal, A. and Glenny, A.-M. (2002). General dental practitioners' knowledge of and attitudes towards evidence based practice. *Br. Dent. J* 193: 587–591. 18.

Sackett, D.L., Rosenberg, W.M., Gray, J.A. et al. (1996). Evidence based medicine: what it is and what it isn't. *BMJ* 312 (7023): 71–72.

Sanz, M., Del Castillo, A.M., Jepsen, S. et al. (2020 February 3). Periodontitis and cardiovascular diseases. Consensus report. *Glob. Heart* 15 (1): 1.

Sbaraini, A., Carter, S.M., and Evans, R.W. (2012). How do dentists understand evidence and adopt it in practice? *Health Educ. J* 71: 195–204.

Straub-Morarend, C.L., Marshall, T.A., Holmes, D.C., and Finkelstein, M.W. (2013). Toward defining dentists' evidence-based practice: influence of decade of dental school graduation and scope of practice on implementation and perceived obstacles. *J. Dent. Educ* 77: 137–145. 17.

Tonetti, M.S. and Van Dyke, T.E. (2013 April). working group 1 of the joint EFP/AAP workshop. Periodontitis and atherosclerotic cardiovascular disease: consensus report of the Joint EFP/AAP Workshop on periodontitis and systemic diseases. *J. Periodontol* 84 (4 Suppl): S24–S29.

Van Dyke, T.E., Kholy, K.E., Ishai, A. et al. (2021 March). Inflammation of the periodontium associates with risk of future cardiovascular events. *J. Periodontol* 92 (3): 348–358.

## 2

## Classification of Periodontal Diseases and Conditions

*Jeremy Kernitsky and Gail McCausland*

### Diagnosis and Classification—AAP 2017

#### History

In 1999 the American Academy of Periodontology assembled an International Workshop for a Classification of Periodontal Diseases and Conditions; this resulted in what became known as the 1999 Armitage Classification. In 2014 an AAP task force looking at the classification determined three areas of concern; attachment level (although clinical attachment level (CAL) is important for research it proved to be overly time consuming in everyday clinical practice); chronic versus aggressive periodontitis; and localized versus generalized periodontitis. In 2017 World Workshop on the Classification of Periodontal Disease and Peri-Implant Conditions was formed to update and standardize the previous 1999 classification and to develop a similar classification for peri-implant diseases and conditions.

The main differences between the 1999 and the 2017 classifications are: Firstly, different statuses of periodontal and gingival health were described. Secondly, that three forms of periodontitis were identified: necrotizing periodontitis, periodontitis as a manifestation of systemic disease, and periodontitis (comprising the forms of disease previously recognized as "chronic" or "aggressive"). Thirdly, this new classification system encompasses a multidimensional view of periodontitis using a staging and grading system. Fourthly, a change in the classification gingival recessions, and the change of terminology of periodontal biotype for periodontal phenotype. Finally, there was a significant expansion in the descriptions of peri-implant health, peri-implant mucositis, and peri-implantitis.

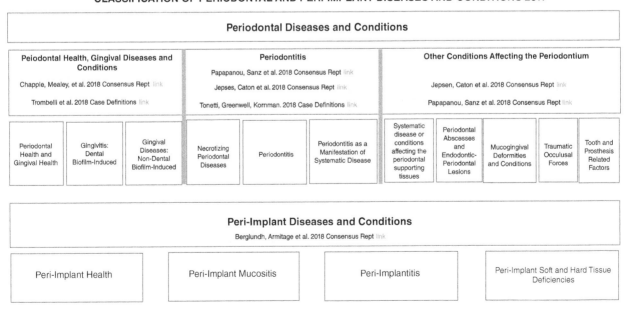

Figure 2.1   Classification of periodontal and peri-implant diseases and conditions 2017 (Caton et al., 2018). Adapted from AAP, Journal of Periodontology.

*Practical Periodontal Diagnosis and Treatment Planning*, Second Edition. Edited by Serge Dibart and Thomas Dietrich.
© 2024 John Wiley & Sons, Inc. Published 2024 by John Wiley & Sons, Inc.

1) **Periodontal Health, Gingival Diseases and Conditions**

   a) Periodontal Health and Gingival Health

   The 2017 world workshop for the classification of periodontal diseases (Chapple et al. 2018) defined periodontal health and gingival health into three different entities based on the history of periodontal disease of the patient and presence or absence of clinical attachment level: intact periodontium, reduced periodontium in a non-periodontitis patient, and reduced periodontium in a successfully treated stable periodontitis patient (Table 2.1).

   It is important to mention that there is certain level of tolerance between the definition of periodontal health on an intact periodontium and gingivitis (dental plaque induced) of less than 10% bleeding on probing on all the sites. If there is any presence of loss in the clinical attachment level the correct term to use would be of a reduced periodontium while the differences on bleeding on probing will determine the health status of the periodontium.

   Interestingly, patients with a reduced periodontium due to periodontitis successfully treated previously can present with increased probing depths of up to 4 mm, this is due that probing depths of <3 mm are rarely achieved on a 100% of treated sites, therefore it could lead to overtreatment as any non-bleeding site of >3 mm would not be considered "health" and would require further treatment instead of monitoring and supportive care. Yet, in the case of gingivitis patients the maximum allowed probing depth was set to 3 mm irrespective of the previous periodontal history of the patient.

   b) **Gingivitis: Dental Biofilm-Induced**

   I) Associated with dental biofilm **alone**

   As explained before, based on the history of periodontal disease of the patient, there are three possible entities to diagnose dental biofilm-induced gingivitis which can be seen in Table 2.1.

   Whether they are associated with hormonal imbalances, mediations, systemic disorders, or malnutrition, these gingival diseases have the following characteristics in common (Mariotti 1999; Trombelli et al. 2018):

**Table 2.1** Diagnostic guideline for periodontal health and gingivitis. Based on 2017 world workshop. Adapted from Chapple et al. 2018.

| Intact Periodontium | Health | Gingivitis |
| --- | --- | --- |
| Probing attachment loss | No | No |
| Probing pocket depths (assuming no pseudo pockets) | ≤3 mm | ≤3 mm |
| Bleeding on probing | <10% | Yes (>10%) |
| Radiological bone loss | No | No |
| **Reduced periodontium Non-periodontitis patient** | **Health** | **Gingivitis** |
| Probing attachment loss | Yes | Yes |
| Probing pocket depths (assuming no pseudo pockets) | ≤3 mm | ≤3 mm |
| Bleeding on probing | <10% | Yes (>10%) |
| Radiological bone loss | Possible | Possible |
| **Successfully treated stable periodontitis patient** | **Health** | **Gingivitis in a patient with history of periodontitis** |
| Probing attachment loss | Yes | Yes |
| Probing pocket depths (assuming no pseudo pockets) | ≤4 mm (no site ≥4 mm with BOP) | ≤3 mm |
| Bleeding on probing | <10% | <10% |
| Radiological bone loss | Possible | Possible |

- The signs and symptoms are confined to the gingiva.
- Plaque is the main etiological factor which will initiate or exacerbate the gingival lesions.
- Inflammation of the gingival tissues will produce changes in color (transition to a red/bluish-red hue), shape (enlarged gingival contours due to edema or fibrosis), texture, bleeding upon stimulation, and elevated sulcular temperature (Figure 2.2).
- There is no alveolar bone loss and pocket depth; clinical attachment levels around teeth are stable.
- This is a reversible condition which resolves upon removal of the etiological factors.
- Possible role as a precursor to attachment loss around teeth.

Gingivitis primarily induced by dental plaque includes the following disease subdivisions:

1) Gingivitis associated with dental biofilm only: Signs and symptoms typical of gingivitis can be observed at all ages of dentate populations and this disease has been considered to be the most common form of periodontal disease (Page 1985). The disease can be observed in a child as young as five years of age, progress with a peak during puberty, and remain present throughout life at various extents. Plaque is present at the gingival margin and a positive correlation exists between gingivitis and plaque accumulation.

   There is no pathognomonic flora associated with gingivitis, although the dental plaque in gingivitis differs from that present in gingival health (Ranney 1993). Note that gingivitis may also occur on a reduced periodontium (decreased amount of alveolar bone height and connective tissue support around teeth) which was previously surgically treated for a periodontitis. This situation is encountered when there is a recurrence of inflammation of the marginal gingiva on a periodon-

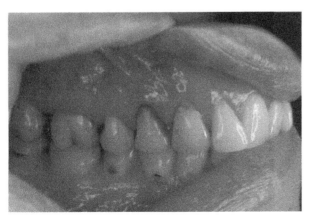

**Figure 2.2** Localized gingivitis, characterized by bleeding upon probing. There is no attachment loss.

tium with previous attachment loss but without any evidence of progressive attachment loss (no indication of active disease) (Mariotti 1999; Trombelli et al. 2018).

II) Mediated by systemic or local risk factors
   a) Systemic risk factor (modifying factors)
      i) Smoking
         Smoking is one of the major risk factors for periodontitis, due to its effects upon gingival tissues. Among the effects we can identify: microvascular vasoconstriction and fibrosis. These can mask clinical signs of inflammation, such as bleeding on probing, despite the presence of a significant underlying pathological inflammatory response in the gingival tissues.
      ii) Hyperglycemia
         Diabetes-mellitus-associated gingivitis: Diabetes mellitus is a complex disease with varying degrees of systemic and oral complications involving abnormalities in insulin production, fat, proteins, and sugar metabolism, and resulting in an impaired vascular and immune system as well as an inadequate inflammatory response. Diabetes mellitus is categorized as Type 1 and Type 2. Type 1 develops due to impaired production of insulin and Type 2 is caused by deficient utilization of insulin. There is evidence to suggest that uncontrolled Type 1 diabetes in children is associated with exaggerated response of the gingival tissues to dental plaque (Lindhe 2003). It is a reversible condition once the diabetes is under control and the dental plaque is removed.
      iii) Nutritional factors
         Ascorbic acid deficiency gingivitis: Nutritional deficiencies such as ascorbic acid (vitamin C deficiency) can significantly exacerbate the response of the gingiva to plaque bacteria (Mariotti 1999). The clinical description of severe vitamin C deficiency or scurvy consists of bulbous, spongy, hemorrhagic, swollen, and erythematous gingival lesions (Charbeneau et al. 1983). The result of compromised antioxidant micronutrient defenses to oxidative stress and impacts negatively collagen synthesis, resulting in weakened capillary blood vessel walls and consequent enhanced gingival bleeding. This condition is unusually seen in areas of adequate food supply but can potentially affect infants of low socioeconomic families, institutionalized elderly individuals, and alcoholics.
      iv) Pharmacological agents (prescription, non-prescription and recreational)

1) Oral contraceptives: Studies have shown that women taking oral contraceptive drugs have a higher incidence of gingival enlargement in comparison to women who do not take the medications (Kaufman 1969). Pronounced inflammation (change in gingival contour, color, exudate) is seen and is reversible upon removal of medications (Figure 2.3).

2) Other. In general any drug that may alter the salivary flow, impact endocrine function, and/or produce gingival enlargement (Trombelli et al. 2018).

v) Sex steroid hormones

1) Puberty

Puberty-associated gingivitis: A rise in gingival inflammation and gingival volume is noted during puberty in both sexes without necessarily seeing a rise in the quantity of plaque (Sutcliffe 1972). The incidence of the severity of gingivitis in adolescence is not only related to the rise in steroid hormones but is also influenced by a variety of factors such as dental caries, mouth breathing, teeth crowding, and tooth eruption (Stamm 1986). These changes are reversible after puberty. More specifically, hyperplastic gingivitis often seen during the adolescence period can be associated with:

— Orthodontic treatment: Note that fibrotic tissue tends to recur if surgical removal is attempted during orthodontic treatment. It is recommended to wait until orthodontic appliances are removed before surgically removing excess tissue (Figure 2.4).

— Mouth breathing: Mouth breathing, which often accompanies Angle's classification 2 division 1 malocclusion, is considered to be an exacerbating factor to gingivitis (Lindhe 2003). Gingival hyperplasia tends to affect

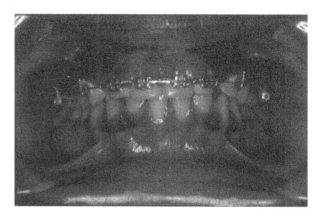

**Figure 2.4** Maxillary generalized gingivitis following the placement of braces. Notice the difference with the mandibular arch, which does not have braces.

mostly the anterior superior region and is also prone to recurrence if surgical removal is performed without any correction of the actual mouth breathing through orthodontic treatment or cessation of habit.

2) Menstrual cycle

Menstrual-cycle-associated gingivitis: The most common sign is a minor gingival inflammation during ovulation; gingival exudate has been shown to increase at least 20% in 75% of women (Hugoson 1971). This situation is reversible after ovulation.

**Note:** Hormonal gingivitis or postmenopausal gingivitis can be seen in women taking hormone replacement therapy. Signs and symptoms may involve atrophic, thin, erythematous gingival tissues, and patient complaints of gingival sensitivity to spicy foods and acidic beverages. Palliative treatment is suggested.

3) Pregnancy

a) Gingivitis: A combination of pregnancy hormones and dental plaque may increase the severity of gingivitis in women sensitive to local irritants. In addition to the typical gingivitis signs, severe inflammation can develop in the presence of relatively low amounts of dental plaque (Hugoson 1971). It will usually affect pregnant women in their second or third trimester, and is reversible after child delivery.

b) Pyogenic granuloma: This refers to a mass of hyperplastic gingival tissue principally found in the interdental maxillary regions. It is not a tumor but an exaggerated inflammatory response to irritation resulting in a solitary

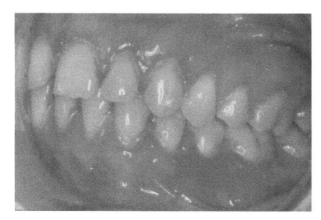

**Figure 2.3** Oral-contraceptive-induced gingivitis in a female patient. Notice the "red patch" in the lower left quadrant. Courtesy of Iain Chapple.

polyploid capillary hemangioma which can easily bleed upon mild provocation (Sills et al. 1996). Pregnancy-associated pyogenic granuloma presents clinically as a painless protuberant exophytic mass attached by a sessile or pedunculated base from the gingival margin. It has been reported to occur in 0.5–5% of pregnancies and can develop as early as the first trimester (Mariotti 1999). It usually regresses or completely disappears following parturition. If needed, surgical excision can be performed postpartum. The treatment for pregnancy-associated gingivitis and pyogenic granuloma during pregnancy is an impeccable control of the etiological factors (scaling, prophylaxis, and chlorhexidine rinses). This condition can also be classified under Epulides in the Reactive processes of non-dental plaque associated gingival conditions (Holmstrup et al. 2018).

4) Oral contraceptives
iv) Hematological conditions
1) Leukemia-associated gingivitis: Leukemia is a progressive malignant hematological disease characterized by the development of abnormal leukocytes and leukocytes precursors in the blood and bone marrow. Leukemia is classified according to disease progression (acute or chronic), cell types involved (myeloid or lymphoid), and cell numbers in blood (leukemic or aleukemic). The oral manifestations are acute, consisting of cervical adenopathies, petechia, gingival enlargements, and mucous ulcers. Dental plaque can exacerbate the gingival inflammatory changes which include swelling, redness/blueness, sponginess, and glazed appearance of the gingiva which is infiltrated with leukemic cells (Lindhe 2003). Persistent and unexplained gingival bleeding may indicate an underlying thrombocytopenia associated with the leukemic condition. Lesions are often found in the acute monocytic type, and consist of a modified gingival volume and bleeding of gingiva upon touch. Symptoms lessen when antiseptic mouthwashes are used and plaque volume is reduced.

2) Other
   b) Local risk factors
      i) Dental plaque biofilm retention factors
      ii) Oral dryness
      iii) Drug-influenced gingival enlargement

Drug-induced gingival enlargement: Three commonly used classes of medications create these lesions:

- Anti-convulsant drug used for treatment of epilepsy: Dilantin (Phenytoin sodium), 50% incidence (Angelopoulos et al. 1972)
- Immunosuppressant drug used to avoid host rejection of grafted tissues: Cyclosporine A, 25–30% incidence (Over time, this drug is tapered and the gingival enlargements become easier to control.) (Romito et al. 2004)
- Calcium channels blocking agents used as hypertensive drugs: Nifedipine, Verapamil, Diltiazem, 15–20% incidence (Barclay et al. 1992)

Over the years more medications have been described to induce gingival enlargement, such as (Bharti et al. 2013):

**Anticonvulsants**
- Ethosuximide
- Ethotoin
- Mephenytoin
- Methsuximide
- Phenobarbital
- Phenytoin
- Primidone
- Sodium valproate
- Vigabatrin

**Immunosuppressants**
- Cyclosporine
- Sirolimus
- Tacrolimus

**Calcium channel blockers**
- Amlodipine
- Diltiazem
- Felodipine
- Manidipine
- Nicardipine
- Nifedipine
- Nimodipine
- Nisoldipine
- Nitrendipine
- Verapamil

Individuals taking these medications may develop gingival enlargements leading to pseudopockets. Characteristics of drug-influenced gingival enlargement include (Mariotti 1999):

- Predilection of anterior gingiva; starts interproximally and expands
- Higher prevalence in children

- Onset within the first three months of taking the drug
- Enlargement of the gingival contours appears
- Stippling is present in the gingiva
- Pronounced inflammatory response in relation to the plaque volume
- Not associated with attachment loss but can be found in periodonitums with and without bone loss

Treatment consists of control of etiological factors followed by full mouth gingivectomy. Gingivectomy (full mouth or local) may need to be performed annually. If possible, the drugs can also be changed or dosages adjusted to improve the oral condition.

c) **Gingival Diseases: Non-Dental Biofilm-Induced**

Although these gingival lesions are not produced by plaque and do not disappear when plaque is removed, it should be noted that the severity of the clinical manifestation can often be related to the presence of bacterial plaque (Holmstrup et al. 2018).

a) Genetic/developmental disorders

   i) Hereditary gingival fibromatosis

   This gingival hyperplasia (gingival overgrowth) is an uncommon condition of genetic origin. Of idiopathic etiology, this condition develops irrespective of effective plaque removal. Hereditary gingival fibromatosis can be an isolated condition or part

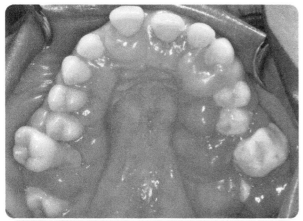
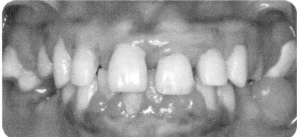

Figure 2.5   Gingival fibromatosis.

of a syndrome or systemic condition (Gorlin et al. 1990) (Figure 2.5).

b) Specific infections

   i) Bacterial origin

   These types of gingivitis and stomatitis can be found in immunocompromised and immunocompetent individuals. They occur when the microorganisms surpass innate host resistance. Clinical signs may range from painful, edematous ulcerations to asymptomatic cancers, mucosal patches, or atypical non-ulcerated inflamed gingiva. Lesions elsewhere on the body may also be present. Gingival lesions may occur due to infections with *Neisseria gonorrhea, Treponema pallidum*, streptococci, or other organisms.

   1) Neisseria gonorrhoeae (Gonorrhea)

   Gonorrhea is a sexually transmitted disease which can affect the oropharyngeal region in approximately 20% of infected individuals (Neville 2002). Diffuse erythema, small erosive pustules, and edema can be seen in this region as well as on tonsils and uvula. Gingivitis and stomatitis, as well as a sore throat and a cervical or submandibular lymphadenopathy, may also be present.

   2) Treponema pallidum (Syphilis)

   Syphilis is a chronic infection produced by *Treponema pallidum*. The primary modes of transmission are sexual contact or mother to fetus. The infection undergoes a characteristic evolution that classically proceeds through three stages: In primary syphilis, an asymptomatic contagious chancre appears three to four weeks post contact at the site of inoculation. When affecting the oral cavity, it can affect the lips, gingiva, tonsils, tongue, and palate. It leaves a scar and heals spontaneously. In secondary syphilis, whitish mucous patches as well as maculopalular cutaneous rashes are often present and are still contagious at this point. In tertiary syphilis, a noncontagious granulomatous inflammation (gumma) reaction appears which can often cause necrosis and perforation of the tongue or palate. Serious systemic conditions are involved (Neville et al. 2002).

   3) Mycobacterium tuberculosis (Tuberculosis)

4) Streptococcal gingivitis

An upper respiratory tract infection usually causes fever and accompanies a diffuse gingivitis, tonsillitis, pharyngitis, and ulceration of the oral mucosa. One of the most common species involved is the group A, β-hemolytic streptococci (Neville et al. 2002).

ii) Viral origin

Several viral infections are known to cause gingivitis. Most of them enter the body during childhood and may give rise to the disease followed by periods of latency.

1) Coxsackie virus (Hand-Foot-Mouth disease)

2) Herpes simplex I and II (primary or recurrent)

   - Primary herpetic gingigostomatitis: Herpes simplex virus type 1 (and occasionally type 2) is responsible for causing the primary infection which involves painful severe gingivitis with ulcerations (on keratinized and non-keratinized tissues) and edema followed by stomatitis. High fever and malaise is generally present. Vesicles on lips can produce a crusty lips appearance after rupturing (Miller 1992) (Figure 2.6).

     Palliative treatment only is required. The infection lasts approximately 10 days. During this period, the patient must be well hydrated with liquids and topical application of anesthetic agents is also indicated. Chlorhexidine and an antibiotic may be needed to prevent a super-infection. In the adult

infection, antiviral drugs such as Zovirax, #70, 200 mg, 1 tabqid, for 2 weeks can be prescribed.

   - Recurrent oral herpes: Reactivation of the virus resulting in recurrent infections occurs in 20–40% of individuals with the primary infection (Greenberg 1996). These lesions (vesicles which become ulcers) usually only affect the keratinized tissues and are usually present unilaterally or locally. The treatment, if any, can consist of topical antiviral ointment or tablets.

3) Varicella zoster (chickenpox—Shingles—V nerve)

Varicella-zoster virus causes varicella (chickenpox) as the primary self-limiting infection. The virus then remains latent and can be reactivated resulting in the herpes zoster infection. This painful unilateral infection is often seen in older individuals and is accompanied by cutaneous lesions of the affected nervous territory (Miller 1996).

4) Molluscum contagiosum

5) Human papilloma virus (squamous cell papilloma, condyloma acuminatum, verruca vulgaris, focal epithelial hyperplasia)

iii) Fungal origin

The most frequent oral fungal infections consist of candidosis and histoplasmosis.

1) Candidosis

Candida-species infections: *C. albicans* is one of the most frequent candida species affecting the oral cavity. It is considered an opportunistic infection occurring when the host resistance is diminished. Most subtypes of candidosis can be treated with antifungal medications (Ketoconazole 200 mg, 1 tab/day, 10 days, or Fluconazole 100 mg, 1 tab/ day, 14 days).

1) Generalized gingival candidosis include:

- Acute types:
  - Pseudomembranous candidosis: This type of infection produces soft white patches disseminated throughout the oral mucosa. These patches can be removed with an instrument leaving behind an erythematous mucosal surface.
  - Atrophic or erythematous candidosis: This type of infection produces red lesions spreading all over the oral mucosa. They are associated with severe pain and discomfort.

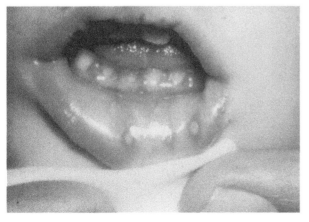

**Figure 2.6** Primary herpetic gingivostomatitis in a child. Notice the characteristic lesions on the lower lip. Courtesy of Iain Chapple.

- Chronic types:
  - Hyperplasic candidosis: Typically, the lesion is long-standing and presents itself as a thick white patch which cannot be rubbed off (leukoplakia correlation).
- Mucocutaneous: This type of candidosis mostly affects the skin, scalp, and nails; much more rarely it affects the gingiva.
- Prosthetic stomatitis (types 1,2,3)
- Linear gingival erythema: This disease was initially termed "HIV-related gingivitis." It mostly affects immunocompromised individuals or HIV patients. The unusual pattern of inflammation appears as a distinctive linear band of erythema which involves 2–3 mm of marginal gingival (Neville et al. 2002). Redness can be circumscribed or diffused and can spread until it passes the mucogingival junction. It is often generalized in the oral cavity, but can be localized to just a few teeth. The main characteristic is that it does not respond to conventional treatment (SRP and plaque control).

**Note:** the HIV patient is also more prone to:
- Hyperplasic candidosis
- Pseudomembranous candidosis
- Cheilitis
- Ulcerative necrotizing gingivitis, ulcerative necrotizing periodontitis
- Hairy leukoplakia
- Kaposi's sarcoma

2) Other mycoses (Histoplasmosis; Aspergillosis)

Histoplasmosis is a granulomatous disease caused by *Histoplasma capsulatum* and represents one of the most frequent systemic mycoses in the United States. The frequently seen subclinical development of infection usually includes either a pulmonary chronic histoplasmosis (30% have oral manifestations) or a disseminated form found primarily in HIV patients (60% have oral manifestations). Oral findings can consist of painful granulomatous ulcerations (Holmstrup 1999).

c) Inflammatory and immune conditions
  i) Hypersensitivity reactions
    1) Contact allergy

Contact allergy is a rare condition, but it is an inflammatory reaction of the gingival tissue mostly to dental restorative materials, dentifrices, mouthwashes, and foods. Their presentation is associated to a type IV hypersensitivity reaction.

    2) Plasma cell gingivitis

Clinically it presents as an erythematous gingival with velvety texture, usually affecting the maxillary anterior gingiva, and histopathologically presents a dense infiltrate of plasma cells in the lamina propia. It is of uncertain etiology.

3) Erythema multiforme

Erythema multiforme is an acute vesiculobullous disease affecting mucous membranes and skin. This inflammatory reaction produces bullae which rupture and leave extensive ulcers covered by yellowish fibrinous exudates, sometimes described as pseudomembranes, on the gingival tissues. Another characteristic oral lesion is the typically swollen lips with crust formation of the vermillion border. "Target lesions," which can be described as a central bulla surrounded by an erythematous halo, can be found on the skin of the hands and feet (Lozada-Nur et al. 1989). The pathogenesis of this disease remains obscure, but an autoimmune reaction is suspected as the main underlying etiological factor. Two main forms of the disease have been described, minor form (limited affection) and major form (Stevens-Johnson syndrome).

ii) Autoimmune diseases of the skin and mucus membranes

Mucocutaneous disorders: Many dermatologic diseases present with gingival manifestations in the form of desquamative, ulcerative, or erythematous gingival lesions. The most relevant ones are presented as follows:

1) Pemphigus vulgaris

Pemphigus is a group of autoimmune diseases characterized by the formation of intraepithelial bulla in skin and mucous membranes. One of the most common and serious subtypes of this disease is pemphigus vulgaris. Clinically, it presents as painful desquamative lesions of the gingiva, as erosions or ulcerations which are remains of ruptured bullae (Sciubba 1996). As a diagnostic tool, the histological analysis can reveal that the bullae contain non-adhering free epithelial cells (Tzank cells). It also will respond positively to the Nicholski test. Direct immunofluorescence will reveal presence of immunoglobulin G (IgG) antibodies and occasionally components of the complement system, more specifically component complement 3 (C3), in the intercellular spaces between the epithelial cells resulting in a "chicken wire" pattern. This disease can be fatal if left untreated.

2) Pemphigoid

Pemphigoid is a group of disorders in which autoantibodies are directed toward components of the basement membrane, resulting in the detachment of the epithelium from the connective tissue. This may occur on the skin (bullous pemphigoid) and mucous membranes. When only mucous membranes are involved, it is termed benign mucous membrane pemphigoid. The main manifestation is desquamative lesions of the gingiva, presenting intensely erythematous lesions. This type of benign epithelial lesion arises from underneath the basement membrane, producing a desquamation more resistant to detachment during the clinical examination. Direct immunofluorescence will reveal a linear deposition of IgG, IgA, or C3 along the epithelial basement membrane zone.

3) Lichen planus

Lichen planus is one of the most common dermatological diseases affecting the oral cavity. Of autoimmune etiology, it can be classified according to the following subtypes: reticular, atrophic, plaque, erosive, and bullous. The characteristic clinical

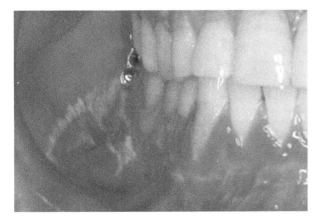

Figure 2.7 Lichen-planus-associated gingivitis. Notice the white striation—a characteristic reticular pattern.

appearance resembles desquamative chronic gingivitis with the presence of white papules and white striations which often form a reticular pattern, also known as the Wickam striae (Thorn et al. 1988) (Figure 2.7). Histopathologic analysis will reveal epithelial rete ridges with a pointed or "saw-toothed" shape, additionally there will be degenerating keratinocytes (civatte bodies) and presence of a band of inflammatory infiltrate (mainly lymphocytes) in the superficial part of the connective tissue.

4) Lupus erythematosus

Lupus erythematosus represents a group of autoimmune connective tissue disorders in which antibodies are directed toward the individual's cellular components. Two major forms exist: the discoid form (chronic type) and the systemic form. The typical lesions that can be seen on the gingiva appear as small, white dots of central atrophy surrounded by irradiating fine white striae with a periphery of telangiectasia. The characteristic "butterfly" skin lesions are photosensitive, scaly, erythematous macules located on the bridge of the nose and cheeks (Schiodt 1984).

a) Systemic lupus erythematosus

b) Discoid lupus erythematosus

iii) Granulomatous inflammatory condition (orofacial granulomatosis)

1) Chron disease

2) Sarcoidosis

d) Reactive processes

i) Epulides

Epulides is a nonspecific term defined as an exophytic process originating from the gingiva, therefore histopathology is necessary to define a more specific diagnosis. Usually it does not have symptoms associated to it, and it affects most frequently the attached gingiva (64%) (Holmstrup et al. 2018).

1) Fibrous epulis

Also known as focal fibrous hyperplasia or irritation fibroma, it presents as an exophytic smooth surfaced pink mass of fibrous consistency. The primary etiologic factor is presumably continued physical trauma/irritation.

2) Calcifying fibroblastic granuloma

Also described as ossifying fibroid epulis or peripheral ossifying fibroma. Clinically it presents as a pedunculated or sessile red to pink mass usually originating from the interproximal papilla. It occurs exclusively in the gingiva. Histopathologic it is characterized by a highly fibroblastic tissue with a lobulated mass of calcified cementum-like tissue.

3) Pyogenic granuloma (vascular epulis)

In the literature it has also been described as telangietatic granuloma, pregnancy granuloma, pregnancy tumor, and vascular epulis. It is common, often associated to pregnancy, and with a high predilection for gingiva. Clinically presents as a pedunculated mass, often ulcerated, smooth, red to pink, and variable in size. Histopathologically presents as a discontinuous hyperplasic parakeratinized stratified squamous epithelium and an increased amount of endothelial cells in the connective tissue.

4) Peripheral giant cell granuloma (or central)

Other names attributed to this lesion are giant cell epulis and peripheral giant cell reparative granuloma. Clinically, presents as a well-defined sessile or pedunculated mass, soft in consistency, sometimes ulcerated, and with a wide variety of color (purple, bluish to brown). Its name is attributed to the histopathological finding of multiple giant cells.

e) Neoplasms
  i) Premalignant
    1) Leukoplakia
    2) Erythroplakia
  ii) Malignant
    1) Squamous cell carcinoma
    2) Leukemia
    3) Lymphoma (Hodgkin and non-Hodgkin)

f) Endocrine, nutritional, and metabolism diseases
  i) Vitamin deficiencies
    1) Fat soluble vitamins (Vitamins A, D, and E)
    2) Water soluble vitamins (Complex B and Vitamin C)

g) Traumatic lesions
  i) Physical/mechanical insults

Physical or mechanical trauma: Gingival recessions or artefacta gingivitis can be the

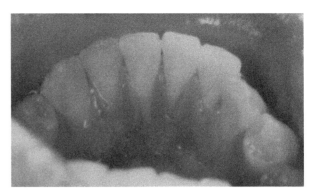

Figure 2.8 Lingual gingival recessions on teeth number 24 and 25 due to chronic trauma from repeated contact with metallic barbell (tongue piercing).

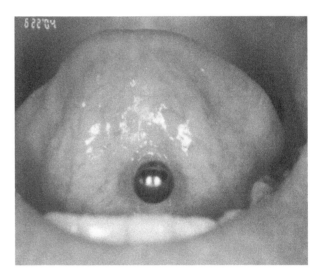

Figure 2.9 Metallic barbell inserted after tongue piercing.

result of physical traumatic events or bad oral habits (Figures 2.8, 2.9, and 2.10).

1) Frictional keratosis
2) Mechanical induced gingival ulceration
3) Factitious injury (self-harm)

  ii) Chemical

Chemical injury or toxic reaction: Toxic gingival reaction can be caused by chemical injury of the mucosa as seen in surface etching of the tissue by toxic products. For example, chlorhexidine can cause desquamation of mucosa; paraformaldehyde can give rise to inflammation and tissue necrosis. Other reactions can be attributed to aspirin, cocaine, or toothpaste rubbed on the gingival tissues (Figure 2.11).

1) Etching
2) Chlorhexidine
3) Acetylsalicylic acid
4) Cocaine

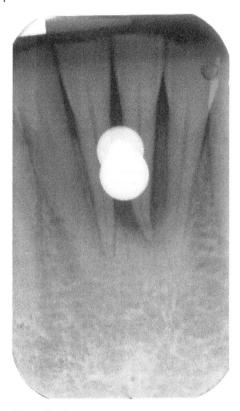

**Figure 2.10** Radiograph of teeth number 24 and 25. Notice the extensive bone loss and periodontal ligament (PDL) enlargement following chronic exposure to the deleterious effects of tongue piercing.

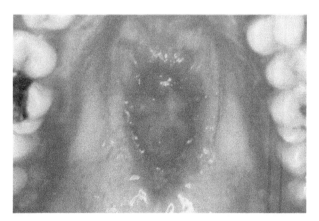

**Figure 2.11** Aspirin-induced chemical injuries to the palate and gingiva. This is characteristic of patients sucking on and keeping the aspirin tablets in their mouths instead of swallowing them. Courtesy of Iain Chapple.

5) Hydrogen peroxide
6) Dentifrice detergents
7) Paraformaldehyde or calcium hydroxide
iii) Thermal insults
Thermal trauma: Minor burns on the oral mucosa can frequently produce painful, vesicle-like lesions of the gingival tissues and palatal and labial mucosa.
1) Burn of the mucosa
h) Gingival pigmentation
i) Gingival pigmentation/melanoplakia
ii) Smoker's melanosis
iii) Drug-induced pigmentation (antimalarials; Minocycline)
iv) Amalgam tattoo

2) Periodontitis
a) **Necrotizing Periodontal Diseases**
Necrotizing periodontal diseases have a unique presentation and development with the manifestation of necrotic lesions occurring concomitantly with the immune system depression.

According to the 2017 world workshop classification (Papapanou et al. 2018) two different categories for necrotizing periodontal diseases exist based on the compromised severity of the patient, as seen in Table 2.2. The main described predisposing factors for severely compromised patient to develop necrotizing diseases are: low counts of CD4 cells and a detectable viral load, other systemic conditions that lead to immunosuppression, severe malnourishment, extreme living conditions, and stress. While the described predisposing factors for temporarily compromised patients are: uncontrolled factors such as stress, nutrition, and smoking; previous necrotizing periodontal disease; local factors such as root proximity and tooth malposition; among others (Herrera et al. 2018).
a) Necrotizing gingivitis

Necrotizing gingivitis (NG): This disease is a type of periodontal disease in which the necrosis is limited to the gingival tissues. It has been known for many centuries and has other names such as Vincent's angina, fusospirochetes gingivitis, and trench mouth disease. NG is an infectious, noncontagious disease, which can undergo dramatic resolution of signs and symptoms once the microbial plaque is eliminated. The following clinical characteristics must be present for diagnosis:

1) Spontaneous bleeding
2) Severe pain
3) Necrosis of gingival papilla (interdental necrosis) leaving crater, NG may also present (Figure 2.12):
4) Formation of white pseudomembranes on gingiva
5) Fever, malaise, lymphadenopathy
6) Increase in salivary flow, submandibular gland enlargement
7) Presence of metallic taste in mouth and oral malodor

Table 2.2  Classification of necrotizing periodontal disease (NPD).

| Category | Patients | Predisposing conditions | Clinical condition |
|---|---|---|---|
| Necrotizing periodontal disease in chronically, severely compromised patients | In adults | HIV+/AIDS with CD4 counts <200 and detectable viral load | NG, NP, NS, Noma. Possible progression |
| | | Other severe systemic conditions (immunosuppression) | |
| | In children | Severe malnourishments [a] | |
| | | Extreme living conditions [b] | |
| | | Severe (viral) infections [c] | |
| Necrotizing periodontal disease in temporarily and/or moderately compromised patients | In gingivitis patients | Uncontrolled factors: stress, nutrition, smoking, habits | Generalized NG. Possible progression to NP |
| | | Previous NPD; residual craters | Localized NP. Possible progression to NP |
| | | Local factors: root proximity, tooth malposition | NG. Infrequent progression |
| | In periodontitis patients | Common predisposing factors for NPD (Refer to Papapanou et al. 2018) | NP. Infrequent progression |

NG: Necrotizing gingivitis; NP: Necrotizing periodontitis; NS: Necrotizing stomatitis.

a)  Mean plasma and serum concentrations of retinol, total ascorbic acid, zinc, and albumin markedly reduced, or very marked depletion of plasma retinol, zinc, and ascorbate; and saliva levels of albumin and cortisol, as well as plasma cortisol concentrations, significantly increased.

b)  Living in substandard accommodations, exposure to debilitating child diseases, living near livestock, poor oral hygiene, limited access to potable water, and poor sanitary disposal of human and animal fecal waste.

c)  Measles, herpes viruses (cytomegalovirus, Epstein-Barr virus-1, herpes simplex virus), chickenpox, malaria, febrile illness.

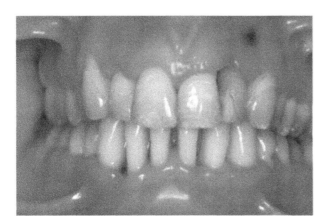

Figure 2.12  Post-necrotizing ulcerative gingivitis/periodontitis oral condition. Notice the typical gingival architecture and the "punched out" papillae.

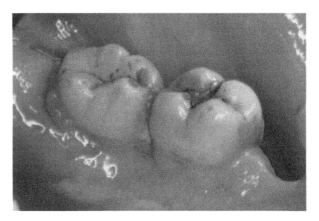

Figure 2.13  Necrotizing periodontitis in an HIV-positive patient. Notice the denuded mandibular bone. Courtesy of Iain Chapple.

**Note:** Necrosis is limited to the gingival tissues and does not extend to the alveolar bone or outside the periodontium. When the alveolar bone is affected, it is called a necrotic/ulcerative stomatitis or periodontitis.

The epidemiologic and etiologic factors related to NG are as follows (Herrera et al. 2018; Rowland 1999):

— Adolescents and young adults which present poor oral hygiene and a low immunitary defense system are most often affected because of emotional stress, malnutrition, viral infections, smoking, lack of sleep, or concomitant

systemic disease (AIDS), or after taking immunosuppressant medications (Figure 2.13).

— *Prevotella intermedia* and spirochetes are characteristic of the microbial flora isolated in these lesions.

b)  Necrotizing periodontitis

Necrotizing periodontitis (NP):
Although less frequent than NG, NP presents severe erythema of the marginal gingiva and alveolar mucosa accompanied by extensive interproximal tissulary necrosis covered with white

pseudomembranes. Spontaneous bleeding and severe loss of attachment around teeth result in the formation of craters interproximally, affecting both hard and soft tissues. Pain, oral malodor, fever, malaise, and lymphadenopathy remain present. NP can occur after an NG or in areas in which there already is a chronic periodontitis.

**Note:** In patients with AIDS, severe bone destruction can produce loss of teeth within three to six months and present bony sequestrum if the disease is not treated. Also, this condition may recur if left untreated.

A combination of antibiotic therapy (Metronidazole 250 mg, 2 tabs stat, 1 tabqid for 7–10 days, or Amoxicillin 500 mg, 1 tabtid for 7 days), mechanical debridement (scaling and root planing with hand instruments), and antiseptic mouth rinses (chlorhexidine and peroxide) is the treatment of choice for both NUG and NUP (Herrera et al. 2018; Rowland 1999).

c) Necrotizing stomatitis

Based on the definition by Papapanou et al. (2018): It is a severe inflammatory condition of the periodontium and oral cavity in which soft tissue necrosis extends beyond the gingiva and bone denudation may occur through the alveolar mucosa, with larger areas of osteitis and alveolar sequestrum. It typically occurs in severely systemically compromised patients.

d) Noma

### b) **Periodontitis**

Periodontitis is defined as an infectious disease resulting in inflammation within the supporting tissues of the teeth, progressive attachment loss, and alveolar bone loss (Armitage 1999). On the previous classification two main identities of this disease existed: chronic and aggressive periodontitis. For the purpose of this chapter a brief description of both will be done, although currently there is no distinction in terms of diagnosis terminology between them.

In regards to chronic periodontitis, the amount of tissulary destruction is proportional to the quantity of local etiological factors. Subgingival calculus is a frequent finding and variable microbial patterns have been associated with the disease. This disease is often associated with local predisposing factors (dental anatomy or iatrogenous factors) as well as multiple systemic diseases (diabetes mellitus and HIV) and disorders in which the host defense mechanisms play an important role in its pathogenesis. Slow to moderate rates of progression are seen and are usually associated with good prognoses and responses after treatment. The adequate therapy involves the removal of etiological factors by scaling and root planing and reevaluation for periodontal surgery and/or maintenance.

On the other hand, aggressive periodontitis, presented with a distinguishable different clinical and radiographical presentation in comparison to chronic periodontitis. This can be summarized as:

- Except for the presence of periodontitis, these individuals are otherwise clinically healthy
- Attachment loss and bone destruction is rapid
- Familial (genetic) aggregation. Secondary features that are generally, but not universally present are:
- Amounts of microbial deposits are inconsistent with the severity of the periodontal destruction
- Elevated proportions of *Actinobacillus Actinomycetemcomitans* and, in some populations, *porphyromonas gingivalis*
- Abnormal phagocytary cells and hyper-responding macrophages (elevated levels of PGE2 and IL-1B)
- Progression of attachment bone loss can be self-arresting

The new classification of periodontitis makes emphasis on the staging and grading of the disease (Needleman et al. 2018; Papapanou et al. 2018; Tonetti et al. 2018). The stage intends to classify the severity and extend extent of the disease, while also to assess the complexity of the case management. On the other hand, the grading provides information on the disease progression rate, potential responsiveness to standard treatment, and modifying factors and their relation to systemic health (Tables 2.3 and 2.4).

In order to diagnose periodontitis there must be clinical radiographic evidence of periodontal loss of attachment, deep probing depths (commonly over $\geq$ 4 mm) with bleeding on probing, and presence of loss of periodontal tissue support (clinical attachment loss) due to inflammation seen as:

1) Interdental clinical attachment loss (CAL) of $\geq$ 2 nonadjacent teeth, or
2) Buccal or oral CAL $\geq$ 3 mm with pocketing $\geq$ 3 mm is detectable at $\geq$ 2 teeth

Additionally the CAL cannot be ascribed to non-periodontitis causes, such as:

1) Gingival recession of traumatic origin
2) Dental caries extending in the cervical area of the tooth
3) Presence of CAL on distal surface of a second molar associated to a malposition or extraction of a third molar
4) Endodontic lesion draining through the marginal periodontium, or root resorption
5) Vertical root fracture

It is important to mention that the most severe site will determine the diagnosis of the mouth, while determining the extent of the disease is also crucial. Three different patterns of extent and distribution can be described as

Table 2.3 Periodontitis—staging.

| | Periodontitis | Stage I | Stage II | Stage III | Stage IV |
|---|---|---|---|---|---|
| Severity | Interdental CAL (at site of greater loss) | 1–2 mm | 3–4 mm | ≥5 mm | ≥5 mm |
| | Radiographically bone loss | Coronal third (<15%) | Coronal third (15–33%) | Extending to middle third of root and beyond | Extending to middle third of root and beyond |
| | Tooth loss (due to periodontitis) | No tooth loss | | ≤4 teeth | ≥5 teeth |
| Complexity | Local | Max. probing depth ≤4 teeth<br><br>Mostly horizontal bone loss | Max. probing depth ≤5 teeth<br><br>Mostly horizontal bone loss | In addition to Stage II complexity:<br>Probing depths ≥6 mm<br>Vertical bone loss ≥3 mm<br>Furcation involvement class II or III<br>Moderate ridge defects | In addition to Stage III complexity:<br>Need for complex rehabilitation due to:<br>Masticatory dysfunction<br>Secondary occlusal trauma (tooth mobility degree ≥2)<br>Severe ridge defect<br>Bite collapse, drifting, flaring<br><20 remaining teeth (10 opposing pairs) |
| Extent and distribution | Add to stage as descriptor | For each stage, describe extent as localized (<30% of teeth involved), generalized, or molar/incisor pattern | | | |

Table 2.4 Periodontitis—grading.

| | Progression | | Grade A: Slow rate | Grade B: Moderate rate | Grade C: Rapid rate |
|---|---|---|---|---|---|
| Primary criteria | Direct evidence of progression | Radiographic bone loss or CAL | No loss over 5 years | <2 mm over 5 years | ≥2 mm over 5 years |
| | Indirect evidence of progression | % bone loss/age | <0.25 | 0.25–1.0 | >1.0 |
| | | Case phenotype | Heavy biofilm deposits with low levels of destruction | Destruction commensurate with biofilm deposits | Destruction exceeds expectations given biofilm deposits; specific clinical patterns suggestive of periods of rapid progression and/or early onset disease |
| Grade modifiers | Risk factors | Smoking | No smoker | <10 cigarettes/day | ≥10 cigarettes/day |
| | | Diabetes | Normoglycemic/no diagnosis of diabetes | HbA1c <7% in patients with diabetes | HbA1c ≥7.0% in patients with diabetes |

**Grading aims to indicate the rate of periodontitis progression, responsiveness to standard therapy, and potential impact on systemic health.**
Clinicians should initially assume grade B disease and seek specific evidence to shift to grade A or C.

1) Localized (≤30% of sites are involved)
2) Generalized
3) Molar/incisor pattern

The molar/incisor pattern has a well-recognized and distinct clinical presentation, previously diagnosed as localized aggressive periodontitis. Yet, due that the specific etiologic factors or pathological elements are not clearly defined it was determine to diagnose it just as a specific distribution of a periodontitis case under the new classification.

As said, this localized form of aggressive periodontitis was characterized by:

- Begins at puberty, at around 10–12 years of age
- Affects mostly individuals with black-colored skin; males and females are equally affected
- Can often be characterized by small quantities of bacterial plaque in relation to bone destruction, showing limited signs of inflammation (Figure 2.14)
- High immune response (increased immunoglobulin production) to infectious agents
- Higher proportions of *Actinobacillus Actinomycetemcomitans*, serotype b (leukotoxin producing)
- Localized bone loss on first molars and incisors with interproximal attachment loss on at least two permanent teeth, one of which is a first molar, and involving no more than two teeth other than first molars and incisors (Figures 2.15 and 2.16)

The adequate treatment is to combine systemic antibiotics (Doxicyclin, 200 mg the first day and 100 mg/day for 10 days, or Tetracyclin, 250 mg, qid for 10 days) with scaling and root planing, followed by periodontal surgery if needed, and/or maintenance (Figures 2.17, 2.18, 2.19, and 2.20).

In general the stage for a periodontitis case does not regress or move to a lower stage, with one exception to this rule: If a case was defined as a Stage III due to the presence of a vertical defect greater than 3 mm or a furcation involvement class II, and a guided tissue regeneration procedure proof to be successful and the initial CAL and probing depth regresses to 4 mm or less and 5 mm or less, respectively, the case could be newly defined as a stage II.

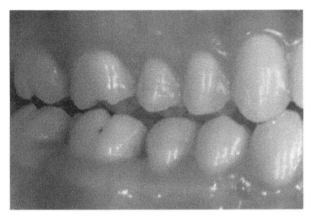

**Figure 2.14** Periodontitis with a molar/incisor pattern (old terminology localized aggressive periodontitis) in a 15-year-old. Notice the lack of obvious etiology (plaque).

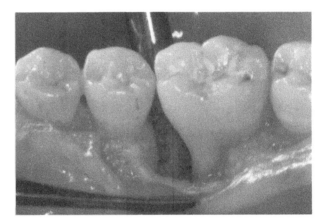

**Figure 2.15** Typical bone loss associated with periodontitis with a molar/incisor pattern (old terminology localized aggressive periodontitis) and affecting the permanent first molars.

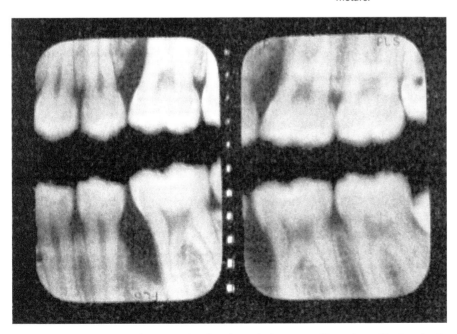

**Figure 2.16** Bite wing radiographs showing the typical pattern of bone loss affecting the first permanent molars.

Figure 2.17 One year post therapy (associated with tetracycline intake); notice partial fill of bony defect.

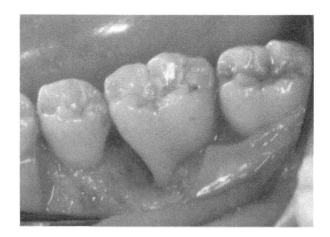

Figure 2.18 Periapical radiographs, before and after treatment at one-year interval.

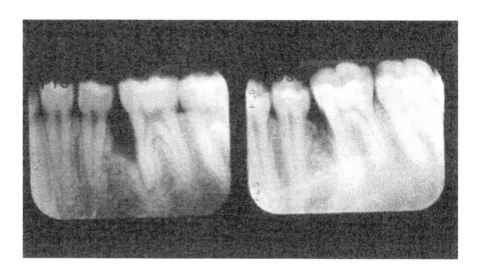

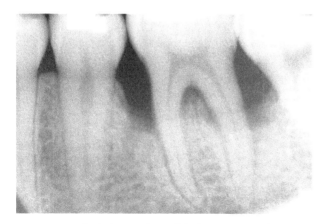

Figure 2.19 Periapical radiograph before treatment in conjunction with antibiotherapy.

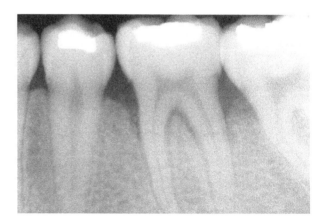

Figure 2.20 Periapical radiograph one year after treatment; notice again the healing of the osseous defect.

Nevertheless, the stage could always progress to a higher stage. For instance, if a patient was successfully treated for periodontitis and is now clinically stable at maintenance, this patient would be diagnose, most likely, as gingival health in a previously treated periodontitis patient. Yet, if this patient demonstrates further advancement of the disease during the maintenance appointments, then it is possible that the stage could further progress from the previous initial diagnosis.

Staging intends to classify the severity and extent of a patient's disease based on the measurable amount of destroyed and/or damaged tissues as a result of periodontitis and to assess the specific factors that may attribute to the complexity of long-term case management.

Initial stage should be determined using clinical attachment loss (CAL). If CAL is not available, radiographic bone loss should be used. Tooth loss due to periodontitis may modify stage definition. One or more complexity factors may shift the stage to a higher level.

c) **Periodontitis as a Manifestations of Systemic Diseases (seen in Table 2.5)**

Bacterial plaque is the original etiologic factor for periodontal disease, but what determines the actual presence or progression of the disease is the immune response of the host. Systemic factors can affect all forms of periodontal diseases by modifying the host's immune and defense mechanisms. Periodontitis forms classified under this category include:

– Associated with hematological disorders: The blood cells have a vital role in supplying oxygen and assuring hemostasis and protecting of the periodontal tissues. Systemic hematological disorders can have profound effects on the periodontium by denying any of these essential functions. Polymorphonuclear leukocytes (PMN cells) are crucial in the defense of the periodontium. They have protective functions by integrating the following activities: chemotaxis, phagocytosis, and killing/neutralizing the ingested organisms or substances. Individuals with either quantitative (neutropenia or agranulocytosis) or qualitative (chemotactic or phagocytic) PMN deficiencies exhibit severe destruction of the periodontium. The quantitative deficiencies generally affect the periodontium of all teeth, whereas the qualitative ones are associated with the destruction of the periodontium of certain teeth only (Lindhe 2003).

1) Acquired neutropenia: Neutropenia refers to a decrease in the number of the circulating neutrophils below 1,500/mm$^3$ in an adult, which is also associated with an increased susceptibility to infections (Neville et al. 2002). Different forms of neutropenia (malignant, chronic, benign, cyclic, and slowly progressing neutropenia) produce variable effects on the periodontium. Generally, oral lesions consist of chronic gingival ulcers which characteristically lack an erythematous periphery and leave a scar once healed.

Cyclic neutropenia is a specific idiopathic disorder (an autosomal dominant pattern of inheritance has been described in a few cases) characterized by regular periodic reductions in the neutrophil population of the affected patient. The underlying cause seems to be related to a defect in the hematopoietic stem cells in the marrow. Beginning in early childhood, the signs and symptoms of cyclic neutropenia last for three to six days and occur in rather uniformly spaced episodes, which usually have a 21-day cycle (Neville et al. 2002). Patients typically present with fever, anorexia, cervical lymphadenopathy, malaise, pharyngitis, oral mucosal ulcerations, and severe periodontal bone loss with marked gingival recessions and tooth mobility. This alveolar bone loss of both primary and permanent dentitions becomes more accentuated at every recurring episode, leading to the loss of primary teeth at 5 years of age instead of 11.

2) Leukemias: Leukemias produce excessive numbers of leukocytes in the blood and tissues and also cause a greatly depleted bone marrow function with associated anemia, thrombocytopenia, neutropenia, and reduced range of immune cells. Periodontal bone loss is a consequence of neutrophil functional alterations and deficiencies.

3) Other

– Associated with genetic disease:

1) Familial cyclic neutropenia
2) Down syndrome
3) Leukocyte adhesion deficiency syndrome (LADS)
4) Papillon-Lefevre syndrome
5) Chediak-Higashi syndrome
6) Histiocytosis syndrome
7) Glycogen storage disease
8) Infantile generalized agranulocytosis
9) Cohen syndrome
10) Ehlers-Danlos syndrome
11) Hypophosphatasia
12) Other

3) **Other Conditions Affecting the Periodontium**

a) **Systemic disease or conditions affecting the periodontal supporting tissues. (Albandar et al. 2018)**

b) **Periodontal abscesses and endodontic periodontal lesions**

a) Periodontal abscesses

Previously, the classification of periodontal abscesses is primarily based on the location of the infective lesion, in the current classification no specific distinction is made based on the location (Herrera et al. 2018; Jepsen et al. 2018). It can be defined as a cavity filled with a collection of pus, formed by disintegrated tissue. Abscesses of the periodontium can show various combinations of the following clinical features:

- Pain and sensitivity to touch
- Color change
- Swelling
- Purulence and sinus tract formation

Table 2.5 Classification of systemic disease and condition that affect the periodontal supporting tissues. Albandar et al., 2018 / John Wiley & Sons.

| Classification | Disorders | ICD-10 code |
|---|---|---|
| 1. | Systemic disorders that have a major impact on the loss of periodontal tissues by influencing periodontal inflammation | |
| 1.1 | Genetic disorders | |
| 1.1.1 | Diseases associated with immunologic disorders | |
| | Down syndrome | Q90.9 |
| | Leukocyte adhesion deficiency syndromes | D72.0 |
| | Papillon-Lefèfre syndrome | Q82.8 |
| | Haim-Munk syndrome | Q82.8 |
| | Chediak-Higashi | E70.3 |
| | Severe neutropenia | |
| | - Congenital neutropenia (Kostmann syndrome) | D70.0 |
| | - Cyclic neutropenia | D70.4 |
| | Primary immunodeficiency diseases | |
| | - Chronic granulomatous disease | D71.0 |
| | - Hyperimmunoglobulin E syndromes | D82.9 |
| | Cohen syndrome | Q87.8 |
| 1.1.2 | Diseases affecting the oral mucosa and gingival tissue | |
| | Epidermolysis bullosa | |
| | - Dystrophic epidermolysis bullosa | Q81.2 |
| | - Kindler syndrome | Q81.8 |
| | Plasminogen deficiency | D68.2 |
| 1.1.3 | Diseases affecting the connective tissues | |
| | Ehlers-Danlos syndromes (type IV, VIII) | Q79.6 |
| | Angioedema (CI-inhibitor deficiency) | D84.1 |
| | Systemic lupus erythematosus | M32.9 |
| 1.1.4 | Metabolic and endocrine disorders | |
| | Glycogen storage disease | E74.0 |
| | Gaucher disease | E75.2 |
| | Hypophosphatasia | E83.30 |
| | Hypophosphatemic rickets | E83.31 |
| | Hadju-Cheney syndrome | Q78.8 |
| 1.2 | Acquired immunodeficiency diseases | |
| | Acquired neutropenia | D70.9 |
| | HIV infection | B24 |
| 1.3 | Inflammatory diseases | |
| | Epidermolysis bullosa acquisita | 1.12.3 |
| | Inflammatory bowel disease | K50, K51.9, K52.9 |
| 2. | Other systemic disorders that influence the pathogenesis of periodontal diseases | |
| | Diabetes mellitus | E10 (type 1), E11 (type 2) |
| | Obesity | E66.9 |
| | Osteoporosis | M81.9 |
| | Arthritis (rheumatoid arthritis, osteoarthritis) | M05, M106, M15–M16 |
| | Emotional stress and depression | F32.9 |
| | Smoking (nicotine dependence) | F17 |
| | Medications | |

- Pulsative pain, lasting
- Tooth is sensitive to percussion
- Teeth mobility and extrusion
- Fever, lymphadenopathy, and possible radiolucency of the affected alveolar bone

Although the 2017 classification no longer does a distinction in the diagnosis based on the location, it is still practical to know the application of the 1999 classification as this is an important factor that will determine the treatment of the lesion. Therefore, according to the 1999 classification, the lesions can be classified as short-lasting (acute: quickly developing) or long-lasting (chronic: developing slowly). They can be further divided into the following three classes:

A) Gingival abscess: Localized purulent infection involving the marginal gingival or the papilla. Generally quickly developing, it becomes fluctuant after 24–48 hours and leads to the formation of a purulent orifice. Pulpal hypersensitivity may occasionally be found. No periodontal pockets or alveolar bone loss surround these lesions, although a pseudopocket (gingival pocket) may be present. These lesions are usually rare and are often caused by a foreign body.

Treatment consists of eliminating local etiological factors (see treatment for periodontal abscess).

B) Periodontal abscess: A periodontal abscess is a localized infection within the tissues adjacent to a periodontal pocket that may lead to the destruction of the periodontal ligament and the alveolar bone. These lesions are commonly found in patients suffering from moderate to severe periodontitis. They are precipitated by a change in the subgingival flora, a decrease of host resistance, or both. The tooth is usually vital (Figure 2.21).

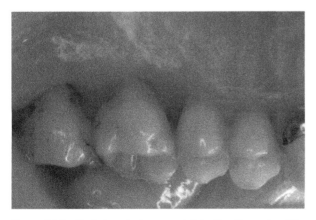

Figure 2.21 Periodontal abscess palatal of tooth number 15. The tooth is vital.

The following factors may be associated with periodontal abscesses:

1) Occlusion of the orifice of a periodontal pocket caused by the introduction of food or foreign body or by the incomplete removal of calculus deposits
2) Furcation involvement of periodontal infection
3) Systemic antibiotic therapy given to patients who are untreated for their periodontitis. This situation may lead to a supra-infection by opportunistic microorganisms resulting in a periodontal abscess
4) Diabetic patients have a tendency to develop purulent infections because of their decreased host immune response and their vascular abnormalities
5) Other predisposing factors (enamel pearls, lateral endodontic perforations, etc.) should be evaluated

The appropriate therapy consists of alleviating the pain by either establishing drainage by incision or by local debridement with surgical flap reflected if needed. An antibiotic can be prescribed and the lesion should be reevaluated after the acute phase has passed to detect any underlying periodontal condition.

C) Pericoronaritis (pericoronal abscess): A pericoronal abscess is a localized purulent infection within the tissues surrounding the crown of a partially erupted or difficultly erupting tooth. These abscesses are often seen adjacent to a mandibular third molar. Not only are these teeth difficult to access for proper hygiene, they frequently have difficulty erupting due to their malposition or lack of space. In addition, the already compromised area is often traumatized by occlusion of the opposing antagonist teeth. The recommended immediate treatment is to prescribe a systemic antibiotic and perform a local debridement if possible. Extraction of the tooth (and possibly the antagonist tooth as well) is recommended in the subsequent weeks.

Currently, the 2017 world workshop has classified periodontal abscesses as (Table 2.6):

– Periodontal abscess in periodontitis patients (in a preexisting periodontal pocket)
– Periodontal abscess in non-periodontitis patient (not mandatory to have a preexisting periodontal pocket)

  b) Endodontic-Periodontal Lesions
     Endodontic-periodontal lesions: Lesions of the periodontal ligament and adjacent alveolar bone may originate from infections of the periodontium or tissue of the dental pulp. A pulpal infection may cause a tissue-destructive process that proceeds from the apical region of a tooth to the marginal gingiva. The term retrograde periodontitis is often used to differentiate this type of lesion from a marginal

Table 2.6 Classification of periodontal abscesses based on the etiologic factors involved.

| | | | |
|---|---|---|---|
| Periodontal abscess in periodontitis patient (in a preexisting periodontal pocket) | Acute exacerbation | Untreated periodontitis | |
| | | Nonresponsive to therapy | |
| | | Supportive periodontal therapy | |
| | After treatment | Post scaling | |
| | | Post-surgery | |
| | | Post-medication | Systemic antimicrobials |
| | | | Other drugs: Nifedipine |
| Periodontal abscess in non-periodontitis patients (not mandatory to have a preexisting periodontal pocket) | Impaction | | Dental floss, orthodontic elastic, toothpick, rubber dam, or popcorn hulls |
| | Harmful habits | | Wire or nail biting and clenching |
| | Orthodontic factors | | Orthodontic forces or a cross-bite |
| | Gingival overgrowth | | |
| | Alteration of root surface | Severe anatomic alterations | Invaginated tooth, dens evaginatus, or odontodysplasia |
| | | Minor anatomic alterations | Cemental tears, enamel pearls, or developmental grooves |
| | | Iatrogenic conditions | Perforations |
| | | Severe root damage | Fissure or fracture, cracked tooth syndrome |
| | | External root resorption | |

periodontitis in which the infection spreads from the gingival margin toward the root apex. Another term, pulpodontic-periodontic syndrome, is also used to describe this type of combined lesion in which a tooth suffers from a pulpal/endodontic lesion and periodontitis at the same time (Herrera et al. 2018; Jepsen et al. 2018) (Figure 2.22).

One reason why these lesions can travel from one area to the other is that the periodontium communicates with the pulp tissues through many channels or pathways (apical, lateral, and accessory canals). Bacteria causative of endodontic lesions can travel in the blood vessels via the root grooves, vertical root fractures, hypoplastic cementum lesions, and root anomalies/resorptions to reach the marginal gingiva. The effects of endodontic lesions on the periodontium include severe and rapid destruction of the periodontal structures. Once the appropriate endodontic treatment is performed, the lesion should heal uneventfully without any residual defects in the periodontium.

A periodontal abscess and an endodontic abscess have similar clinical manifestations, and differ by the origin of the infection.

**Note:** Root perforation or root fracture during/after root canal therapy can result in an increased periodontal ligament, suppuration,

and increased tooth mobility in an individual with a healthy periodontium. The principal symptoms include pain upon mastication, swelling, periodontal abscess formation, and fistula. The tooth can be vital or not and the formation of a localized deep (narrow) pocket, periodontal ligament, and widening and apical radiolucency may be present. Periodontal pockets, furcation involvement, subgingival calculus, inflammation, deep fillings, past dental trauma, or root canal treatments must be considered to establish the correct diagnosis (Meng 1999a, 1999b).

i) Endo-Periodontal lesion with root damage
ii) Endo-Periodontal lesion without root damage

c) **Mucogingival deformities and conditions**
Mucogingival deformities and conditions: The presence of mucogingival deformities often has an impact on patients in terms of esthetics and function. Mucogingival deformities may be congenital, developmental, or acquired defects and may be localized to soft tissues or associated with defects in the underlying bone. Mucogingival deformities may be classified in the following conditions (Jepsen et al. 2018; Pini Prato 1999):

According to the 2017 world workshop (Jepsen et al. 2018) the following conditions can be classified as Mucogingival conditions: gingival

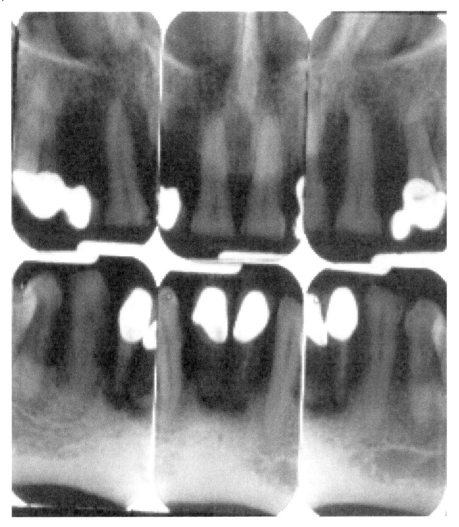

Figure 2.22 Perio-endo lesion affecting teeth number 24 and 25. There are lesions of endodontic origin as well as periodontal probings surrounding these teeth.

phenotype, gingival tissue recession, lack of gingiva, decreased vestibular depth, aberrant frenum/muscle position, gingival excess, abnormal color, condition of the exposed root surface.
Phenotype classification

The 2017 workshop suggested the change of "biotype" for phenotype, this is due that phenotype describes a characteristic that may change overtime due to environmental factors or clinical intervention while also can be site specific. On the other hand, biotype is associated to the genotype or genetics.

Periodontal phenotype is determined by gingival phenotype which includes gingival thickness and keratinized tissue width, and bone morphotype which describes the thickness of the buccal bone plate (Jepsen et al. 2018).

As described by (Zweers et al. 2014), the periodontal phenotype can be identified as:

"Thin scalloped"—Clear thin delicate gingiva, narrow zone of keratinized tissue, slender triangular shaped crowns, subtle cervical convexity, interproximal contacts close to the incisal edge and a relatively thin alveolar bone.

"Thick scalloped"—Clear thick fibrotic gingiva, high gingival scallop, narrow zone of keratinized tissue, and slender teeth.

"Thick flat"—Clear thick fibrotic gingiva, broad zone of keratinized tissue, more square shaped crowns, pronounced cervical convexity, large interproximal contact located more apically, and a comparatively thick alveolar bone.

1) Gingival soft tissue recession: Gingival soft tissue recessions are noted when the free gingival margin is positioned apically to the cementoenamel junction. They can occur in two different locations:
   - Buccal or lingual surfaces
   - Interproximal surfaces

Etiologic factors predisposing to gingival recessions include:

- Dehiscence or bone fenestration
- Thin, bony plate
- Thin or absent keratinized gingiva
- Tooth malposition
- Frenum traction

Etiological factors stimulating a recession:

- Traumatic brushing
- Cervical abrasion
- Inflammation
- Violation of biological width
- Extraction
- Orthodontic movement
- Trauma due to a removable appliance, bad crown shape/margins, habit

Gingival Recession Classification (RT Classification based on Cairo et al. 2011)

i) Recession type 1

Gingival recession with no loss of interproximal attachment. Interproximal CEJ is clinically nondetectable at both mesial and distal aspects of the tooth.

ii) Recession type 2

Gingival recession associated with loss of interproximal attachment. The amount of interproximal attachment loss (measured from the interproximal CEJ to the depth of the interproximal sulcus/pocket) is less than equal to the buccal attachment loss (measured from the buccal CEJ to the apical end of the buccal sulcus/pocket).

iii) Recession type 3

Gingival recession associated with loss of interproximal attachment. The amount of interproximal attachment is higher than the buccal attachment loss.

In addition to the severity of the recession in regards to the location of the clinical attachment loss, it is also important to mention the gingival thickness, keratin-ized tissue width, the presence or absence of an identifiable (Class A or B, respectively), and the presence or absence of a step (Jepsen et al. 2018) (Table 2.7).

## Mucogingival conditions with gingival recessions

As noticed above, if there is presence of a mucogingival condition in presence of gingival recession the following conditions may be considered relevant features to describe the condition: interdental clinical attachment level, gingival phenotype, root surface condition (presence/absence of NCCL or caries), detection of the CEJ, tooth position, aberrant frenum and the number of adjacent recessions.

## Mucogingival conditions without gingival recessions

The following may be considered relevant features to describe the mucogingival condition in absence of gingival recession: gingival phenotype, tooth position, aberrant frenum, vestibular depth.

2) Lack of keratinized tissue: The quantity and quality of keratinized gingiva may be altered in numerous conditions. The following factors may be analyzed to establish the etiology and treatment of the condition:
- Plaque control
- Tooth brushing technique (toothbrush with soft bristles should be used)
- Etiological factors (frenum attachment, occlusion, prominent tooth, irritation or rubbing trauma from removable appliance)
- Age (a younger individual may be treated differently than an older one)
- Quality and quantity of attached gingiva
- Types of periodontium:
  - Type 1: 3–5 mm of keratinized tissue (KT), normal alveolar bone (40% of population)

Table 2.7 Classification of mucogingival conditions (gingival phenotype) and gingival recessions.

| Gingival site | | | | Tooth site | |
| --- | --- | --- | --- | --- | --- |
| | REC Depth | GT | KTW | CEJ (A/B) | Step (±) |
| No recession | | | | | |
| RT1 | | | | | |
| RT2 | | | | | |
| RT3 | | | | | |

**RT**: recession type; **REC Depth**: depth of the gingival recession; **GT**: gingival thickness; **KTW**: keratinized tissue width; **CEJ**: cemento-enamel junction (Class A = Detectable; Class B = undetectable CEJ); **Step**: root surface concavity (Class + = presence of a cervical step > 0.5 mm; Class − = absence of a cervical step > 0.5 mm)

- Type 2: Less than 2 mm of KT, normal alveolar bone (10% of population)
- Type 3: 3–5 mm of KT, thin alveolar bone (20% of population)
- Type 4: Less than 2 mm of KT, thin alveolar bone (30% of population)

● Recession classification (Miller 1985):
  ○ Class I: Recession doesn't pass the mucogingival junction (MCJ), no attachment loss interproximally, 100% success is expected after treatment
  ○ Class II: Recession at or passes MCJ, no attachment loss interproximally, 100% success is expected after treatment
  ○ Class III: Recession at or passes MCJ, attachment loss interproximally or unfavorable tooth position, less than 100% success is expected after treatment
  ○ Class IV: Recession at or passes MCJ, severe attachment loss interproximally and very unfavorable tooth position, no success is expected after treatment

3) Decreased vestibular depth
4) Aberrant frenum, muscle position
5) Gingival excess:
   a) Pseudopocket
   b) Inconsistent gingival margin
   c) Gingival excess
   d) gingival enlargement (1A3, 1B4)

Additionally, there can be mucogingival deformities and conditions on the edentulous ridge:

1) Vertical and horizontal deficiency
2) Lack of gingival keratinized tissue
3) Gingival soft tissue enlargement
4) Aberrant frenum, muscle position
5) Decreased vestibular depth
6) Abnormal color

   d) **Traumatic Occlusal forces**
     a) Occlusal trauma
        Occlusal trauma: This is a histologic term. A defined lesion and response of the attachment apparatus has been demonstrated in association with excessive occlusal forces, and has been termed occlusal trauma (Fan et al. 2018; Jepsen et al. 2018). The effect of traumatogenic occlusion on the progression of periodontitis has been associated with tooth mobility due to occlusal trauma. This creates a pathological state in which the PDL is destroyed and osteoclasts destroy alveolar bone, increasing tooth mobility. Occlusal trauma is due to the occlusal force, direct or indirect, which exceeds the resistance of the supporting tissues. It can be characterized by the following features:

A clinical diagnosis of occlusal trauma may be made in presence of: progressive tooth mobility, adaptive tooth mobility (fremitus), radiographically widened periodontal ligament space, tooth migration, discomfort/pain on chewing, and root resorption. They can be further subdivided into primary or secondary occlusal trauma.

● Hypermobility
● Abnormal PDL widening
● Histological analysis shows cementum tears and radicular resorption

Primary occlusal trauma: Injury resulting in tissue changes from excessive occlusal forces applied to a tooth with a normal periodontal support: 1) normal bone levels, 2) normal attachment levels, and 3) excessive occlusal forces.

Secondary occlusal trauma: Injury resulting in tissue changes from normal or excessive occlusal forces applied to a tooth with reduced periodontal support: 1) bone loss, 2) attachment loss, and 3) normal/excessive occlusal forces.

A traumatic occlusal force is defined as any occlusal force resulting in injury of the teeth and/or the periodontal attachment apparatus. Indications of a traumatic occlusion may present as tooth mobility, fremitus, occlusal interference, wear facettes, tooth migration, tooth fracture, and thermal sensitivity. Radiographs may show widened PDL space, bone loss, radicular resorption, and hypercementosis.

   i) Primary
   ii) Secondary
      b) Orthodontic forces/effect in the periodontium
         Prevalence of gingival recession associated to previous orthodontic treatment has been reported to be between 5% and 12% at the end of the treatment, with an increase of the prevalence up to 47% at 5 years (Renkema et al. 2013). This increase of prevalence may be directly associated to the type of orthodontic movement performed, where teeth that have been moved in a buccal direction or outside of the bony housing will have a higher prevalence of gingival recession (Morris et al. 2017).

         Additionally, there is evidence from animal models that suggest that excessive orthodontic forces can adversely affect the periodontium resulting in root resorption, pulpal disorders, gingival recession, and alveolar bone loss (Wennström et al. 1987). There is also evidence that teeth with a reduced and healthy periodontium and good oral hygiene can undergo successfully orthodontic movements without further compromising the periodontium support (Boyd et al. 1989; Eliasson et al. 1982).

c) Non-carious cervical lesions

In the past they have been described individually as erosion, attrition, corrosion, and abfraction, yet it has been established in the literature that the etiology of this lesions to be multifactorial (Grippo et al. 2012). Abfractions can be defined as a wedge-shaped defect that occurs at the cemento-enamel junction of affected teeth, with a etiology resulting from flexure and fatigue of enamel and dentin. The current evidence, however, does not support the existence of abfraction.

d) Traumatic occlusal forces

e) Tooth and prosthesis related factors

The term "biologic width," commonly used to describe the apico-coronal variable dimensions of the supracrestal attached tissues, has been change to supracrestal tissue attachment. Histologically composed of the junctional epithelium and supracrestal connective tissue attachment (Ercoli et al. 2018; Jepsen et al. 2018).

Localized tooth-related factors that modify or predispose to plaque-induced gingivitis or periodontitis (factors which favor plaque accumulation) (Table 2.8):

1) The tooth-related anatomic factors to consider may be (Matthews et al. 2004):
   - Enamel pearls and projections are related to the attachment loss in furcations of molars. They are enamel deposits located below the CEJ and extending to the furcation area, especially found on maxillary second molars
   - Tooth malposition or tooth inclination can lead to plaque accumulation and attachment loss. A tooth which is positioned more buccally on the dental arch may present a thin, bony plate leading to recession after inflammation. Trauma from abrasion can also occur more easily
   - Root proximity is a problem encountered when the volume of soft tissue and bone is reduced between the two roots of adjacent teeth, leading to more rapid destruction of periodontium during inflammation
   - Open proximal contacts resulting from defective restorations can lead to decreased deflection of food during chewing, causing food impaction interproximally
   - Root anomalies such as palato-gingival grooves are principally found on incisors. Incorrect hygiene can lead to bacterial plaque accumulation, ultimately leading to bone loss along the groove track

2) Dental restorations, appliances: A chronic inflammation or gingival recession may develop when a restoration violates the biological width around a tooth. The minimal desired space needed to preserve the health of periodontal tissues is 3 mm in total, from the crestal bone to the crown margin (Gargiulo 1961). Optimal restoration margins located within the sulcus do not cause gingival inflammation if patients have adequate oral hygiene.

3) Root fractures: Root fractures can be caused by mechanical stress from occlusion, a post, or a root canal treatment. When fractures are vertical, they are hard to distinguish if they are periodontal or endodontic lesions. These problems can lead to attachment loss due to bacterial invasion of the fracture area.

4) Cervical root resorption: Cervical root resorptions in the coronal part of the root (in contact with the oral cavity) may be involved in bacterial plaque accumulation and periodontal destruction.

**Table 2.8** Classification of factors related to teeth and to dental prostheses that can affect the periodontium.

A) Localized tooth-related factors that modify or predispose to biofilm-induced gingival diseases/periodontitis

1) Tooth anatomic factors

2) Root factors

3) Cervical root resorption, cemental tears

4) Root proximity

5) Altered passive eruption

B) Localized dental prosthesis-related factors

1) Restoration margins placed within the supracrestal attached tissues

2) Clinical procedures related to the fabrication of indirect restorations

3) Hypersensitivity/toxicity reactions to dental materials

**5) Altered Passive Eruption (Coslet 1977)**

Altered passive eruption can be defined as a developmental condition that is characterized by the gingival margin (and sometimes bone) located at a more coronal level (Jepsen et al. 2018). This condition can result in formation of pseudo-pockets, and esthetic concerns.

Coslet et al. (1977) classified altered passive eruption into four subtypes, which can be seen in Figure 2.23.

**1) Peri-Diseases and Conditions**
  **a) Peri-Implant Health**
    In order to be considered peri-implant health there must be absence of clinical signs of inflammation, bleeding on probing (not related to mechanical induced trauma while probing), and further bone loss following initial healing (first year in function) greater than 2 mm. Additionally, the implant position and the height of the soft tissues will influence the probing depth around the implant, but in general it should not be greater than 5 mm or increase over time (Berglundh et al. 2018).
  **b) Peri-Implant Mucositis**
    Peri-implant mucositis is a reversible inflammatory condition affecting the supporting tissues around the implant. Histologically it is a well-defined inflammatory lesion lateral to the junctional epithelium with an infil-trate rich in vascular structures, plasma cells, and lymphocytes. This lesion does not extend apically beyond the junctional epithelium into the connective tissue (Heitz-Mayfield et al. 2018; Renvert et al. 2018).

The diagnosis of peri-implant mucositis should be based on the presence of clinical signs of inflammation, bleeding on probing, an increased probing depth compared to the baseline, and absence of additional bone loss after initial remodeling (Renvert et al. 2018).
  **c) Peri-Implantitis**
    Currently peri-implantitis can be defined as a pathological condition occurring in tissues around dental implants, characterized by inflammation in the peri-implant mucosa and progressive loss of supporting bone (Schwarz et al. 2018).

It has been determined that in absence of treatment, peri-implantitis has a nonlinear and accelerating pattern, its conversion from peri-mucositis into peri-implantitis has not been fully understood but it is more prevalent to develop in patients with peri-mucositis that are not enrolled in a regular maintenance program compared to those patients that are (43% vs. 18%) (Costa et al. 2012).

Histologically, the lesion extends apically of the junctional epithelium, are larger than those found in peri-mucositis, and contain large numbers and densities of

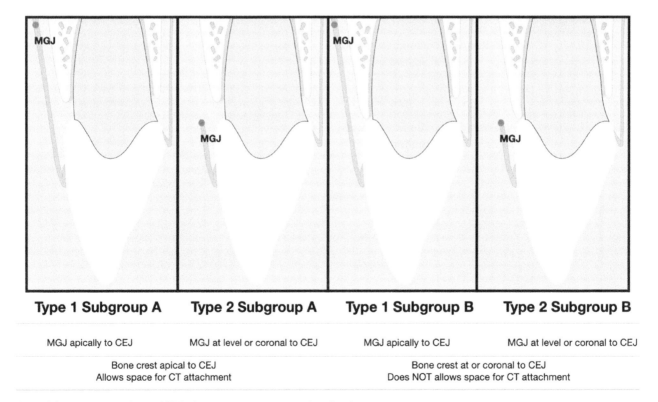

| **Type 1 Subgroup A** | **Type 2 Subgroup A** | **Type 1 Subgroup B** | **Type 2 Subgroup B** |
|---|---|---|---|
| MGJ apically to CEJ | MGJ at level or coronal to CEJ | MGJ apically to CEJ | MGJ at level or coronal to CEJ |
| Bone crest apical to CEJ<br>Allows space for CT attachment | | Bone crest at or coronal to CEJ<br>Does NOT allows space for CT attachment | |

**Figure 2.23** Based on (Coslet 1977) altered passive eruption classification.

inflammatory cells, predominantly plasma cells, macrophages and neutrophils (Berglundh et al. 2018).

The criteria to diagnose peri-implantitis varies significantly in the literature, but according to the 2017 world workshop there has to be presence of inflammatory signs with bleeding on probing or suppuration, increased probing depths compared to previous examinations, and lastly clinical and radiographic signs of progressive bone loss after the initial remodeling (1 year in function) has elapse or greater than 2 mm at any time. In absence of previous examinations, peri-implantitis would be defined as presence of inflammatory signs, probing depths greater than 6 mm, and the bone level is 3 mm or more apical to the most coronal portion of the intraosseous implant. (Renvert et al. 2018).

d) Peri-Implant Soft and Hard Tissue Deficiencies
Peri-implant soft tissue deficiencies to consider are thin peri-implant mucosa, lack of keratinized tissue, reduced papilla height, and peri-implant frenum attachments. While the hard tissue deficiencies are horizontal, vertical or combined ridge deficiencies, pneumatization of the maxillary sinus, and thin/absent buccal/lingual bone plate (Berglundh et al. 2018).

## References

Albandar, J.M., Susin, C., and Hughes, F.J. (2018 June). Manifestations of systemic diseases and conditions that affect the periodontal attachment apparatus: case definitions and diagnostic considerations. *J. Clin. Periodontol.* 45 (Suppl 20): S171–S189. doi: 10.1111/jcpe.12947. PMID: 29926486.

Angelopoulos, A.P. and Goaz, P.W. (1972 December). Incidence of diphenylhydantoin gingival hyperplasia. *Oral Surg. Oral Med. Oral Pathol.* 34 (6): 898–906. doi:10.1016/0030-4220(72)90228-9. PMID: 4509004.

Armitage, G.C. (1999 December). Development of a classification system for peri- odontal diseases and conditions. *Ann. Periodontol.* 4 (1): 1–6.

Barclay, S., Thomason, J.M., Idle, J.R., and Seymour, R.A. (1992 May). The incidence and severity of nifedipine-induced gingival overgrowth. *J. Clin. Periodontol.* 19 (5): 311–314. doi: 10.1111/j.1600-051x.1992.tb00650.x. PMID: 1517474.

Berglundh, T., Armitage, G., Araujo, M.G. et al. (2018 June). Peri-implant diseases and conditions: consensus report of workgroup 4 of the 2017 World Workshop on the classification of periodontal and peri-implant diseases and conditions. *J. Clin. Periodontol.* 45 (Suppl 20): S286–S291. doi: 10.1111/jcpe.12957. PMID: 29926491.

Bharti, V. and Bansal, C. (2013 March). Drug-induced gingival overgrowth: the nemesis of gingiva unravelled. *J. Indian Soc. Periodontol.* 17 (2): 182–187. doi: 10.4103/0972-124X.113066. PMID: 23869123; PMCID: PMC3713748.

Boyd, R.L., Leggott, P.J., Quinn, R.S. et al. (1989 September). Periodontal implications of orthodontic treatment in adults with reduced or normal periodontal tissues versus those of adolescents. *Am. J. Orthod. Dentofacial Orthop.* 96 (3): 191–198. doi:10.1016/0889-5406(89)90455-1. PMID: 2773862.

Cairo, F., Nieri, M., Cincinelli, S. et al. (2011 July). The interproximal clinical attachment level to classify gingival recessions and predict root coverage outcomes: an explorative and reliability study. *J. Clin. Periodontol.* 38 (7): 661–666. doi: 10.1111/j.1600-051X.2011.01732.x. Epub 2011 Apr 20. PMID: 21507033.

Caton J.G., Armitage, G., Berglundh, T. et al. (2018 June). A new classification scheme for periodontal and peri-implant diseases and conditions – Introduction and key changes from the 1999 classification. *J Clin Periodontol.* 45 (Suppl 20): S1–S8. doi: 10.1111/jcpe.12935. PMID: 29926489.

Chapple, I.L.C., Mealey, B.L., Van Dyke, T.E. et al. (2018 June). Periodontal health and gingival diseases and conditions on an intact and a reduced periodontium: consensus report of workgroup 1 of the 2017 World workshop on the classification of periodontal and peri-implant diseases and conditions. *J. Periodontol.* 89 (Suppl 1): S74–S84. doi: 10.1002/JPER.17-0719. PMID: 29926944.

Charbeneau, T.D. and Hurt, W.C. (1983). Gingival findings in spontaneous scurvy. A case report. *J. Periodontol.* 54: 694–697.

Coslet, J.G., Vanarsdall, R., and Weisgold, A. (1977 December). Diagnosis and classification of delayed passive eruption of the dentogingival junction in the adult. *Alpha Omegan* 70 (3): 24–28. PMID: 276255.

Costa, F.O., Takenaka-Martinez, S., Cota, L.O. et al. (2012 February). Peri-implant disease in subjects with and without preventive maintenance: a 5-year follow-up. *J. Clin. Periodontol.* 39 (2): 173–181. doi: 10.1111/j.1600-051X.2011.01819.x. Epub 2011 Nov 23. PMID: 22111654.

Eliasson, L.A., Hugoson, A., Kurol, J., and Siwe, H. (1982 February). The effects of orthodontic treatment on periodontal tissues in patients with reduced periodontal support. *Eur. J. Orthod.* 4 (1): 1–9. doi: 10.1093/ejo/4.1.1. PMID: 6950899.

Ercoli, C. and Caton, J.G. (2018 June). Dental prostheses and tooth-related factors. *J. Periodontol.* 89 (Suppl 1): S223–S236. doi: 10.1002/JPER.16-0569. PMID: 29926939.

Fan, J. and Caton, J.G. (2018 June). Occlusal trauma and excessive occlusal forces: narrative review, case definitions, and diagnostic considerations. *J. Periodontol.* 89 (Suppl 1): S214–S222. doi: 10.1002/JPER.16-0581. PMID: 29926937.

Gargiulo, A.W., Wentz, F.M., and Orban, B. (1961). Dimensions and relations of the dentogingival function in humans. *J. Periodontol.* 32: 261–267.

Gorlin, R.J., Cohen, M.M., and Levis, L.S. (1990). *Syndromes of the Head and Neck*, 3e. 847–855. New York: Oxford University Press.

Greenberg, M.S. (1996). Herpes virus infections. *Dent. Clin. North Am.* 40: 359–368.

Grippo, J.O., Simring, M., and Coleman, T.A. (2012 February). Abfraction, abrasion, biocorrosion, and the enigma of noncarious cervical lesions: a 20-year perspective. *J. Esthet Restor. Dent.* 24 (1): 10–23. doi: 10.1111/j.1708-8240.2011.00487.x. Epub 2011 Nov 17. PMID: 22296690.

Heitz-Mayfield, L.J.A. and Salvi, G.E. (2018 June). Peri-implant mucositis. *J. Clin. Periodontol.* 45 (Suppl 20): S237–S245. doi: 10.1111/jcpe.12953. PMID: 29926488.

Herrera, D., Retamal-Valdes, B., Alonso, B., and Feres, M. (2018 June). Acute periodontal lesions (periodontal abscesses and necrotizing periodontal diseases) and endo-periodontal lesions. *J. Periodontol.* 89 (Suppl 1): S85–S102. doi: 10.1002/JPER.16-0642. PMID: 29926942.

Holmstrup, P. (1999 December). Non-plaque-induced gingival lesions. *Ann. Periodontol.* 4 (1): 20–31.

Holmstrup, P., Plemons, J., and Meyle, J. (2018 June). Non-plaque-induced gingival diseases. *J. Clin Periodontol.* 45 (Suppl 20): S28–S43. doi: 10.1111/jcpe.12938. PMID: 29926497.

Hugoson, A. (1971). Gingivitis in pregnant women. A longitudinal clinical study. *Odontol. Revy* 22: 65–84.

Jepsen, S., Caton, J.G., Albandar, J.M. et al. (2018 June). Periodontal manifestations of systemic diseases and developmental and acquired conditions: consensus report of workgroup 3 of the 2017 world workshop on the classification of periodontal and peri-implant diseases and conditions. *J. Periodontol.* 89 (Suppl 1): S237–S248. doi: 10.1002/JPER.17-0733. PMID: 29926943.

Kaufman, A.Y. (1969). An oral contraceptive as an etiologic factor producing hyperplasic gingivitis and a neoplasm of the pregnancy tumor type. *Oral Surg. Oral Med. Oral Pathol.* 28: 666–670.

Lindhe, J. (2003). *Clinical Periodontology and Implant Dentistry*, 4e. Wiley-Blackwell.

Lozada-Nur, F., Gorsky, M., and Silverman, S. Jr. (1989). Oral erythema multiforme: clinical observation and treatment of 95 patients. *Oral Surg. Oral Med. Oral Pathol.* 67: 36–40.

Mariotti, A. (1999 December). Dental plaque-induced gingival diseases. *Ann. Periodontol.* 4 (1): 7–19.

Matthews, D.C. and Tabesh, M. (2004). Detection of localized tooth-related factors that predispose to periodontal infections. *Periodontol. 2000* 34: 136–150.

Meng, H.X. (1999a December). Periodontal abscess. *Ann. Periodontol.* 4 (1): 79–83.

Meng, H.X. (1999b December). Periodontic-endodontic lesions. *Ann. Periodontol.* 4 (1): 84–90.

Miller, C.S. (1996). Viral infection of the immunocompetent patient. *Dermatol. Clin.* 14: 225–241.

Miller, C.S. and Redding, S.W. (1992). Diagnosis and management of orofacial herpes simplex virus infections. *Dent. Clin. North Am.* 36: 879–895.

Miller, P.D. (1985). Root coverage using the free soft tissue autograft following citric acid application. III. A successful and predictable procedure in areas of deep wide recession. *Int. J. Periodontics Restorative Dent.* 5 (2): 15–37.

Morris, J.W., Campbell, P.M., Tadlock, L.P. et al. (2017 May). Prevalence of gingival recession after orthodontic tooth movements. *Am. J. Orthod. Dentofacial Orthop.* 151 (5): 851–859. doi: 10.1016/j.ajodo.2016.09.027. PMID: 28457262.

Needleman, I., Garcia, R., Gkranias, N. et al. (2018 June). Mean annual attachment, bone level, and tooth loss: a systematic review. *J. Periodontol.* 89 (Suppl 1): S120–S139. doi: 10.1002/JPER.17-0062. PMID: 29926956.

Neville, B.W., Damm, D.D., Allen, C.M., and Bouquot, J.E. (2002). *Oral and Maxil- Lofacial Pathology*, 2e. Saunders LTD.

Page, R.C. (1985). Oral health status in the United States: prevalence of inflammatory periodontal diseases. *J. Dent. Educ.* 49: 354–367.

Papapanou, P.N., Sanz, M., Buduneli, N. et al. (2018 June). Periodontitis: consensus report of workgroup 2 of the 2017 World workshop on the classification of periodontal and peri-implant diseases and conditions. *J. Periodontol.* 89 (Suppl 1): S173–S182. doi: 10.1002/JPER.17-0721. PMID: 29926951.

Pini Prato, G. (1999 December). Mucogingival deformities. *Ann. Periodontol.* 4 (1): 98–101.

Ranney, R.R. (1993). Classification of periodontal diseases. *Periodontol. 2000* 2: 57–71.

Renkema, A.M., Fudalej, P.S., Renkema, A. et al. (2013 February). Development of labial gingival recessions in orthodontically treated patients. *Am. J. Orthod. Dentofacial Orthop.* 143 (2): 206–212. doi: 10.1016/j.ajodo.2012.09.018. PMID: 23374927.

Renvert, S., Persson, G.R., Pirih, F.Q., and Camargo, P.M. (2018 June). Peri-implant health, peri-implant mucositis, and peri-implantitis: case definitions and diagnostic considerations. *J Periodontol* 89 (Suppl 1): S304–S312. doi: 10.1002/JPER.17-0588. PMID: 29926953.

Romito, G.A., Pustiglioni, F.E., Saraiva, L. et al. (2004 July). Relationship of subgingival and salivary microbiota to gingival overgrowth in heart transplant patients following cyclosporin A therapy. *J. Periodontol.* 75 (7): 918–924. doi: 10.1902/jop.2004.75.7.918. PMID: 15341348.

Rowland, R.W. (1999 December). Necrotizing ulcerative gingivitis. *Ann. Periodontol.* 4 (1): 65–73; discussion 78. doi: 10.1902/annals.1999.4.1.65. PMID: 10863376.

Schiodt, M. (1984). Oral discoid lupus erythematus II. Skin lesions and systemic lupus erythematosus in sixty-six patients with 6-year follow-up. *Oral Surg. Oral Med. Oral Pathol.* 57: 177–180.

Schwarz, F., Derks, J., Monje, A., and Wang, H.L. (2018 June). Peri-implantitis. *J. Periodontol.* 89 (Suppl 1): S267–S290. doi: 10.1002/JPER.16-0350. PMID: 29926957.

Sciubba, J.J. (1996 April). Autoimmune aspect of pemphigus vulgaris in mucosal pemphigoid. *Adv. Dent. Res.* 10 (1): 52–56. Review.

Sills, E.S., Zegarelli, S.J., Hoschander, M.M., and Strider, W.E. (1996). Clinical diagnosis and management of hormonally responsive oral pregnancy tumor (pyogenic granuloma). *J. Reprod. Med.* 41: 467–470.

Stamm, J.W. (1986). Epidemiology of gingivitis. *J. Clin. Periodontol.* 13: 360–366.

Sutcliffe, P. (1972). A longitudinal study of gingivitis and puberty. *J. Periodont. Res.* 7: 52–58.

Thorn, J.T., Holmstrup, P., Rindum, J., and Pindborg, J.J. (1988). Course of various clinical forms of oral lichen planus. A prospective follow-up study of 611 patients. *J. Oral Pathol.* 17: 213–218.

Tonetti, M.S., Greenwell, H., and Kornman, K.S. (2018 June). Staging and grading of periodontitis: framework and proposal of a new classification and case definition. *J. Periodontol.* 89 (Suppl 1): S159–S172. doi: 10.1002/JPER.18-0006. Erratum in: *J. Periodontol.* 2018 Dec; 89 (12): 1475.PMID: 29926952.

Trombelli, L., Farina, R., Silva, C.O., and Tatakis, D.N. (2018 June). Plaque-induced gingivitis: case definition and diagnostic considerations. *J. Periodontol.* 89 (Suppl 1): S46–S73. doi: 10.1002/JPER.17-0576. PMID: 29926936.

Wennström, J.L., Lindhe, J., Sinclair, F., and Thilander, B. (1987 March). Some periodontal tissue reactions to orthodontic tooth movement in monkeys. *J. Clin. Periodontol.* 14 (3): 121–129. doi: 10.1111/j.1600-051x.1987.tb00954.x. PMID: 3470318.

Zweers, J., Thomas, R.Z., Slot, D.E. et al. (2014 October). Characteristics of periodontal biotype, its dimensions, associations and prevalence: a systematic review. *J. Clin. Periodontol.* 41 (10): 958–971. doi: 10.1111/jcpe.12275. Epub 2014 Aug 27. PMID: 24836578.

3

# Periodontal Risk Factors and Modification

*Christoph Ramseier, Clemens Walter, and Thomas Dietrich*

## Introduction

As a common chronic disease of the oral cavity, periodontal disease is a set of inflammatory conditions affecting the supporting structures of the dentition (Armitage 1999). After its initiation, the disease progresses with the loss of collagen attachment to the root surface, the apical migration of the pocket epithelium, the formation of deepened periodontal pockets, and the resorption of alveolar bone. Untreated periodontal disease continues with progressive alveolar bone destruction, leading to increased tooth mobility and potential tooth loss (Page and Kornman 1997).

Reports from epidemiological studies, analysis of tissue histology, clinical studies, and animal experiments consistently demonstrate a multifactorial etiology of periodontal disease. Periodontitis is the most prevalent form of destructive periodontal disease (Albandar et al. 1999). Furthermore, cross-sectional and longitudinal data from epidemiological research in periodontology suggest that risk factors can be identified, and that some of these factors could be controlled to prevent the development and progression of the disease. Risk factors are part of the causal chain of a particular disease or can lead to the exposure of the host to a disease ("Consensus Report, Annals of Periodontology," 1996). The presence of a risk factor implies a direct increase in the probability of a disease occurring, and if absent or modified, a reduction in that probability should occur. Risk factors are generally classified as modifiable and non-modifiable. While gender, age, and ethnicity are non-modifiable, insufficient oral hygiene or tobacco use are identified as modifiable risk factors for periodontal disease.

A risk factor may be modified by interventions, thereby reducing the probability that a particular disease will occur. However, the susceptibility to a specific disease will vary among different individuals exposed to a given risk factor over time. Additionally, cumulative interactions between both modifiable and non-modifiable risk factors,

described as "complex risk factors," have been suggested (Stolk et al. 2008).

A variety of interrelated risk factors may influence both the onset of periodontal disease and its progression (Figure 3.1). The detection of periodontal disease progression remains challenging since it typically relies on the comparison of measurements made with a calibrated periodontal probe and non-standardized periapical radiographs over time. Some emphasis should be placed on the early identification of periodontal risk factors to assess the likelihood of periodontal disease progression in susceptible individuals since both methods detect periodontal breakdown only after it has occurred. The goal of this chapter is to discuss known non-modifiable and modifiable risk factors as well as their management in the dental practice to provide prevention and a careful maintenance program for the periodontal patient while following the best available evidence today. The concept of risk factor control is now firmly embedded in periodontal practice and is strongly recommended in the S3 clinical practice guideline by the European Federation of Periodontology (EFP) (Sanz et al. 2020).

## Non-Modifiable Risk Factors

### Genetic and Hereditary Factors

Periodontitis is a complex disease, with multiple causative factors. Immune-mediated inflammatory conditions, such as periodontitis, are complex due to the interplay of several causal components (genetic and environmental factors) which simultaneously interact with each other in an unpredictable manner. Furthermore, due to the nonlinear nature of these complex interactions, the presentation of disease in some individuals may be disproportionately greater than in other individuals with the same causal factors.

When there is a dysbiosis between host and oral microbiome, an atypical response manifesting in altered inflammatory

*Practical Periodontal Diagnosis and Treatment Planning*, Second Edition. Edited by Serge Dibart and Thomas Dietrich.
© 2024 John Wiley & Sons, Inc. Published 2024 by John Wiley & Sons, Inc.

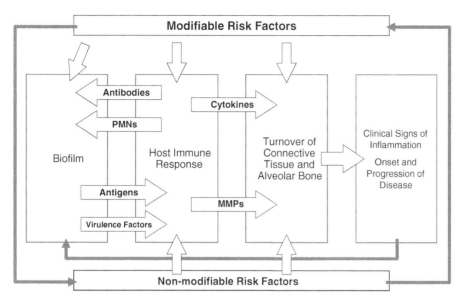

**Figure 3.1** Interplay of modifiable and non-modifiable risk factors with the pathogenesis of periodontal diseases.

reactions may lead to changes in the subgingival environment which elicit further periodontal inflammation and disease progression.

Periodontal diseases have been shown to be affected by genetic factors (Page and Kornman 1997). A number of genetic disorders, such as Down syndrome, leukocyte adhesion deficiency syndrome (LADS), Papillon-Lefevre syndrome, Chediak-Higashi syndrome, chronic neutrophil defects, or cyclic neutropenia are associated with more or less severe periodontal conditions.

The hereditary aggregation was demonstrated in a twin study for periodontitis (Michalowicz et al. 1991) and an epidemiological trial on aggressive periodontitis in a Dutch population (van der Velden et al. 1993). Following the adjustment for environmental factors such as tobacco use, it was estimated that 50% of the variance in disease may be attributed to a genetic background (Michalowicz et al. 2000) in younger patients, with a much lower percentage (<25%) attributed to genetic background in older populations.

**Practical Application of Genetic Susceptibility Testing**

During periodontal inflammation, inflammatory cytokines, including interleukin-1 β (IL-1β) and tumor necrosis factor-α (TNF-α), activate catabolic enzymes such as matrix metalloproteinases, subsequently leading to the breakdown of connective tissue. Any gene polymorphism of such proteins potentially alters the susceptibility of the host to periodontal diseases. A single nucleotide polymorphism (SNP) is a mutation that occurs when a single nucleotide is altered within its genome due to changes in the base pair sequence.

Past periodontal diagnostic research has focused on evaluating several selected candidate gene SNPs including variations of IL-1β or TNF-α.

The evidence-based perspective: Initial evidence suggested that some polymorphisms in the genes encoding interleukins (IL)-1, Fc gamma receptors (FcgR), IL-10, and the vitamin D receptor may be associated with periodontitis in certain ethnic groups (Huynh-Ba et al. 2007; Loos et al. 2005). These findings sparked some enthusiasm and led to the development of commercially available tests for genetic periodontal risk factors.

However, it is now widely accepted that periodontitis as a complex disease is polygenic, i.e., there is a multitude of genetic variations involved. The genetic factors directly associated with, and/or directly contributing to, periodontal pathogenesis are currently poorly validated, with further work needed in this area (Loos and Van Dyke 2020).

Hence, there is currently no role for genetic testing in the management of patients with periodontitis.

### Gender

Hormonal changes in women during menstruation, pregnancy, menopause, or therapy with pharmaceutical supplements have an impact on periodontal health. Disease susceptibility may be increased due to hormone-related alterations of the gingival blood flow (Kovar et al. 1985), the composition and flow rate of saliva (Laine 2002), or the bone metabolism (Lerner 2006). Additionally, data from epidemiological studies interestingly reveal that men may be at greater risk for periodontal diseases: in most clinical trials men are often found with worse periodontal health (Albandar 2002; Meisel et al. 2008). Most often, however, these deteriorations may be explained by an increased prevalence of male tobacco use and men's increased tendency to neglect oral hygiene (Meisel et al. 2008).

**Gender-specific Practical Applications**

Periodontal diseases have been associated with gender-specific complications such as an increased susceptibility for gingivitis during pregnancy (Russell and Mayberry 2008), preterm delivery, or low birth weight (Madianos et al. 2002). Therefore, gender-specific periodontal disease risk factors should be assessed in women by all oral health professionals (Krejci and Bissada 2002). In pregnant women, a rigid recall interval including oral hygiene motivation is recommended. Consequently, it is suggested that existing periodontal inflammation should be treated before pregnancy.

Factors that are increasingly investigated in recent studies include gender-specific diseases such as osteoporosis or metastatic bone disease in relation with hormone substitute therapy or bisphosphonate medication in postmenopausal women (Diel et al. 2007; Payne et al. 1999). Bisphosphonates affect osteoclast functions, leading to the inhibition of physiological bone remodeling. With both surgical and nonsurgical periodontal treatment, a bisphosphonate-associated osteonecrosis of the jaws should be considered as a complication. In one prospective cohort study of osteoporotic women in early menopause, it was found that a supplementation of estrogen may be associated with reduced gingival inflammation and impaired clinical attachment loss (Reinhardt et al. 1999).

## Age

The aging process itself is suggested to be an independent risk factor for periodontal diseases (Papapanou et al. 1989). In contrast, a longitudinal study involving an elderly Scandinavian population (age 75 or older) demonstrated stable periodontal conditions for five years, suggesting a limited impact of the aging process itself in otherwise relatively healthy individuals (Ajwani and Ainamo 2001). However, the extent and severity of periodontal diseases are shown to increase with age (Albandar 2002) as a consequence of the cumulative burden from various risk factors such as tobacco use or plaque accumulation (Albandar 2002; Albandar et al. 1999). Additionally, metabolic disorders, including diabetes mellitus, osteoporosis, rheumatoid arthritis, or vascular diseases, are more likely to develop in the elderly and thus affect periodontal conditions (Persson 2006).

**Age-specific Practical Applications**

Life expectancy has increased significantly over the past few years in industrialized countries (Holm-Pedersen et al. 2005). As compared to previous populations, the elderly population is retaining its natural dentition, potentially leading to more periodontal problems. The presence of various chronic diseases, such as diabetes mellitus or

specific medications (e.g. Vitamin K antagonists), may also interact with the periodontal condition or the treatment. Thus, there is a need for multidisciplinary treatment in many cases, due to the increased likelihood of comorbidity in the elderly (Persson 2006). Aging is often associated with the individual's impaired mobility, probably leading to an incapacity for regular supportive periodontal treatment. A close interplay with nursing homes or public oral healthcare providers may be advisable. Physical or mental disorders may affect the effectiveness of supragingival plaque control. The suggestion of simple interventions, including the weekly use of chlorhexidine-containing mouth rinses in conjunction with cognitive behavioral interventions, might be useful (Hujoel et al. 1997).

# Modifiable Risk Factors

## Insufficient Oral Hygiene

Today, accumulated plaque is considered to be a dental biofilm briefly defined as a complex bacterial structure adherent to wet surfaces (Socransky and Haffajee 2002). For the therapy of periodontal diseases, it is important to consider that biofilms can protect their microorganisms, either from the host immune response or antimicrobial agents, and thus become difficult therapeutic targets (Socransky and Haffajee 2002). So far, only mechanical debridement was shown to be a predictable approach to successfully destruct the dental biofilm. Therefore, mechanical plaque control should be performed supragingivally by the individual on a regular basis and subgingivally, if needed, by the oral health professional.

Any factors that facilitate biofilm formation, such as plaque retention or insufficient supragingival plaque control, are common risk factors for periodontal breakdown due to their causality with gingival inflammation and possibly the onset of periodontitis. This includes several anatomic conditions, such as enamel pearls, tongues, grooves, root furcations, and concavities, as well as root proximities (Roussa 1998; Vermylen et al. 2005). Calculus and acquired iatrogenic factors, such as insufficient restorations, additionally contribute to plaque accumulation (Lang et al. 1983; Oliver et al. 1998).

It was proven some 40 years ago by classical experiments conducted by the work group Löe and Theilade that oral microorganisms are relevant for the development of inflammable periodontal diseases (Theilade et al. 1966). In a longitudinal study of more than 26 years, a further research group examined the influence of plaque-induced gingival inflammation on the subsequent loss of clinical attachment in a periodontally well-maintained Scandinavian population (Schatzle et al. 2003). The supragingival plaque accumulation correlated with the degree of gingival inflammation. However, sites with bleeding on probing at every visit demonstrated about 70% more attachment loss than sites without inflammation for the duration of the study. Moreover, it was shown that the susceptibility of gingivitis seems to be higher among males suffering from periodontitis (Dietrich et al. 2006).

It should therefore come as no surprise that the recent EFP S3 level practice guideline (Sanz et al. 2020) makes several strong recommendations aiming at achieving adequate oral hygiene in patients with periodontitis. These recommendations include continued enforcement of oral hygiene advice throughout all phases of periodontal therapy, engaging the periodontitis patient in behavioral change for oral hygiene improvement, and the performance of supragingival professional mechanical plaque removal and control of retentive factors as part of the first step of therapy (Sanz et al. 2020).

### Practical Application of Microbiological Testing

A multitude of different microbiological tests, based on morphological, enzymatic, cultural, genetic, or antigenetic bacterial properties, are available for both qualitative and quantitative microbiologic risk assessment of periodontitis. In many clinical situations, however, these tests fail to provide evidence-based recommendations for therapy (Sanz et al. 2004). Nevertheless, in a few cases, microbiologic tests can support treatment planning, including cases resistant to combined mechanical-antibiotic therapies, e.g., scaling and root planing, and the prescription of metronidazole and amoxicillin.

### Tobacco Use

Over the past 40 years, robust epidemiologic oral health research has identified cigarette smoking as the most important environmental risk factor, second only to poor oral hygiene. Cigarette smoking has consistently been demonstrated to have a dose- and time-dependent association with periodontitis and tooth loss (Dietrich and Hoffmann 2004; Dietrich et al. 2015), with smokers showing increased clinical attachment loss, deeper periodontal probing depths, and more recession. Paradoxically, the clinical characteristics of gingival inflammation or bleeding on periodontal probing are suppressed in smokers (Dietrich et al. 2004). Smokers show less favorable results after conventional, surgical, and regenerative periodontal therapy. Periodontal plastic surgery has poorer outcomes in smokers (Erley et al. 2006). Moreover, smoking impairs the osseointegration of

oral implants and is at least partly responsible for a majority of biological complications in implant dentistry, such as peri-implantitis (Strietzel et al. 2007). A common clinical observation is delayed wound healing after therapeutic interventions (Figure 3.2) (Silverstein 1992).

The unequivocal evidence for the importance of cigarette smoking as a cause of periodontitis and a factor associated with disease occurrence and treatment outcomes has led to cigarette smoking being included as a "grade modifier" in the current classification of periodontal diseases. Specifically, periodontitis patients who are not classified as grade B or C based on disease progression or bone loss relative to age will be "upgraded" to grades B or C if they are light (<10 cigarettes per day) or heavy (10+ cigarettes per day) smokers, respectively (Tonetti et al. 2018).

There are various potentially significant pathogenic effects of tobacco-related substances on the periodontal tissues, immune response system, or composition of the oral flora. Periodontal destruction associated with tobacco use is caused by a wide multidimensional range of effects on different functions in cells, tissues, and organ systems. Some of these effects are diametric in nature, due to the effects of different tobacco constituents. However, when summarizing the properties of the tobacco-induced alterations in the metabolism of vasculature, connective-tissue, and bone, as well as on cell-mediated and humoral immunity, it is more than likely that tobacco use shifts the physiological balance between anabolic and catabolic mechanisms in a more destructive direction, due to an alteration of protective immune and tissue mechanisms (Johnson and Guthmiller 2007; Palmer 2005; Ryder 2007). Moreover, there is evidence that tobacco consumption may change the genetically determined susceptibility for periodontal diseases (Meisel et al. 2004).

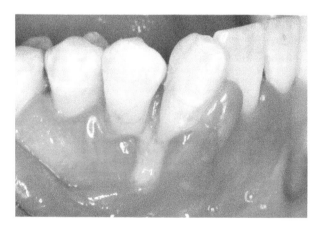

**Figure 3.2** Impaired wound healing in a female smoker (age 44, 45 pack years) seven days following periodontal nonsurgical debridement.

## Diabetes Mellitus

Diabetes mellitus is a metabolic disorder categorized by a hyperglycemia due to impaired insulin production or insulin resistance. Insulin is a pancreatic-hormone-maintaining glucose metabolism. At least two major groups of diabetes mellitus (type 1 and type 2) are differentiated based on their pathogenesis. In addition, some diseases such as hormone-secreting tumors, conditions such as pregnancy (gestational diabetes), or drugs such as corticosteroids can lead to diabetes mellitus. Treatment of diabetes mellitus primarily aims to keep blood sugar levels within a target range. Treatment may include an interview for behavioral change for dietary adjustment, reducing physical inactivity and sedentary time, or several drugs. They usually include oral antihyperglycemic drugs or insulin replacement therapy, as well as drugs for prevention and/or treatment of diabetes complications such as hypertension. If left untreated, serious long-term complications may occur, affecting small and large blood vessels, eyes, kidneys, nerves, or the immune system.

Diabetes mellitus has been associated with increased prevalence and severity of periodontal disease (Figure 3.3) (Emrich et al. 1991; Shlossman et al. 1990). The majority of studies demonstrate a more severe periodontal condition in diabetic adults than in adults without diabetes (Papapanou 1996; Verma and Bhat 2004). The type of diabetes does not affect the extent of periodontitis when the duration of diabetes is similar. However, those living with type 1 diabetes develop the disease at an earlier age, and, hence, have it for longer periods, and may therefore develop a greater extent and severity of periodontitis (Oliver and Tervonen 1994; Thorstensson and Hugoson 1993). Individuals who have optimal time in range (i.e., well-managed diabetes) are more likely to be similar to non-diabetics in their periodontal status (Westfelt et al. 1996).

Diabetes status is also considered in the diagnosis and classification of periodontal disease as a grade modifier. Periodontitis patients who also live with diabetes may be upgraded to grade B or—if exhibiting increased time out of range (HbA1c ≥7.0%)—grade C (Tonetti et al. 2018).

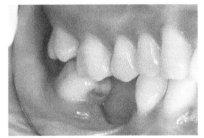
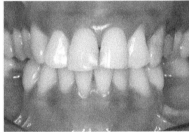
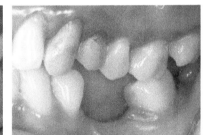

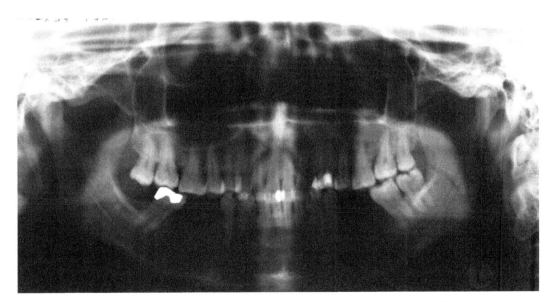

Figure 3.3  Clinical and radiographic images of a 46-year-old female patient with type II diabetes mellitus and periodontitis. The metabolic disease was diagnosed in 1993 and is well managed (level of blood sugar glucose 6, 3 mmol/l). The patient receives oral antidiabetic drugs.

A common complication of diabetes mellitus is the increased susceptibility for microbial infections due to an impaired function of the host immune response. Diabetes mellitus may contribute to periodontal inflammation via specific mechanisms. The hyperglycemia may promote the formation of advanced glycation end products (AGE), i.e., glycated body proteins (Wautier and Guillausseau 1998). Accumulation of AGE may have an impact on periodontal micro-vascularization or may lead to an increased number of monocytes within the site of inflammation (Katz et al. 2005). A modification of physiologic cell functions of certain subtypes of granulocytes is also reported (Manouchehr-Pour et al. 1981a, 1981b). Moreover, some studies suggest an alteration of pro-inflammatory mediators in gingival crevicular fluid, including tumor necrosis factor-α, prostaglandin-E2, and interleukin-1 β (S. P. Engebretson et al. 2004; Salvi et al. 1997a, 1997b). A further research group reported a decreased gene expression of anti-inflammatory and anti-bone-resorptive molecules such as interleukin-10 and osteo-protegerin (Duarte et al. 2007). Collagen is produced by fibroblasts and is an important molecule of the periodontium. In vitro findings indicate a reduction of collagen synthesis in a dose-dependent fashion of glucose concentration (Willershausen-Zonnchen et al. 1991).

Interestingly, there is some evidence for periodontitis as a contributing factor in the pathogenesis of diabetes mellitus (Taylor et al. 1998). Inflammatory markers, including tumor necrosis factor-α, increase with periodontal severity and thus affect the insulin metabolism in in those with diabetes (S. Engebretson et al. 2007). In contrast, their reduction occurs following antimicrobial periodontal therapy, leading to an improvement of glycemic control (Iwamoto et al. 2001).

The evidence-based perspective: Evidence from a systematic review, including meta-analysis, suggests a significantly higher severity but the same extent of periodontal disease in individuals living with diabetes compared with non-diabetics (Khader et al. 2006).

## Stress

Stress may be caused by acute or chronic stressors. A stressor can be intrinsic or extrinsic in origin and is frequently defined as anything that causes an adaptive and nonspecific neurological and physiological response in an individual. Chronic stressors are of relatively longer duration and include several "life events" such as the loss of a family member, splitting of a relationship, long-term illness, miscarriage, or "daily hassles." Events of a relative short duration, such as traffic jams, surgical interventions, dental visits, or unpleasant questions in a medical exam, on the other hand, may act as acute stressors to an individual. The physiologic response is mediated by several immune-to-brain-to-immune regulatory pathways (Breivik et al. 2006). The individual stress coping behavior depends on genetic susceptibility and environmental and developmental factors as well as gathered experiences during the course of life.

Several studies indicated an association of negative stress, depression, anxiety, or poor coping behavior with periodontal diseases (Genco et al. 1999; Hugoson et al. 2002; Wimmer et al. 2002). Negative stress may lead to an increased susceptibility to periodontitis mediated through different pathways.

As one mechanism, it was suggested that due to stress, the oral hygiene may be limited (Deinzer et al. 2001). Additionally, academic stress was shown to cause an enhancement of interleukin-1 secretion detected in gingival crevicular fluid in a study by Deinzer and coworkers (Deinzer et al. 1999). This cytokine is a strong stimulator of osteoclasts leading to destructive bone metabolism. Interleukin-6, another inflammatory cytokine, was found to be elevated in the gingival fluid of depressed women (Johannsen et al. 2006). In addition, a prolonged reduction of the secretion of immunoglobulin A, an important salivary antibody, was observed in students participating in a major medical exam (Deinzer et al. 2000).

Cortisol and the catecholamines adrenaline and noradrenaline are the major stress hormones produced by the cortex of the suprarenal gland in response to stimulation by hypothalamus-releasing hormones. Increased levels of stress-mediated cortisol were found in the gingival crevicular fluid and in saliva (Hugo et al. 2006; Ishisaka et al. 2007; Nakajima et al. 2006). Additionally, stress-induced hypercortisolemia was linked to elevated levels of plaque and gingivitis (Hugo et al. 2006). Moreover, evidence from animal experiments reveals changes in the periodontal tissues following stress exposure (Nakajima et al. 2006). Restraint stress was able to enhance attachment loss after challenge with the putative periodontal pathogen *Porphyromonas gingivalis*. Findings from in vitro experiments suggest an effect of catecholamines on the growth of certain oral bacteria (Roberts et al. 2002). Thus, a stress-induced increase of catecholamine levels in the gingival crevicular fluid may be able to mediate the composition of the subgingival biofilm.

## HIV/AIDS

The acquired immunodeficiency syndrome (AIDS) is caused by infection with the human immunodeficiency virus (HIV), leading to a destruction of the immune system of the affected host. The CD4$^+$ T cells as a subset of T lymphocytes are destroyed in particular. AIDS consists of various (opportunistic) infections including pulmonary and gastrointestinal infections and/or clinical manifestations including neurological and psychiatric involvement as well as tumors and other malignancies.

The current status of immunosuppression, assessed by $CD4^+$ lymphocyte levels and viral load with HIV, are predictors of AIDS as well as HIV-associated complications in the oral cavity (Kroidl et al. 2005). A multitude of oral lesions, including Kaposi's sarcoma, linear gingival erythema (LGE), necrotizing ulcerative gingivitis (NUG), and necrotizing ulcerative periodontitis (NUP), were described in individuals infected with HIV (Figure 3.4). However, the likelihood of HIV-associated oral diseases has decreased in recent years, due to advanced treatment approaches in HIV/AIDS therapy, such as highly active antiretroviral therapy (HAART) (Reichart 2006).

HAART combines the use of several drugs, affecting or inhibiting different stages of the retrovirus life cycle, including viral entry in host cells, syntheses of viral DNA, or activity of viral proteases. A number of studies dealt with the issue of occurrence of periodontal disease in HIV-seropositive subjects and AIDS patients (Lamster et al. 1994; McKaig et al. 1998). After controlling for CD41 counts, HIV-infected people taking HIV-antiretroviral medication were five times less likely to suffer from periodontitis compared with those not taking such medication (McKaig et al. 1998).

The effects of taking HAART on the outcome of periodontal therapy were assessed by Jordan and coworkers (Jordan et al. 2006). Periodontitis patients with HIV can be successfully treated by nonsurgical scaling and root planing, followed by supportive periodontal therapy. However, a close collaboration of oral healthcare providers and general practitioners should become a routine procedure in HIV patients' care.

## Nutrition

Possible consequences of nutrition deficiencies on oral and periodontal health have been reviewed (Dorsky 2001). Several nutrients have been found to have a negative impact on periodontal health when not sufficiently delivered, such as vitamins, trace metals, antioxidants, and proteins (Eklund and Burt 1994; Krall 2001; Nishida et al. 2000a, 2000b). So far, however, there are no reports in the current literature on the effect of nutrition counseling, either on the periodontal status or on the outcome of periodontal therapy.

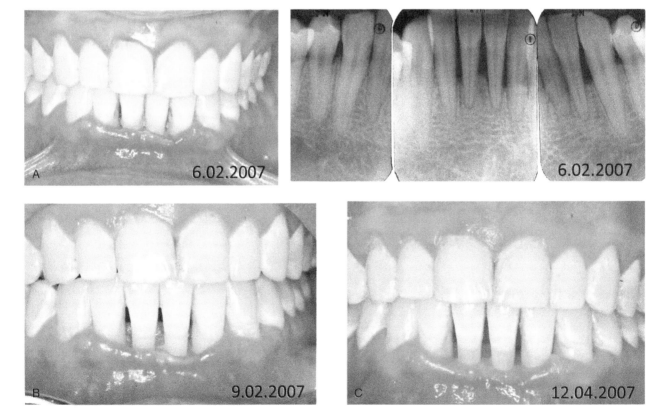

Figure 3.4 Necrotizing ulcerative periodontitis in a 26-year-old HIV-positive male (20 cigarettes per day) with medical observation for virus load and CD4 counts and no further prescription of HIV medication (HAART). (A) Pre-therapeutical clinical and radiographic images, (B) clinical view three days following nonsurgical periodontal therapy, (C) clinical view two months following therapy.

# Risk Factor Modification

## Behavioral Change

Primary and secondary prevention oriented toward the change of inappropriate behavior is about to become a part of daily dental care. Traditional periodontal care includes the instruction of proper oral hygiene methods. Unfortunately, many health education approaches seem to be inefficient in accomplishing long-term change, potentially leading to frustration of both the patient and the clinician. Additionally, there is a shortcoming of evidence in both the dental and psychology literature on effective methods for behavior counseling in periodontal care, particularly regarding:

- Individual oral hygiene instructions for optimal oral hygiene
- Effective tobacco use prevention and cessation counseling to help abstain from tobacco
- Appropriate dietary counseling for a healthy diet

It may be necessary to apply different behavior change counseling methods to target individual behavior to get reliably effective outcomes in periodontal care. According to the best available evidence for oral hygiene instructions, the repeated demonstration of a cleaning device may be applied. For tobacco use cessation, in addition to pharmacotherapy, the method of the five A's (Ask, Advise, Assess, Assist, Arrange) may be used (Fiore 2000). Additionally, type 2 diabetic patients may be referred to nutritionists for dietary counseling. From a practical point of view, however, it may be complicated and even discouraging to approach the periodontal patient with a variety of different methods targeting the same purpose: establishing appropriate behavior to improve the outcomes of both periodontal therapy and long-term supportive periodontal care.

### Brief Motivational Interviewing (BMI)

Aiming for simplicity, it may be preferable to apply one single counseling method for behavior change in periodontal care that is shown to be effective in both primary and secondary prevention of oral diseases. Numerous behavioral research studies have confirmed the success achieved by state-of-the-art motivational interviewing (MI). MI is a patient-centered interviewing technique which was initially used as an auxiliary tool during counseling for smoking cessation and alcohol abuse (Miller and Rollnick 2002). In the context of dentistry, a "short form" of MI known as "brief motivational interviewing" (BMI) appears to be suited for use during health behavior interventions in dental practices. The aim of BMI is to achieve the following objectives within a short amount of time (i.e., less than five minutes):

1) To question the patient concerning her motivation to change her behavior, or
2) To give the patient the self-confidence he may need to accomplish the envisaged change of behavior, and
3) To reach an agreement to discuss behavior change at another appointment.

BMI uses a patient-driven pathway which is reflected by the acronym **OARS**:

**O**pen-ended questions: "Yes" or "no" answers often terminate the topic of a conversation. Using "who," "what," "where," or "why" questions further allow the patient to provide more information for the counseling.

**A**ffirm: Acknowledging the feelings of the patient offers validation and assurance that the counselor is actively listening.

**R**eflection: Playing back the conversation to the patient often demonstrates empathy and may also highlight ambivalent behavior.

**S**ummarize: Providing an overview of the conversation allows confirmation of potential key points in the process of change.

For further information on communication methods for behavioral change counseling, the reader is referred to the textbook of Miller and Rollnick (Miller and Rollnick 2002).

## Supragingival Plaque Control

Proper self-performed mechanical plaque removal and compliance with needs-related recall visits are critical components of successful prevention and therapy of periodontal diseases. Both surgical and nonsurgical periodontal treatments are only shown to be successful along with supragingival plaque control (Magnusson et al. 1984; Rosling et al. 1976). Additionally, periodontal therapy in combination with adequate, self-performed supragingival plaque control has been demonstrated to be effective in maintaining periodontal health for more than 20 years (Axelsson et al. 2004). Consequently, this approach has been considered as the "gold standard" for periodontal care (Figure 3.5) (Carra et al. 2020). It is recognized that the daily removal of the bacterial biofilm represents the most important risk factor control (Figure 3.6). For the detailed instruction of supragingival plaque control for the prevention and treatment of gingivitis and periodontitis, the reader is referred to textbooks on periodontal therapy.

The evidence-based perspective: Evidence from a review suggests that an optimal level of self-performed oral hygiene can have major effects on the subgingival biofilm composition and thus lead to significant therapeutic implications for the treatment of periodontal diseases (Ower 2003; Sanz et al. 2020).

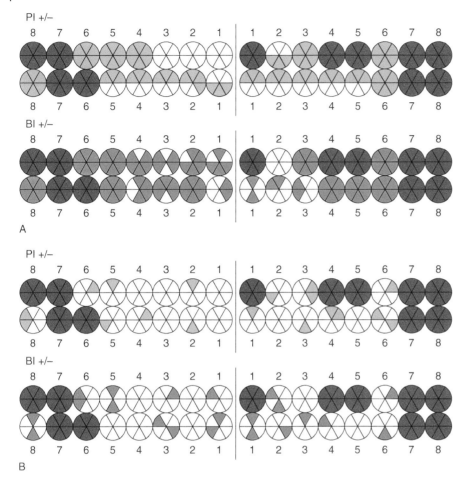

**Figure 3.5** Oral hygiene motivation. Oral hygiene assessment: Visibility of supragingival plaque (Pl, green) and gingival bleeding (Bl, red) is analyzed on six sites per tooth; missing teeth are colored black. The initial scores (A) indicate insufficient supragingival plaque control as well as gingival inflammation. Following oral hygiene instruction (toothbrush and interdental brushes) the plaque control improved (B).

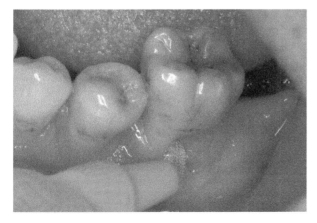

**Figure 3.6** Oral hygiene aids (interdental brushes).

## Tobacco Use Cessation

Recent reports reveal short-term effects after quitting smoking as well as long-term results of smoking cessation on the periodontal and peri-implant status (Bain 1996; Bergstrom 2004; Heasman et al. 2006). Generally, the periodontal status of former smokers is found to be intermediate between that of people who never smoked and current smokers (Bergstrom et al. 2000). Furthermore, smoking cessation has been shown to be beneficial for periodontal conditions: former smokers show less alveolar bone loss (Bergstrom et al. 2000; Bolin et al. 1993; Paulander et al. 2004) and reduced tooth loss (Krall et al. 1997) and present better outcomes after periodontal therapy (Kaldahl et al. 1996; Preshaw et al. 2005).

The potential benefit of smoking cessation is likely to be mediated through a number of different pathways. They may include shifts toward a less pathogenic subgingival flora; recovery of the gingival microcirculation; restoration of neutrophil function, metabolism, and viability; damping of the enhanced immune response; and reestablishment of any imbalance in the local or systemic production of cytokines (Heasman et al. 2006). The duration of the recovery of periodontal and peri-implant tissues following tobacco use cessation has not been determined yet. However, with the National Health and Nutrition Examination Survey (NHANES) of 12,623 patients in the USA, periodontal recovery was shown to be influenced by intensity, duration, and recency of smoking. Additionally, with this data, a half-time (50% risk reduction) of one and a half years has been computed (Dietrich and Hoffmann 2004).

The evidence-based perspective: One systematic review and one narrative review summarizing data from epidemiological, cross-sectional, and case control studies strongly suggest that smoking cessation is beneficial to patients following periodontal treatments (Heasman et al. 2006; Ramseier et al. 2020). The periodontal status of former smokers following treatment demonstrates that quitting smoking is beneficial. However, there are only limited data from long-term longitudinal clinical trials to demonstrate unequivocally the periodontal benefit of quitting smoking. Despite the lack of data from intervention studies, these findings suggest that smoking cessation may generally result in a long-term benefit to the periodontal condition. In addition, there is no need for randomized, controlled trials of the effectiveness of smoking cessation on oral health outcomes because such trials would not be feasible and would be too costly. However, well-designed observational studies are needed to fill the knowledge gaps.

Based on this body of evidence, tobacco use cessation becomes an important factor in daily dental care. Every member of the dental practice team plays an important role in the teamwork of smoking cessation counseling. With an appropriate assignment of tasks for every team member, patients are welcomed professionally, asked regularly about their smoking status, and continuously monitored.

A comprehensive model for smoking prevention and cessation applicable for both dental and dental hygiene education has been presented by Ramseier (2003) (Figure 3.7) (Ramseier 2003). This tobacco use cessation strategy is based on: (1) the model "stages of change" (or transtheoretical model) (Prochaska and DiClemente 1983); (2) the five A's using nicotine replacement therapy (NRT) (Fiore et al. 1996); and (3) the main principles of motivational interviewing techniques (Miller and Rollnick 2002).

In brief, the model includes recording every patient's tobacco use history, followed by a brief interview of no more than five minutes. The main aim of these interviews is to help tobacco using patients to move from pre-contemplation to contemplation, and further to preparation, action, and maintenance stages. The routine use of a tobacco use history form as well as a record sheet to monitor tobacco use intervention is suggested (Figure 3.8). Patients' tobacco use history may be recorded on this form

regarding intensity, time since cessation, and duration of each period, and they may be asked about their readiness to quit. According to a number of authors, current and former tobacco users should be asked about (1) the type of tobacco used, (2) the intensity of use (quantity per day), (3) the duration of use (years), and (4) time since cessation (years) (Dietrich and Hoffmann 2004; Ramseier 2003).

The evidence-based perspective: Evidence from a systematic review (Carr and Ebbert 2007) suggests that behavioral interventions for tobacco use conducted by oral health professionals incorporating an oral exam component in the dental office and community setting increase tobacco abstinence rates.

This is also reflected in the EFP S3 level practice guidelines, which include a strong recommendation for tobacco smoking cessation interventions to be implemented in patients undergoing periodontitis therapy (Sanz et al. 2020).

### Behavioral Support

People who want to kick the smoking habit do not always take part in state-of-the-art nicotine withdrawal programs in linear fashion from start to finish. Nevertheless, simple instructions, such as those offered in the "Assist" and "Arrange" programs, can be a valuable tool for physicians supporting patients in their attempts to quit smoking.

Some smokers are so euphoric about stopping smoking that they tend to move from one step to the next in a premature, i.e., unprepared manner. Even if this approach works for some smokers, others require varying amounts of behavioral support. This behavioral support can be given in an individual manner by adopting the following steps:

1) Asking the patient to complete a tobacco use journal (Figure 3.9): Every smoker has his individual smoking habits. To pinpoint the behavioral changes required in the particular case, it is advisable to keep a tobacco use journal for several days.

2) Evaluate the tobacco use journal: Reading through the journal entries later, the patient will notice smoking patterns and assessments of which she was previously unaware. These can serve as the basis for deciding which habits she must change to give up smoking (ideally without withdrawal symptoms) and replace the old habit with new patterns of behavior. During the control period, it is advisable to reduce nicotine consumption only down to a level where the "sacrifice" is bearable.

3) Behavioral changes: The process of successfully replacing smoking habits with other activities can be difficult and time consuming. Each patient should name an action that is good for him. It might be wise to arrange additional consultations at this point so that enough time can be devoted to this important step.

# Tobacco Use Cessation (TUC) care pathway for dental practice

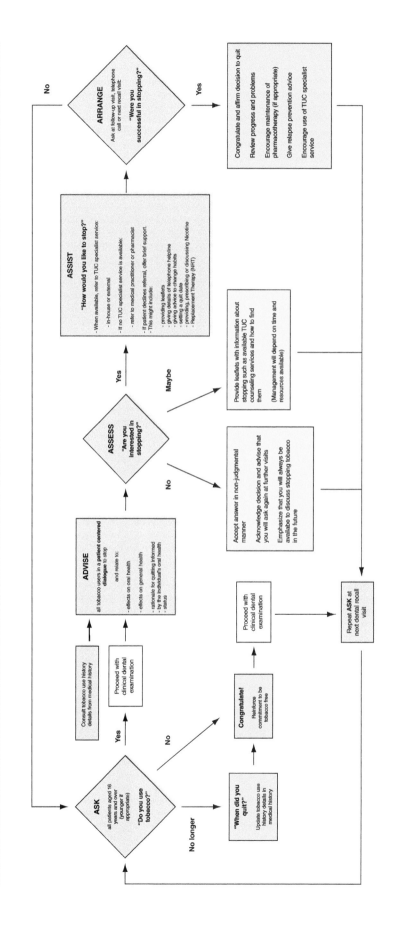

Figure 3.7  Tobacco use cessation care pathway for the dental practice.

## Tobacco use history

Last / first name: _____     Date: _____

| | | |
|---|---|---|
| 1. | **Have you ever smoked more than 200 cigarettes?** | ☐ yes<br>☐ no (go on with question 6) |
| 2. | **At what age did you start to smoke regularly?** | _____ years |
| 3. | **Are you currently smoking cigarettes?** | ☐ yes (go on with question 5)<br>☐ no |
| 4. | **In which year did you quit smoking?** | _____ |
| 5. | **How many cigarettes do you smoke per day?** | _____ |
| 6. | **Have you used other tobacco products regularly?** | ☐ no (go on with question 8)<br>☐ yes, the following:<br><br>**Cigar**  ☐ never  ☐ in the past  ☐ now<br>**Pipe**  ☐ never  ☐ in the past  ☐ now<br>**Chewing tobacco** ☐ never  ☐ in the past  ☐ now<br>**Other**  ☐ never  ☐ in the past  ☐ now |
| 7. | **How often have you already tried quitting tobacco use?** | ☐ never<br>☐ once<br>☐ 2 - 4 times<br>☐ more than _____ times |
| 8. | **Are you currently thinking of quitting tobacco use?** | ☐ no<br>☐ yes, within the next _____ months |
| 9. | **Personal information**<br><br>a.  **Age**<br><br>b.  **Sex** | Date of birth: _____<br><br>☐ female<br>☐ male |

**Figure 3.8**  Tobacco use history form.

**Pharmacotherapy**

Kotlyar and Hatsukami (2002) have reviewed the management of nicotine addiction (Kotlyar and Hatsukami 2002). The use of nicotine replacement therapy in dental tobacco use cessation was recently reviewed by Ramseier (2003) and Christen et al. (2003) (Christen et al. 2003; Ramseier 2003). On the quit date, the patients should be sent home from the dental practice as "former smokers." It may be worthwhile to give each individual patient a written recommendation concerning the use of nicotine replacement products during the next three months (Figure 3.10).

There are various nicotine replacement products on the market such as gum, patches, sublingual tablets, inhalators, and nasal sprays. For the use of each product available, the reader is referred to the manufacturers' instructions.

The evidence-based perspective: There is strong evidence from a systematic Cochrane review that different commercially available forms of NRT can help people to quit smoking (Hartmann-Boyce et al. 2018). NRTs increase the rate of quitting by 50–70%. The effectiveness of NRT seems to be largely independent of the intensity of additional support provided to the individual.

## TOBACCO USE JOURNAL

Date: _____

| Cig. | Time | Place or activity | Accompanied by | Importance | Alternative |
|------|------|-------------------|----------------|------------|-------------|
| 1 | | | | | |
| 2 | | | | | |
| 3 | | | | | |
| 3 | | | | | |
| 4 | | | | | |
| 5 | | | | | |
| 6 | | | | | |
| 7 | | | | | |
| 8 | | | | | |
| 9 | | | | | |
| 10 | | | | | |

Front

## TOBACCO USE JOURNAL

Date: _____

| Cig. | Time | Place or activity | Accompanied by | Importance | Alternative |
|------|------|-------------------|----------------|------------|-------------|
| 11 | | | | | |
| 12 | | | | | |
| 13 | | | | | |
| 13 | | | | | |
| 14 | | | | | |
| 15 | | | | | |
| 16 | | | | | |
| 17 | | | | | |
| 18 | | | | | |
| 19 | | | | | |
| 20 | | | | | |

Back

Figure 3.9 Tobacco use journal.

# Recommendation for use of Nicotine Replacement Therapy

Last name: _____    First name: _____

**Level of nicotine dependency:**

☐  very high
☐  high
☐  moderate
☐  low

**Smoking behavior:**

☐  smokes regularly through the day:
    recommendations: use of patch

☐  smokes only at specific times:
    recommendations: use of gum

**From Day 1 of quitting:**

|  | **Patch**<br>(mg per day) | **Gum**<br>(number per day) | **others**<br>(number per day) |
|---|---|---|---|
| 1$^{st}$ month |  |  |  |
| 2$^{nd}$ month |  |  |  |
| 3$^{rd}$ month |  |  |  |
| After month 4 |  |  |  |

Place, Date: _____    Signature: _____

| Nicotine replacement | Low nicotine dependency | Moderate nicotine dependency | High nicotine dependency | Very high nicotine dependency |
|---|---|---|---|---|
| Patch |  | ■ | ■<br>in combination with another nicotine preparation | ■<br>in combination with another nicotine preparation |
| Gum | ■ 2 mg | ■ 2 mg | ■ 4 mg | ■ 4 mg |
| Sublingual tablets | ■ | ■ | ■<br>in combination with patch | ■<br>in combination with patch |

Figure 3.10   Recommendations for use of nicotine replacement therapy.

## Other Risk Factor Modifications

### Metabolic Control

The effects of metabolic control of diabetes mellitus on the periodontal status were mainly evaluated in cross-sectional studies and a few prospective cohort studies, with some conflicting results (Bridges et al. 1996; Sastrowijoto et al. 1990; Taylor et al. 1998). From a clinical perspective, it is important to note that prevalence and severity of periodontal disease vary greatly within the diabetes mellitus population, just as it does in the non-diabetic population. Some individuals living with diabetes may suffer from periodontitis because of inadequate oral hygiene and tobacco use rather than their diabetic condition (Haber et al. 1993).

To appoint the risk factor diabetes mellitus and the metabolic control of blood sugar levels in a periodontitis patient seems to be important for the understanding of the pathogenesis or the outcome of periodontal treatment. Once a patient is identified as having diabetes by a medical history, a close collaboration with the diabetologist is advisable (Sanz et al. 2020; Thorstensson et al. 1996).

The 2017 World Workshop "Classification of Periodontal and Peri-implant Diseases and Conditions" highlights metabolic control as an exposure which impacts on the severity and management of periodontitis. As such a patient's time out of ideal metabolic range will influence their periodontitis diagnostic statement, specifically the grading component. Grading of periodontitis relates to the rate of disease progression and enables clinicians to incorporate individual patient factors into the diagnosis, which are deemed crucial to comprehensive case management (Caton J et al. 2018).

The EFP practice guideline has a strong recommendation for diabetes control interventions to be undertaken in patients undergoing periodontal therapy. These may include patient education as well as brief dietary counseling and/or referral to a diabetologist (Sanz et al. 2020).

### Stress Reduction Therapy

An interesting approach on depression-related enhanced susceptibility of periodontitis was introduced by Breivik et al. (Breivik et al. 2006). According to this approach, treatment with an antidepressant drug inhibited periodontal bone loss in an animal model of depression. Additionally, the individual coping behavior with stress in humans is shown to interfere with periodontal conditions (Genco et al. 1999; Wimmer et al. 2005). Coping behavioral training is likely to have a positive impact on disease severity or periodontal treatment outcomes. However, meaningful longitudinal clinical studies assessing the influence of psychological stress-related therapy on the outcome of periodontal treatment are currently not available.

Both risk factors for stress and poor coping behavior must be considered to achieve positive treatment outcomes in periodontitis patients (Ramseier and Suvan 2015). Once a patient is identified with stress or poor coping behavior, a close collaboration with a psychiatrist or psychologist may be advisable.

## Summary

Clinical research data indicate that risk factors associated with periodontitis can be identified. While certain non-modifiable factors are found, modifiable factors when amended may improve both periodontal conditions and the outcome of treatment. According to recent data, it appears reasonable to suggest that second to the removal of the bacterial biofilm, smoking cessation is the most important measure in periodontitis management. Consequently, periodontal health is to be supported by appropriate behaviors such as regular self-performed supragingival plaque control, avoidance of tobacco, and consumption of a healthy diet. The dental community involved with oral healthcare should gain an understanding of the health effects from inappropriate behavior to successfully target prevention and disease control. As a consequence, services for primary and secondary prevention on an individual level oriented toward the change of inappropriate behavior become a professional responsibility for all oral healthcare providers.

## References

Ajwani, S. and Ainamo, A. (2001). Periodontal conditions among the old elderly: five-year longitudinal study. *Spec. Care Dentist.* 21 (2): 45.

Albandar, J.M. (2002). Global risk factors and risk indicators for periodontal diseases. *Periodontol. 2000* 29: 177.

Albandar, J.M., Brunelle, J.A., and Kingman, A. (1999). Destructive periodontal disease in adults 30 years of age and older in the United States, 1988–1994. *J. Periodontol.* 70 (1): 13.

Armitage, G.C. (1999). Development of a classification system for periodontal diseases and conditions. *Ann. Periodontol.* 4 (1): 1.

Axelsson, P., Nystrom, B., and Lindhe, J. (2004). The long-term effect of a plaque control program on tooth mortality, caries and periodontal disease in adults. Results after 30 years of maintenance. *J. Clin. Periodontol.* 31 (9): 749.

Bain, C.A. (1996). Smoking and implant failure–benefits of a smoking cessation protocol. *Int. J. Oral Maxillofac. Implants* 11 (6): 756–759.

Bergstrom, J. (2004). Influence of tobacco smoking on periodontal bone height. Long-term observations and a hypothesis. *J. Clin. Periodontol.* 31 (4): 260–266.

Bergstrom, J., Eliasson, S., and Dock, J. (2000). A 10-year prospective study of tobacco smoking and periodontal health. *J. Periodontol.* 71 (8): 1338–1347.

Bolin, A., Eklund, G., Frithiof, L., and Lavstedt, S. (1993). The effect of changed smoking habits on marginal alveolar bone loss. A longitudinal study. *Swed. Dent. J.* 17 (5): 211–216.

Breivik, T., Gundersen, Y., Myhrer, T. et al. (2006). Enhanced susceptibility to periodontitis in an animal model of depression: reversed by chronic treatment with the anti-depressant tianeptine. *J. Clin. Periodontol.* 33 (7): 469.

Bridges, R.B., Anderson, J.W., Saxe, S.R. et al. (1996). Periodontal status of diabetic and non-diabetic men: effects of smoking, glycemic control, and socioeconomic factors. *J. Periodontol.* 67 (11): 1185.

Carr, A.B. and Ebbert, J.O. (2007). Interventions for tobacco cessation in the dental setting. A systematic review. *Community Dent. Health* 24 (2): 70–74.

Carra, M.C., Detzen, L., Kitzmann, J. et al. (2020). Promoting behavioural changes to improve oral hygiene in patients with periodontal diseases: a systematic review. *J. Clin. Periodontol.* doi: 10.1111/jcpe.13234.

Caton J.G., Armitage G., Berglundh T. et al. (2018 June). A new classification scheme for periodontal and peri-implant diseases and conditions – Introduction and key changes from the 1999 classification. *J. Clin. Periodontol.* 45 (Suppl 20): S1-S8. doi: 10.1111/jcpe.12935. PMID: 29926489.

Christen, A.G., Jay, S.J., and Christen, J.A. (2003). Tobacco cessation and nicotine replacement therapy for dental practice. *Gen. Dent.* 51 (6): 525–532.

Consensus report (1996). Periodontal diseases: epidemiology and diagnosis. *Ann. Periodontol.* 1 (1): 216.

Deinzer, R., Forster, P., Fuck, L. et al. (1999). Increase of crevicular interleukin 1beta under academic stress at experimental gingivitis sites and at sites of perfect oral hygiene. *J. Clin. Periodontol.* 26 (1): 1.

Deinzer, R., Hilpert, D., Bach, K. et al. (2001). Effects of academic stress on oral hygiene—a potential link between stress and plaque-associated disease? *J. Clin. Periodontol.* 28 (5): 459.

Deinzer, R., Kleineidam, C., Stiller-Winkler, R. et al. (2000). Prolonged reduction of salivary immunoglobulin A (sIgA) after a major academic exam. *Int. J. Psychophysiol.* 37 (3): 219.

Diel, I.J., Bergner, R., and Grotz, K.A. (2007). Adverse effects of bisphosphonates: current issues. *J. Support. Oncol.* 5 (10): 475.

Dietrich, T., Bernimoulin, J.P., and Glynn, R.J. (2004). The effect of cigarette smoking on gingival bleeding. *J. Periodontol.* 75 (1): 16–22.

Dietrich, T. and Hoffmann, K. (2004). A comprehensive index for the modeling of smoking history in periodontal research. *J. Dent. Res.* 83 (11): 859–863.

Dietrich, T., Kaye, E.K., Nunn, M.E. et al. (2006). Gingivitis susceptibility and its relation to periodontitis in men. *J. Dent. Res.* 85 (12): 1134.

Dietrich, T., Walter, C., Oluwagbemigun, K. et al. (2015). Smoking, smoking cessation, and risk of tooth loss: the EPIC-Potsdam study. *J. Dent. Res.* 94 (10): 1369–1375. doi: 10.1177/0022034515598961.

Dorsky, R. (2001). Nutrition and oral health. *Gen. Dent.* 49 (6): 576–582.

Duarte, P.M., Neto, J.B., Casati, M.Z. et al. (2007). Diabetes modulates gene expression in the gingival tissues of patients with chronic periodontitis. *Oral Dis.* 13 (6): 594.

Eklund, S.A. and Burt, B.A. (1994). Risk factors for total tooth loss in the United States; longitudinal analysis of national data. *J. Public Health Dent.* 54 (1): 5–14.

Emrich, L.J., Shlossman, M., and Genco, R.J. (1991). Periodontal disease in non-insulin-dependent diabetes mellitus. *J. Periodontol.* 62 (2): 123.

Engebretson, S., Chertog, R., Nichols, A. et al. (2007). Plasma levels of tumour necrosis factor-alpha in patients with chronic periodontitis and type 2 diabetes. *J. Clin. Periodontol.* 34 (1): 18.

Engebretson, S.P., Hey-Hadavi, J., Ehrhardt, F.J. et al. (2004). Gingival crevicular fluid levels of interleukin-1beta and glycemic control in patients with chronic periodontitis and type 2 diabetes. *J. Periodontol.* 75 (9): 1203.

Erley, K.J., Swiec, G.D., Herold, R. et al. (2006). Gingival recession treatment with connective tissue grafts in smokers and non-smokers. *J. Periodontol.* 77 (7): 1148–1155.

Fiore, M.C. (2000). US public health service clinical practice guideline: treating tobacco use and dependence. *Respir. Care* 45 (10): 1200–1262.

Fiore, M.C., Bailey, W.C., and Cohen, S.J. (1996). *Smoking Cessation: Clinical Practice Guideline, No. 18.* Rockville, MD: U.S. Department for Health Care Policy and Research.

Genco, R.J., Ho, A.W., Grossi, S.G. et al. (1999). Relationship of stress, distress and inadequate coping behaviors to periodontal disease. *J.Periodontol.* 70 (7): 711.

Haber, J., Wattles, J., Crowley, M. et al. (1993). Evidence for cigarette smoking as a major risk factor for periodontitis. *J.Periodontol.* 64 (1): 16.

Hartmann-Boyce, J., Chepkin, S.C., Ye, W. et al. (2018 May 31). Nicotine replacement therapy versus control for smoking cessation. *Cochrane Database Syst. Rev.* 5 (5): CD000146. doi: 10.1002/14651858.CD000146.pub5. PMID: 29852054; PMCID: PMC6353172.

Heasman, L., Stacey, F., Preshaw, P.M. et al. (2006). The effect of smoking on periodontal treatment response: a review of clinical evidence. *J. Clin. Periodontol.* 33 (4): 241–253.

Holm-Pedersen, P., Vigild, M., Nitschke, I., and Berkey, D.B. (2005). Dental care for aging populations in Denmark, Sweden, Norway, United Kingdom, and Germany. *J. Dent. Educ.* 69 (9): 987.

Hugo, F.N., Hilgert, J.B., Bozzetti, M.C. et al. (2006). Chronic stress, depression, and cortisol levels as risk indicators of elevated plaque and gingivitis levels in individuals aged 50 years and older. *J. Periodontol.* 77 (6): 1008.

Hugoson, A., Ljungquist, B., and Breivik, T. (2002). The relationship of some negative events and psychological factors to periodontal disease in an adult Swedish population 50 to 80 years of age. *J. Clin. Periodontol.* 29 (3): 247.

Hujoel, P.P., Powell, L.V., and Kiyak, H.A. (1997). The effects of simple interventions on tooth mortality: findings in one trial and implications for future studies. *J. Dent. Res.* 76 (4): 867.

Huynh-Ba, G., Lang, N.P., Tonetti, M.S., and Salvi, G.E. (2007). The association of the composite IL-1 genotype with periodontitis progression and/or treatment outcomes: a systematic review. *J. Clin. Periodontol.* 34 (4): 305–317.

Ishisaka, A., Ansai, T., Soh, I. et al. (2007). Association of salivary levels of cortisol and dehydroepiandrosterone with periodontitis in older Japanese adults. *J. Periodontol.* 78 (9): 1767.

Iwamoto, Y., Nishimura, F., Nakagawa, M. et al. (2001). The effect of antimicrobial periodontal treatment on circulating tumor necrosis factor-alpha and glycated hemoglobin level in patients with type 2 diabetes. *J. Periodontol.* 72 (6): 774.

Johannsen, A., Rylander, G., Soder, B., and Asberg, M. (2006). Dental plaque, gingival inflammation, and elevated levels of interleukin-6 and cortisol in gingival crevicular fluid from women with stress-related depression and exhaustion. *J. Periodontol.* 77 (8): 1403.

Johnson, G.K. and Guthmiller, J.M. (2007). The impact of cigarette smoking on periodontal disease and treatment. *Periodontol. 2000* 44: 178–194.

Jordan, R.A., Gangler, P., and Johren, H.P. (2006). Clinical treatment outcomes of periodontal therapy in HIV-seropositive patients undergoing highly active antiretroviral therapy. *Eur. J. Med. Res.* 11 (6): 232–235.

Kaldahl, W.B., Johnson, G.K., Patil, K.D., and Kalkwarf, K.L. (1996). Levels of cigarette consumption and response to periodontal therapy. *J. Periodontol.* 67 (7): 675–681.

Katz, J., Bhattacharyya, I., Farkhondeh-Kish, F. et al. (2005). Expression of the receptor of advanced glycation end products in gingival tissues of type 2 diabetes patients with chronic periodontal disease: a study utilizing immunohistochemistry and RT-PCR. *J. Clin. Periodontol.* 32 (1): 40.

Khader, Y.S., Dauod, A.S., El-Qaderi, S.S. et al. (2006). Periodontal status of diabetics compared with nondiabetics: a meta-analysis. *J. Diabetes Complicat.* 20 (1): 59–68.

Kotlyar, M. and Hatsukami, D.K. (2002). Managing nicotine addiction. *J. Dent. Educ.* 66 (9): 1061–1073.

Kovar, M., Jany, Z., and Erdelsky, I. (1985). Influence of the menstrual cycle on the gingival microcirculation. *Czech. Med.* 8 (2): 98.

Krall, E.A. (2001). The periodontal-systemic connection: implications for treatment of patients with osteoporosis and periodontal disease. *Ann. Periodontol.* 6 (1): 209–213.

Krall, E.A., Dawson-Hughes, B., Garvey, A.J., and Garcia, R.I. (1997). Smoking, smoking cessation, and tooth loss. *J. Dent. Res.* 76 (10): 1653–1659.

Krejci, C.B. and Bissada, N.F. (2002). Women's health issues and their relationship to periodontitis. *J. Am. Dent. Assoc.* 133 (3): 323.

Kroidl, A., Schaeben, A., Oette, M. et al. (2005). Prevalence of oral lesions and periodontal diseases in HIV-infected patients on antiretroviral therapy. *Eur. J. Med. Res.* 10 (10): 448–453.

Laine, M.A. (2002). Effect of pregnancy on periodontal and dental health. *Acta Odontol. Scand.* 60 (5): 257.

Lamster, I.B., Begg, M.D., Mitchell-Lewis, D. et al. (1994). Oral manifestations of HIV infection in homosexual men and intravenous drug users. Study design and relationship of epidemiologic, clinical, and immunologic parameters to oral lesions. *Oral Surg. Oral Med. Oral Pathol.* 78 (2): 163–174.

Lang, N.P., Kiel, R.A., and Anderhalden, K. (1983). Clinical and microbiological effects of subgingival restorations with overhanging or clinically perfect margins. *J. Clin. Periodontol.* 10 (6): 563.

Lerner, U.H. (2006). Inflammation-induced bone remodeling in periodontal disease and the influence of post-menopausal osteoporosis. *J. Dent. Res.* 85 (7): 596.

Loos, B.G., John, R.P., and Laine, M.L. (2005). Identification of genetic risk factors for periodontitis and possible mechanisms of action. *J. Clin. Periodontol.* 32 (Suppl 6): 159.

Loos, B.G. and Van Dyke, T.E. (2020). The role of inflammation and genetics in periodontal disease. *Periodontol. 2000* 83: 26–39.

Madianos, P.N., Bobetsis, G.A., and Kinane, D.F. (2002). Is periodontitis associated with an increased risk of coronary heart disease and preterm and/or low birth weight births? *J. Clin. Periodontol.* 29 (Suppl 3): 22.

Magnusson, I., Lindhe, J., Yoneyama, T., and Liljenberg, B. (1984). Recolonization of a subgingival microbiota following scaling in deep pockets. *J. Clin. Periodontol.* 11 (3): 193.

Manouchehr-Pour, M., Spagnuolo, P.J., Rodman, H.M., and Bissada, N.F. (1981a). Comparison of neutrophil chemotactic response in diabetic patients with mild and severe periodontal disease. *J. Periodontol.* 52 (8): 410.

Manouchehr-Pour, M., Spagnuolo, P.J., Rodman, H.M., and Bissada, N.F. (1981b). Impaired neutrophil chemotaxis in diabetic patients with severe periodontitis. *J. Dent. Res.* 60 (3): 729.

McKaig, R.G., Thomas, J.C., Patton, L.L. et al. (1998). Prevalence of HIV-associated periodontitis and chronic periodontitis in a southeastern US study group. *J. Public Health Dent.* 58 (4): 294–300.

Meisel, P., Reifenberger, J., Haase, R. et al. (2008). Women are periodontally healthier than men, but why don't they have more teeth than men? *Menopause* 15 (2): 270–275.

Meisel, P., Schwahn, C., Gesch, D. et al. (2004). Dose-effect relation of smoking and the interleukin-1 gene polymorphism in periodontal disease. *J. Periodontol.* 75 (2): 236–242.

Michalowicz, B.S., Aeppli, D., Virag, J.G. et al. (1991). Periodontal findings in adult twins. *J. Periodontol.* 62 (5): 293–299.

Michalowicz, B.S., Diehl, S.R., Gunsolley, J.C. et al. (2000). Evidence of a substantial genetic basis for risk of adult periodontitis. *J. Periodontol.* 71 (11): 1699–1707.

Miller, W.R. and Rollnick, S. (2002). *Motivational Interviewing*. New York: Guilford Press.

Nakajima, K., Hamada, N., Takahashi, Y. et al. (2006). Restraint stress enhances alveolar bone loss in an experimental rat model. *J.Periodontal Res.* 41 (6): 527.

Nishida, M., Grossi, S.G., Dunford, R.G. et al. (2000a). Calcium and the risk for periodontal disease. *J. Periodontol.* 71 (7): 1057–1066.

Nishida, M., Grossi, S.G., Dunford, R.G. et al. (2000b). Dietary vitamin C and the risk for periodontal disease. *J. Periodontol.* 71 (8): 1215–1223.

Oliver, R.C., Brown, L.J., and Loe, H. (1998). Periodontal diseases in the United States population. *J. Periodontol.* 69 (2): 269.

Oliver, R.C. and Tervonen, T. (1994). Diabetes–a risk factor for periodontitis in adults? *J. Periodontol.* 65 (5 Suppl): 530.

Ower, P. (2003). The role of self-administered plaque control in the management of periodontal diseases: i. A review of the evidence. *Dent. Update* 30 (2): 60–64, 66, 68.

Page, R.C. and Kornman, K.S. (1997). The pathogenesis of human periodontitis: an introduction. *Periodontol. 2000* 14: 9.

Palmer, R.M. (2005). Should quit smoking interventions be the first part of initial periodontal therapy? *J. Clin. Periodontol.* 32 (8): 867–868.

Papapanou, P.N. (1996). Periodontal diseases: epidemiology. *Ann. Periodontol.* 1 (1): 1.

Papapanou, P.N., Wennstrom, J.L., and Grondahl, K. (1989). A 10-year retrospective study of periodontal disease progression. *J. Clin. Periodontol.* 16 (7): 403.

Paulander, J., Wennstrom, J.L., Axelsson, P., and Lindhe, J. (2004). Some risk factors for periodontal bone loss in 50-year-old individuals. A 10-year cohort study. *J. Clin. Periodontol.* 31 (7): 489–496.

Payne, J.B., Reinhardt, R.A., Nummikoski, P.V., and Patil, K.D. (1999). Longitudinal alveolar bone loss in postmenopausal osteoporotic/osteopenic women. *Osteoporos. Int.* 10 (1): 34.

Persson, G.R. (2006). What has ageing to do with periodontal health and disease? *Int. Dent. J.* 56 (4 Suppl 1): 240–249.

Preshaw, P.M., Heasman, L., Stacey, F. et al. (2005). The effect of quitting smoking on chronic periodontitis. *J. Clin. Periodontol.* 32 (8): 869–879.

Prochaska, J.O. and DiClemente, C.C. (1983). Stages and processes of self-change of smoking: toward an integrative model of change. *J. Consult Clin. Psychol.* 51 (3): 390–395.

Ramseier, C.A. (2003). Smoking prevention and cessation. *Oral Health Prev. Dent.* 1 (Suppl 1): 427–439. discussion 440–422.

Ramseier, C.A. and Suvan, J.E. (2015). Behaviour change counselling for tobacco use cessation and promotion of healthy lifestyles: a systematic review. *J. Clin. Periodontol.* 42 (Suppl 16): S47–58. doi: 10.1111/jcpe.12351.

Ramseier, C.A., Woelber, J.P., Kitzmann, J. et al. (2020). Impact of risk factor control interventions for smoking cessation and promotion of healthy lifestyles in patients with periodontitis: a systematic review. *J. Clin. Periodontol.* doi: 10.1111/jcpe.13240.

Reichart, P. (2006). US1 HIV - changing patterns in HAART era, patients' quality of life and occupational risks. *Oral Dis.* 12 (Suppl 1): 3.

Reinhardt, R.A., Payne, J.B., Maze, C.A. et al. (1999). Influence of estrogen and osteopenia/osteoporosis on clinical periodontitis in postmenopausal women. *J. Periodontol.* 70 (8): 823.

Roberts, A., Matthews, J.B., Socransky, S.S. et al. (2002). Stress and the periodontal diseases: effects of catecholamines on the growth of periodontal bacteria in vitro. *Oral Microbiol. Immunol.* 17 (5): 296.

Rosling, B., Nyman, S., and Lindhe, J. (1976). The effect of systematic plaque control on bone regeneration in infrabony pockets. *J. Clin. Periodontol.* 3 (1): 38.

Roussa, E. (1998). Anatomic characteristics of the furcation and root surfaces of molar teeth and their significance in the clinical management of marginal periodontitis. *Clin. Anat.* 11 (3): 177.

Russell, S.L. and Mayberry, L.J. (2008). Pregnancy and oral health: a review and recommendations to reduce gaps in practice and research. *MCN Am. J. Matern. Child Nurs.* 33 (1): 32–37.

Ryder, M.I. (2007). The influence of smoking on host responses in periodontal infections. *Periodontol. 2000* 43: 267–277.

Salvi, G.E., Collins, J.G., Yalda, B. et al. (1997a). Monocytic TNF alpha secretion patterns in IDDM patients with periodontal diseases. *J. Clin. Periodontol.* 24 (1): 8.

Salvi, G.E., Yalda, B., Collins, J.G. et al. (1997b). Inflammatory mediator response as a potential risk marker for periodontal diseases in insulin-dependent diabetes mellitus patients. *J. Periodontol.* 68 (2): 127.

Sanz, M., Herrera, D., Kebschull, M. et al. (2020). Treatment of stage I-III periodontitis-The EFP S3 level clinical practice guideline. *J. Clin. Periodontol.* 47 (Suppl 22): 4–60. doi: 10.1111/jcpe.13290.

Sanz, M., Lau, L., Herrera, D. et al. (2004). Methods of detection of Actinobacillus actinomycetemcomitans, Porphyromonas gingivalis and Tannerella forsythensis in periodontal microbiology, with special emphasis on advanced molecular techniques: a review. *J. Clin. Periodontol.* 31 (12): 1034.

Sastrowijoto, S.H., Abbas, F., Abraham-Inpijn, L., and van der Veiden, U. (1990). Relationship between bleeding/plaque ratio, family history of diabetes mellitus and impaired glucose tolerance. *J. Clin. Periodontol.* 17 (1): 55.

Schatzle, M., Loe, H., Burgin, W. et al. (2003). Clinical course of chronic periodontitis. I. Role of gingivitis. *J. Clin. Periodontol.* 30 (10): 887.

Shlossman, M., Knowler, W.C., Pettitt, D.J., and Genco, R.J. (1990). Type 2 diabetes mellitus and periodontal disease. *J. Am. Dent. Assoc.* 121 (4): 532.

Silverstein, P. (1992). Smoking and wound healing. *Am. J. Med.* 93 (1A): 22S–24S. doi: 10.1016/0002-9343(92)90623-j.

Socransky, S.S. and Haffajee, A.D. (2002). Dental biofilms: difficult therapeutic targets. *Periodontol. 2000* 28: 12.

Stolk, R.P., Rosmalen, J.G., Postma, D.S. et al. (2008). Universal risk factors for multifactorial diseases: lifeLines: a three-generation population-based study. *Eur. J. Epidemiol.* 23 (1): 67.

Strietzel, F.P., Reichart, P.A., Kale, A. et al. (2007). Smoking interferes with the prognosis of dental implant treatment: a systematic review and meta-analysis. *J. Clin. Periodontol.* 34 (6): 523–544.

Taylor, G.W., Burt, B.A., Becker, M.P. et al. (1998). Glycemic control and alveolar bone loss progression in type 2 diabetes. *Ann. Periodontol.* 3 (1): 30.

Theilade, E., Wright, W.H., Jensen, S.B., and Loe, H. (1966). Experimental gingivitis in man. II. A longitudinal clinical and bacteriological investigation. *J. Periodontal. Res.* 1: 1.

Thorstensson, H. and Hugoson, A. (1993). Periodontal disease experience in adult long-duration insulin-dependent diabetics. *J. Clin. Periodontol.* 20 (5): 352.

Thorstensson, H., Kuylenstierna, J., and Hugoson, A. (1996). Medical status and complications in relation to periodontal disease experience in insulin-dependent diabetics. *J. Clin. Periodontol.* 23 (3 Pt 1): 194.

Tonetti, M.S., Greenwell, H., and Kornman, K.S. (2018). Staging and grading of periodontitis: framework and proposal of a new classification and case definition. *J. Periodontol.* 89 (Suppl 1): S159–S172. doi: 10.1002/JPER.18-0006.

van der Velden, U., Abbas, F., Armand, S. et al. (1993). The effect of sibling relationship on the periodontal condition. *J. Clin. Periodontol.* 20 (9): 683–690.

Verma, S. and Bhat, K.M. (2004). Diabetes mellitus—a modifier of periodontal disease expression. *J. Int. Acad. Periodontol.* 6 (1): 13.

Vermylen, K., De Quincey, G.N., Wolffe, G.N. et al. (2005). Root proximity as a risk marker for periodontal disease: a case-control study. *J. Clin. Periodontol.* 32 (3): 260.

Wautier, J.L. and Guillausseau, P.J. (1998). Diabetes, advanced glycation endproducts and vascular disease. *Vasc. Med.* 3 (2): 131.

Westfelt, E., Rylander, H., Blohme, G. et al. (1996). The effect of periodontal therapy in diabetics. Results after 5 years. *J. Clin. Periodontol.* 23 (2): 92.

Willershausen-Zonnchen, B., Lemmen, C., and Hamm, G. (1991). Influence of high glucose concentrations on glycosaminoglycan and collagen synthesis in cultured human gingival fibroblasts. *J. Clin. Periodontol.* 18 (3): 190.

Wimmer, G., Janda, M., Wieselmann-Penkner, K. et al. (2002). Coping with stress: its influence on periodontal disease. *J. Periodontol.* 73 (11): 1343.

Wimmer, G., Kohldorfer, G., Mischak, I. et al. (2005). Coping with stress: its influence on periodontal therapy. *J. Periodontol.* 76 (1): 90.

# 4

# Scaling and Root Planing
*Raman Kohli*

## Introduction

Ever since Loe demonstrated the role that plaque plays in the development of gingivitis (Loe et al. 1965; Theilade et al. 1966) there has been an emphasis on plaque removal as the primary goal of nonsurgical periodontal therapy. With the confirmation that microorganisms are involved in the initiation and progression of periodontal infections, studies have examined the efficacy of various modalities of treatment to eliminate or suppress these microorganisms and reverse the inflammatory changes or damage to the periodontium. Manual scaling and root planing (SRP) are considered the basis of periodontal treatment and as such are often the control to which other modalities are compared. This chapter provides an evidence-based understanding of what can and cannot be achieved with scaling and root planing and how its effectiveness can be optimized.

Scaling refers to the removal of hard and soft deposits from the crown and root surfaces. Root planing denotes the removal of cementum and dentin that is rough or impregnated with bacteria, endotoxins, and calculus to produce a root surface that is smooth and hard. SRP can be performed as either a closed or open procedure. An open procedure differs from a closed one in that it denotes reflection of the gingival tissues, allowing direct visualization of the root surface—this is also known as surgical scaling.

The general purpose of SRP is to reduce or eliminate plaque-associated gingival inflammation (Figure 4.1). Specifically, this is achieved by mechanical instrumentation of the affected root surfaces. The result of this instrumentation is a reduction of bacterial plaque via disruption and/or removal of the microbial biofilm, the removal of accretions from the root surface, and ultimately a shift in the ecology of the pocket from one that favors disease to one that is conducive to health.

Instruments that can be used for scaling can be either manual or power-driven. Power-driven types can be sonic or ultrasonic, rotating instruments such as fine-grained diamonds, reciprocating instruments represented by the

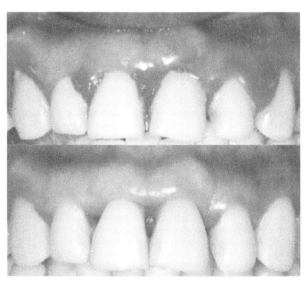

**Figure 4.1** One month follow-up demonstrating resolution of gingival inflammation after scaling and root planing.

Profin Directional System, or lasers. The most commonly used and studied instruments for mechanical debridement are manual scalers and sonic or ultrasonic scalers.

## Instrumentation

### Manual Scalers

All manual instruments have three sections: (1) the handle, (2) the shank, which can have bends, and (3) the working end or blade (Figure 4.2). The various scalers differ primarily in the number and angle of bends at the shank, and the shape, curvature, and number of cutting edges at the blade. There are five major classifications: sickle, curette, file, hoe, and chisel. The most commonly used are the sickle and curette. The design of a sickle scaler enables it to be used effectively for supragingival calculus removal, while curettes are better suited for subgingival application.

*Practical Periodontal Diagnosis and Treatment Planning,* Second Edition. Edited by Serge Dibart and Thomas Dietrich.
© 2024 John Wiley & Sons, Inc. Published 2024 by John Wiley & Sons, Inc.

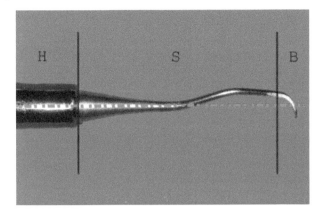

Figure 4.2   Scaler design. H: handle, S: shank, B: blade. Note that the blade is centered to the handle for ideal force transmission.

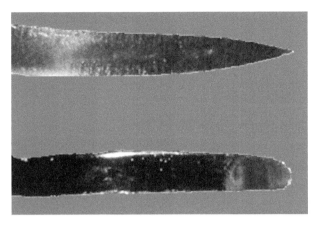

Figure 4.3   Contrast between the sharp tip of a sickle scaler (above) and the rounded toe of a curette (below).

The working end of a sickle scaler is triangular in cross-section, coming to a point at the tip. The blade faces up and is angled 90 degrees to the terminal shank with cutting edges on both sides of the face. This shape facilitates removal of heavy calculus and access to the area associated with the gingival embrasure and the proximal contact, which can be quite narrow. It is also very useful as an initial instrument to remove large, heavy deposits of supragingival calculus, thus improving access to the subgingival areas with the curettes. While sickle-type scalers are very effective at supragingival sites, they are not designed to be used at subgingival sites because the sharp tip can easily traumatize gingival tissues and gouge the root surface. Furthermore, the blade shape does not adapt well against the often concave, subgingival root anatomy (Figure 4.3).

Accessing the complex subgingival anatomy and minimizing damage to the delicate sulcular tissues is better achieved with curettes. Curettes are subdivided into two types, universal and Gracey. The main difference is that Gracey curettes are area specific; this specificity is realized via differences in the working ends. Gracey curettes have bends in the shank to facilitate access to either of the four sides of a tooth: mesial, distal, oral, or facial. In addition, the face of the blade is angled down 120 degrees to the terminal shank and only the lower side of the blade is sharpened. Thus, the Gracey 11/12 curette is designed to scale only the mesial surfaces of molars and premolars, while the Gracey 13/14 is specific to the distal surfaces (Figure 4.4). On the other hand, the universal curettes are not area-specific; the same instrument can be used anteriorly or posteriorly and for any of the four sides of the tooth. This is because both sides of the blade are sharpened and the angle of the face to the terminal shank is 90 degrees (Figure 4.5). Neither is objectively better than the other and thus operator preference based on an understanding of

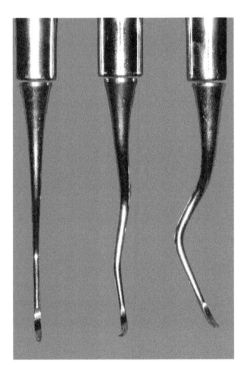

Figure 4.4   Series of Gracey scalers from left to right: 1/2 (anteriors), 11/12 (mesial of posteriors), and 13/14 (distal of posteriors). Note the increasing angle of bends in the shank to allow access to more posterior sites.

the instrument's design and the dental anatomy being scaled determines which instrument is best for any particular circumstance.

### Power-driven Scalers

Power-driven scalers are classified as either sonic or ultrasonic; the ultrasonic variety are subclassified as magnetostrictive or piezoelectric. They are broadly distinguished

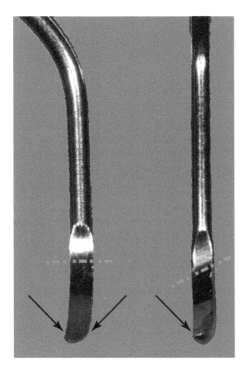

Figure 4.5    Key differences in blade design between universal and Gracey curettes. Universal: the face of the blade is 90 degrees to the shank (red dotted line) with both sides sharpened (arrows). Gracey: the face is angled 120 degrees to the shank (red dotted line) with only the lower side of the blade sharpened (arrow).

according to the type of tip movement and tip vibration frequency. The sonic scalers operate at low frequencies ranging from 3,000 to 8,000 cycles per second (Cps) with a tip movement that is generally orbital, while both types of ultrasonic scalers operate at much higher frequencies. The magnetostrictive range is from 18,000 to 45,000 Cps with an elliptical tip movement, while piezoelectric units have a Cps in the 25,000–50,000 range and a tip movement that is generally linear.

Sonic and ultrasonic instruments were originally only used for supragingival plaque, calculus, and stain removal. They were found to leave an uneven root surface, and thus it was thought that manual root planing was required following ultrasonic scaling to smooth the root surface. Over the years, there have been many modifications in the instruments, including smaller tip diameters, longer working lengths, different angles, and diamond coatings. These developments, along with a better, evidence-based understanding of the root surface alterations, have allowed powered scalers to be used safely and effectively in deep subgingival probing depths and difficult anatomy such as furcations, without having to be supplemented with subsequent manual instrumentation.

It should be noted that manual and sonic/ultrasonic scalers are used in a very different manner. The blade of a curette is inserted within the sulcus apical to the deposit at

the base of the pocket. The calculus is then engaged and removed as the scaler is pulled coronally out of the sulcus. On the other hand, sonic and ultrasonic scalers engage the deposit at its coronal extent. The instrument is inserted within the pocket like a dental probe, with the working end parallel to the root surface and the tip pointing into the sulcus. Calculus is removed with multiple, light apically directed strokes. It is beyond the scope of this chapter to discuss how each instrument is used and maintained. However, it should be understood that all scalers are technique sensitive. It is critical that the clinician be fully aware of an instrument's design and its proper use because incorrect application of a scaler will result in poor calculus removal and damage to the root surface or gingival tissues.

## Manual vs. Power-driven Scalers

The advances in ultrasonic and sonic instrument design and the expansion of their use to subgingival sites have resulted in a body of literature that compares their effectiveness with hand scalers. These studies have examined the efficacy of the debridement to bring about improvements in clinical endpoints such as probing depth and bleeding on probing, as well as shifts in the microbiological profile of the sulcus. Researchers have also considered alterations to the root surface and whether there is any advantage with powered scalers in accessing difficult anatomy or reducing the time required to effect this debridement.

## Clinical Endpoints

Generally, the studies show that there is no statistical difference in clinical endpoints such as reduction in bleeding on probing, pocket depth reduction, attachment level gain, and reduction in sites with plaque (Badersten et al. 1984; Boretti et al. 1995; Copulos et al. 1993; Laurell and Pettersson 1988; Loos et al. 1987). The reduction in probing depths with sonic or ultrasonic instruments ranges from 1.2 mm to 2.7 mm (Drisko et al. 1996). This compares favorably with the reductions achieved with manual scalers of 1.29–2.16 mm (Cobb 1996). The microbiological changes are related to the clinical outcomes. Here, as well, there does not appear to be a clear difference between the two types of debridement; both treatments result in similar shifts in the microbial flora (Baehni et al. 1992; Oosterwaal et al. 1987).

## Access to the Base of the Pocket or Difficult Anatomy

In relation to the similarity in clinical and microbiological endpoints achieved, it should be noted that in their systematic review, Tunkel et al. point out that most studies comparing powered and manual scaling are either done on single-rooted teeth or they group the results of single- and multi-rooted teeth, and that more research is required to assess the efficacy of powered instrumentation on multi-rooted teeth (Tunkel et al. 2002). In this regard there is evidence that suggests that ultrasonic instruments have an advantage over hand scalers for the debridement of furcations (Leon et al. 1987; Oda et al. 1989). These studies have found that both types of instruments are equally efficacious in Class I furcations, but in Class II and III situations the ultrasonic scalers are more effective. If one considers that anatomical studies have found that the entrance to a furcation is often smaller than the width of a curette (Bower 1979), then it is not surprising that specialized ultrasonic tips with widths of 0.55 mm or less would have an advantage (Figure 4.6).

Other modifications of ultrasonic tips are designed to allow improved penetration into the base of deep pockets. These tips, which are slimmer and probe-like in shape, can reach closer to the base of the pocket (0.78 mm) than manual curettes (1.25 mm) (Dragoo 1992). This result was confirmed recently by Barendregt et al., who also found that ultrasonic tips penetrated deeper, particularly in moderate (4–6 mm) and severe (≥7 mm) pockets (Barendregt et al. 2008).

In both of these papers, the greater penetration depth for ultrasonic scalers was on untreated periodontitis patients. The relevance of this point is highlighted by the Barendregt

paper, which found that unlike the results observed for the periodontitis group, the maintenance group (less inflamed gingival tissue) showed equal penetration depth for manual curettes and ultrasonic instruments. It is likely that in the periodontitis group some of the greater depth reached by the ultrasonic scaler could be explained as ingress of the ultrasonic tip through the epithelial attachment and into the connective tissue. This has been observed when using a periodontal probe to measure pocket depth in inflamed tissues where the difference in probing depths between treated and untreated pockets amounted to approximately 1.2 mm (Fowler et al. 1982). Even if all of the deeper access cannot be explained by connective tissue invasion, it has yet to be established if greater penetration translates to improved calculus and plaque removal.

Where studies have shown clear differences is in the time required to clean the root surface. A review of the evidence indicates that manual instrumentation takes 20–50% longer to achieve the same clinical results as with powered scaling (Cobb 1996).

## Surface Roughness and Cementum Removal

Since the introduction of sonic/ultrasonic instruments there have been investigations to determine if these instruments remove less or more root surface than hand scalers, as well as the smoothness of the resultant surface. Recent evidence suggests that ultrasonic scalers remove less cementum (Ritz et al. 1991; Vastardis et al. 2005) but leave a rougher surface than curettes (Kocher et al. 2001; Schlageter et al. 1996). However, as will be discussed later, the clinical significance of a rougher surface has yet to be elucidated. Irrespective, sonic and ultrasonic instrumentation can result in excessive cementum removal if used improperly. Increasing instrument pressure, contact time, or tip to tooth angle can all cause more root damage. In this regard it has been suggested that the ultrasonic scaler be used at low or medium power with multiple, *light* overlapping strokes and with the tip angled parallel to the root surface (Flemmig et al. 1997). The importance of light strokes is underlined by a study which found that increasing the application force from 0.3 N to 0.7 N resulted in a twofold increase in root surface loss (Jespen et al. 2004).

## Summary

In general, studies have found that a comparison of clinical endpoints shows manual and power-driven instruments to be equally effective. Thus, if the desired therapeutic outcome is reduction in inflammation, reduction in probing depth, and removal of root surface accretion, then either manual or powered instruments can be used. Despite these

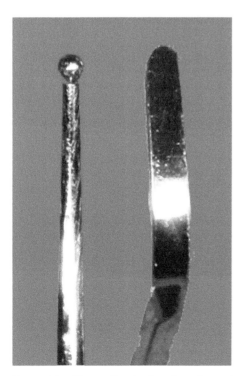

**Figure 4.6** The smaller tip size of an ultrasonic scaler (left), designed for access into a furcation, contrasted with a curette (right).

findings, powered scalers demonstrate some advantages, particularly with respect to time efficiency and access to challenging root anatomy. It remains to be seen if continued advances in tip design and ultrasonic energy generators will further improve the efficacy of these instruments.

## Scaling and Root Planing

### Objectives

As indicated above, effective scaling and root planing can be achieved by either powered or manual instrumentation. Although advances in technology may engender advantages to one instrument or the other, the focus of the therapy remains constant: the primary objective of mechanical nonsurgical therapy is the removal of bacterial plaque from the tooth surface. This is affected by removal of the soft microbial biofilm on the root surface as well as the hard accretions or calculus that harbor bacteria within their structure. With this mechanical reduction or disturbance of the microbial community, we expect resolution of the inflammatory changes in the tissues of the periodontium, which in turn precipitate a change in the local environment of the sulcus from one that supports inflammatory destruction to one that is conducive to the maintenance of periodontal health.

To gain a holistic understanding of mechanical nonsurgical therapy we need to consider not only the response of the periodontium to our hygiene efforts but also the factors that modify this response. In this way we can better optimize our results as well as understand the limits of and limitations on this form of therapy.

### Changes in Clinical Endpoints

The most common endpoints used to evaluate the clinical outcome of mechanical therapy are probing pocket depth and clinical attachment level. Although there is only a weak correlation between bleeding on probing and continued disease activity (Lang et al. 1990), decreases in the percentage of bleeding sites continue to be considered a surrogate indicator for the resolution of gingival inflammation. In this regard it is useful to note that collectively, studies investigating all forms of mechanical therapy show reductions in gingival inflammation by 45% in 4–6.5-mm pockets (Cobb 2002). In addition, this resolution of inflammation is affected largely by subgingival instrumentation, with supragingival plaque control alone providing little or no benefit (Cobb 2002).

Many researchers have investigated the effect of scaling and root planing on probing depth and clinical attachment

level. Cobb conducted a review of these papers and presented the results of the collective data reported in these studies (Figure 4.7). He found that in sites with initial probing depths of 1–3 mm there was a pocket depth reduction of 0.03 mm with a loss in clinical attachment of 0.34 mm. At sites measuring 4–6 mm the probing depth reduction was 1.3 mm with a gain of 0.55 mm in the clinical attachment level. The greatest improvements were gained at pocket depths ≥7 mm with probing depth reductions of 2.16 mm and gains in the clinical attachment level of 1.19 mm (Cobb 1996). A systematic review by Van der Weijden reported that in sites measuring ≥5 mm the reduction in probing depth was 1.18 mm with an attachment gain of 0.64 mm (Van der Weijden et al. 2002). Both studies found that the effect of treatment on clinical outcome measures was related to the initial pocket depth; improvements in sites with initially deeper probing depths were greater than in those that were initially shallower. They also found that half of the decrease in probing depth could be attributed to attachment gain and thus the remaining decrease was the result of a change in the gingival margin position.

As a caveat, it should be noted that in many of the classic scaling studies very proficient clinicians spent 10 minutes or more per tooth. Thus, the gains achieved represent an ideal result rather than the usual clinical reality, in which considerably less time is spent and possibly with less proficient operators. Additionally, most studies group molar and non-molar sites. There is limited evidence to suggest that the improvements obtained at multi-rooted furcation involved teeth with probing depths measuring ≥4 mm are less than those achieved at single-rooted teeth (Claffey et al. 1990; Kalkwarf et al. 1988; Loos et al. 1989). In these studies pocket depth changes at moderately deep sites (4–6 mm) ranged from 0 mm to 1.02 mm, and at deep (≥7 mm) sites the range was 0–1.52 mm, which is considerably less than the 2.16-mm decrease observed when all teeth are grouped.

| Initial PPD | Δ PD | Δ CAL |
|:---:|:---:|:---:|
| 1–3 | −0.03 | −0.34 |
| 4–6 | −1.3 | +0.55 |
| ≥7 | −2.16 | 1.19 |

**Δ**: change **PD**: pocket depth **CAL**: clinical attachment level

all measurements in millimeters *adapted from Cobb 1996*

Figure 4.7 Summary of pocket depth and attachment level changes following SRP.

## Microbiological Changes

In general, studies show that subgingival debridement results in a decrease in gram-negative microbes with an accompanying increase in the numbers of gram-positive cocci and rods. This shift in the composition of subgingival plaque from one with many pathogenic bacteria to one dominated by beneficial species usually results in a decrease in gingival inflammation, resulting in an improvement in clinical outcome measures such as pocket depth and bleeding on probing (Cobb 2002).

Cugini et al., in a recent study using DNA probe counts, found that SRP resulted in decreased prevalence and levels of *Porphyromonas gingivalis, Tannerella forsythensis,* and *Treponema denticola.* This decrease in pathogenic species was concomitant with an increase in prevalence and levels of beneficial species such as *Actinomyces* species, *Fusobacterium nudeatum* subspecies, *Streptococci* species, and *Veillonella parvula.* It should be noted, however, that while SRP appeared to be effective in lowering the numbers of selected periodontal pathogens, none of these species was completely eliminated from any subject by this therapy. Another important observation is that SRP was only effective in reducing a specific subset of the subgingival microflora. Specifically, reductions in pocket depth were most strongly associated with decreases in *Tannerella forsythensis,* which suggests that individuals with non-susceptible (to scaling) species or low numbers of susceptible pathogenic species would experience limited benefits from nonsurgical mechanical treatment (Cugini et al. 2000). This finding correlates well with a number of other studies (Haffajee et al. 1997; Mombelli et al. 2000; Shiloah et al. 1994; van Winkelhoff et al. 1988) that have found that *Actinomyces Actinomycetemcomitans* and *Porphyromonas gingivalis* are more resistant to removal by nonsurgical mechanical means and that the persistence of these bacteria has been associated with poor response to scaling and root planing.

To better understand these findings it is useful to know that bacteria exist at three areas within the pocket: the tooth surface, on and within the gingival tissues of the sulcus wall, and in planktonic form in the pocket space between the tooth and sulcus wall. It may be that the ability of particular bacteria to invade the gingival tissues allows them to evade removal by mechanical means.

Another limitation in microbiological changes is pretreatment pocket depth. Haffajee et al. found that although the greatest reduction in counts of periodontal pathogens was found at deep (greater than 6 mm) sites, the counts at all-time points (three, six, nine, and 12 months) were always higher in deep sites than at the shallow sites (less than 4 mm). Deep sites continue, even after treatment, to be an environment conducive to certain pathogenic bacteria (Haffajee et al. 1997). Thus, gingival health does not necessarily follow thorough debridement. In this regard, Haffajee et al. reported that mechanical nonsurgical therapy resulted in improving clinical parameters only 68% of the time and that 32% of the time there was no benefit.

Additionally, it should be noted that the shifts in the microbial flora are transient, particularly in pockets with residual probing depths of >6 mm, with reestablishment of a pathogenic microflora at varied time points depending largely on the frequency of supportive periodontal therapy and proficiency of oral hygiene. Various mechanisms have been proposed for the transient character of this shift, including recolonization from other intraoral niches such as tongue and mucosa (Quirynen et al. 1999), recolonization from tissue-invading bacteria, particularly *Actinomyces Actinomycetemcomitans* and to a lesser extent *Porphyromonas gingivalis* (Cugini et al. 2000), high post-treatment plaque levels due to incomplete eradication of the pathogenic bacteria (Sbordone et al. 1990), and the level of patient oral hygiene (Sbordone et al. 1990).

## Efficacy of Plaque and Calculus Removal

A review of the literature indicates that although scaling and root planing is effective for the reduction of plaque and calculus, it cannot affect the complete removal of deposits. Rather, what we find is varying degrees of success in producing calculus-free teeth depending on a variety of factors. Variables that have been investigated are: (1) initial probing depth, (2) surgical access, (3) furcation involvement, (4) level of operator training, and (5) manual vs. machine-driven scalers.

The most significant limitations on the residual amount of plaque or calculus following mechanical therapy are the depth of the pocket and furcation involvement. Although studies demonstrate a wide range of residual calculus left on roots, from 5% to 80%, the general trend is that as probing depth increases the effectiveness of mechanical debridement diminishes. In probing depths measuring 3 mm or less there is a good chance of removing all of the subgingival plaque. But in pocket depths ranging from 3 mm to 5 mm, the chance of failure to completely debride the root exceeds the chance of success. Furthermore, in pockets measuring 5 mm or more, failure becomes the dominant result (Rabbani et al. 1981; Stambaugh et al. 1981).

Studies investigating the concept of visualizing the root surface to improve the efficacy of scaling and root planing have found that surgical (open) access allows the operator to be much more effective in achieving calculus-free teeth but only in ≥4 mm depths. In shallow pockets of less than 4 mm, nonsurgical debridement is as effective or only slightly less effective than surgical debridement (Brayer et al. 1989; Buchanan et al., 1987; Caffesse et al.

1986). Nevertheless, even with direct visualization, scaling efficacy was reduced with increasing pocket depth. Furthermore, most of the residual calculus was found in grooves, fossae, and furcations (Caffesse et al. 1986). Together, these observations suggest that root anatomy has a significant influence on the thoroughness of debridement.

The effect of anatomy on treatment results was also investigated by Wylam et al., who found that although the effectiveness of scaling and root planing on multi-rooted teeth was significantly improved with open access over closed (54.3% vs. 33%), if the results were restricted to an examination of the furcation areas there remained heavy residual calculus regardless of the type of access. In addition, increased time spent did not correlate with improved calculus removal (Wylam et al. 1993). Fleischer also found that even with open access difficult areas such as furcations often had more residual calculus than other surfaces after scaling and root planing (Fleischer 1989).

These findings are not surprising when one considers that the width of a molar furcation is often not large enough to allow insertion of a standard Gracey curette. Bower observed that 58% of molar furcation entrances had a width of less than 0.75 mm and 81% were less than 1 mm, while an average curette was 0.75–1.1 mm wide (Bower 1979). It should be noted that both the Wylam and Fleischer papers used manual instruments, and while the Fleischer study did use ultrasonic instrumentation, it was with a P-10 tip, which is indicated for supragingival use. Their results are not transferable to powered scalers using tips designed for subgingival and furcation sites. In fact, it is in these areas that ultrasonic instruments with tips measuring .55 mm or less have shown an advantage (Oda and Shikawa 1989).

Operator experience also appears to play a role in the efficacy of root surface debridement. Studies have found that inexperienced dentists (Kocher et al. 1997) and periodontists in training (Brayer et al. 1989; Fleischer et al. 1989) left residual calculus on a greater number of root surfaces than trained periodontists. These studies also found that experienced periodontists took more time to scale, suggesting either a better understanding of the time required to scale teeth or a more sensitive tactile endpoint.

An interesting finding was that use of ultrasonic instead of hand instruments does not improve results for inexperienced operators, and thus the ultrasonic scaler should not be considered an instrument for less skilled operators.

### Summary

Regardless of the variables affecting the efficacy of mechanical therapy, complete debridement of the root surface does not appear to be a realizable goal. Even surgical access only makes a slight improvement, and thus it seems a likely inference from all of the studies that the limitations on the effectiveness of scaling are related only in part to operator experience, instrument type, and direct visualization, and that ultimately efforts to completely remove calculus are hampered by difficulty in accessing both the macroscopic anatomy such as furcations, concavities, and grooves, and the microscopic anatomy such as erosions and porosities. In any event, healing following scaling and root planing is a clinical reality, which raises questions regarding which aspects of mechanical debridement are important to success. It may be that all are required, at least in the short term, to cause a disturbance of a pathogenic subset of the microbial biofilm or achieve an as yet undetermined threshold of debridement, and that thoroughness of debridement is more relevant to long-term maintenance of the initial resolution of inflammation.

## Root Surface Smoothness

Another aspect of scaling and root planing that has been explored is posttreatment root surface changes and their effect on plaque accumulation and resolution of inflammation. A smooth root surface is often used as a clinical endpoint for thorough debridement. At a microscopic level it has been found that the different root planing instruments achieve varying degrees of root surface smoothness. Although these differences cannot be detected clinically, they have been investigated for their effect on rate of plaque accumulation and ultimately tissue healing.

It is generally agreed that rougher surfaces promote and increase the rate of plaque accumulation (Leknes et al. 1994; Quirynen et al. 1995). However, with respect to root surface smoothness following root planing, no instrument leaves behind a smooth surface. An in vivo study on root surface roughness following scaling by various instruments found that 15 nm rotating diamonds and Gracey curettes left the smoothest surface followed by the piezo-electric, 75 μm diamond, and sonic scalers with roughness values ($R_a$) ranging from 1.64 μm to 2.1 μm (Schlageter et al. 1996). The point of the paper that is relevant to this discussion is that all of the tested instruments left a root surface that was 8–13 times rougher than the smoothness threshold of 0.2 μm, which was determined in a literature review to be the $R_a$ value above which plaque accumulation is facilitated (Quirynen and Bollen 1995). Thus, it appears that even if we accept that the rate of biofilm formation decreases with smoother surfaces, the root surface roughness subsequent to scaling, regardless of instrument choice, will always facilitate plaque accumulation.

Furthermore, despite the correlation between surface smoothness and plaque accumulation, it has not been established that a rougher surface is significant for healing.

An early study using closed scaling failed to find an effect on gingival inflammation (Rosenberg and Ash 1974) and later, in vivo studies using direct visualization (surgical access) failed to find differences in healing after flap surgery between root surfaces that were smoothed after being cleaned and those that were intentionally roughened with a diamond (Khatiblou and Ghodossi 1983; Oberholzer et al. 1996).

These findings reinforce a point previously made, that healing subsequent to SRP is not dependent on complete removal of plaque but rather a disruption of the biofilm sufficient to change a pathogenic microbial profile to one that is conducive to periodontal health.

## Full-Mouth Debridement

An area that has received recent attention is the difference in clinical and microbiological results when standard therapy—defined as four quadrants of root planing, each separated by one or two—is compared to full-mouth root planing, whereby all four quadrants are scaled within 24 hours. The philosophy behind this alternative treatment regimen is that it prevents recolonization of instrumented sites by bacteria from non-instrumented sites. It is also claimed that multiple scalings within 24 hours can stimulate an immune response, supplementing the mechanical effect of debridement on plaque.

A number of papers from a group of researchers based out of the Catholic University of Leuven, Belgium, have demonstrated additional gains in pocket depth reduction of about 1 mm at moderately deep pockets (4–6 mm) and 1.6–1.9 mm at deep (≥7 mm) sites. In addition, these studies found greater reductions in proportions of spirochetes and motile rods, although these differences were no longer statistically significant after two months (De Soete et al. 2001; Mongardini et al. 1999; Quirynen et al. 1999). In contrast, studies from other centers have all failed to find any statistically significant differences (Apatzidou et al. 2004a; Jervoe-Storm et al. 2006; Nagata et al. 2001). Thus, although the concept behind full-mouth scaling may seem reasonable, conflicting results have been reported in the literature. Regardless, both treatment regimens seem to provide at least comparable gains and thus the choice of modality may be better based on practical concerns for the patient such as convenience, comfort, and financial considerations.

## Practical Aspects

Given the plethora of instruments on the market, with new ones being continually introduced, it is imperative to use the literature to make educated practical decisions regarding both instrument selection and their correct application. Taking the studies collectively, it appears that the most important factors influencing complete debridement are instrument access and dental anatomy. Root concavities and grooves, the cementoenamel junction, interproximal areas, deep pockets, and furcations all complicate the debridement process and are the sites most likely to exhibit residual calculus.

Many advances in scaling instrument design are intended to improve access to the complex root anatomy that impedes calculus removal. Thus, maximizing the quality of debridement requires both an understanding of an instrument's design and an intimate knowledge of root anatomy. Knowing the physical characteristics of the working end of a scaler enables the practitioner to choose the instrument most appropriate for the anatomy being scaled. For example, when scaling a root groove or through a constricted entrance in class II and III furcation involvements, the narrow tip of an ultrasonic scaler would be more efficacious than a curette. There may also be an advantage of ultrasonics in deep, narrow pockets. Here the thin, probe-like shape can provide less traumatic calculus removal than the larger blade of curettes. Because there is individual variation in root shape, even among similar teeth, an experienced tactile sense also plays an important part.

Considering that manual instrumentation requires more complex hand movements (with respect to firm, stable fulcrums and specific blade angulations against the root surface), increased chair time, and greater stamina, it may be that ultrasonic scalers will become the instrument of choice. Nevertheless, whether the clinician prefers manual or powered scalers, a dogmatic adherence to one type of scaler limits the armamentarium of the clinician. An integrated approach with both powered and manual scalers enables the clinician to approach each tooth individually and use the advantages of any instrument to reach the desired endpoint.

As discussed, increasing pocket depth greatly diminishes the efficacy of debridement, and although surgical access is not immune to the variable of pocket depth, it does nevertheless significantly enhance results over closed scaling in pocket depths measuring greater than 4 mm. An interesting twist is introduced into our decision-making process when a paper by Lindhe is considered. Lindhe et al. looked at the surgical modality from the perspective of critical probing depth, defined as the pocket depth above which there was an improvement in clinical attachment level for surgical over nonsurgical scaling. The value was 4.5 mm for molars, compared to 6–7 mm for incisors and premolar teeth; a shallower depth was required for molars before surgery provided a better result (Lindhe et al. 1982). These results can be understood in the context of access and root anatomy, both of which are generally more complicated at molar teeth. Thus, when considering improving visualization with surgery, the pocket depth must be considered in the context of the tooth with which it is associated.

A final important practical aspect is the matter of how one determines if a root surface has been adequately debrided. Originally, roots were scaled and planed aggressively to a hard, glossy finish. This was intended to completely remove plaque, calculus, and cementum contaminated by bacteria and their endotoxins. This practice has recently been called into question due to observations that endotoxins form a superficial layer on cementum that can be removed with gentle scaling (Cheetham et al. 1988) or ultrasonic debridement (Smart et al. 1990). In 1996, the consensus report of the World Workshop in Periodontics stated that the removal of cementum for the purposes of endotoxin removal was no longer considered prudent (Cobb 1996). However, it is still relevant to plane roots to some degree because short of using endoscopy or surgical visualization, without smoothing roots we cannot evaluate the completeness of calculus removal. Although scaling is certainly indicated for the removal of plaque and calculus, root planing should be used judiciously to avoid unnecessary and excessive removal of root substance.

In this respect it is advantageous to use ultrasonic scalers for the bulk of the debridement because although manual scalers produce a smoother surface than sonic/ultrasonic scalers, they do so at the expense of greater root substance removal. One may consider the difference to be small (in the order of microns) and not of clinical consequence, but years of repeated root planing at regular maintenance visits will add up to a clinically significant amount.

## Conclusion

Although it is well accepted that plaque biofilms are the main etiologic factor for periodontal disease, we now understand that there are other considerations that need to be taken into account if we are to fully understand the pathogenesis of periodontal disease. Genetic, environmental, and host systemic factors all play an important role in modulating the progression of periodontal disease and the response to periodontal therapy. Nevertheless, scaling and root planing remain the primary therapy for dealing with periodontal infections. Mechanical debridement can affect the composition of the bacterial plaque directly, affect the host response to bacteria, or alter the habitat; alterations of any of these factors can have an impact on the remaining factors in this triad.

To successfully use scaling and root planing in the armamentarium to combat periodontal disease, the trained professional must gain a thorough understanding of the evidence for what can be realistically achieved, how one can optimize those gains, and what factors can limit the efficacy of this modality of treatment. As discussed, due to microbial, environmental, or anatomical limitations, mechanical debridement alone is not always successful in controlling periodontal disease or its progression. Thus, although scaling and root planing is the predominant form of periodontal therapy, it should be understood from the outset that it is to be regarded as a component of an overall treatment plan and, if required, may be supplemented by other forms of nonsurgical therapy such as local or systemic antimicrobials or surgical means. The determination can be made on a patient-by-patient basis at the reevaluation appointment or at subsequent maintenance visits.

When considering the evidence on the benefits of scaling and root planing we must take into account the endpoints being evaluated. Most commonly our attention is directed toward clinical changes in inflammation, probing depth, and attachment level. As important as these changes are, a holistic approach to patient care must also take into account other factors including efficiency, costs, compliance issues, and a host of others. Thus, when planning treatment, consideration should be given not only to the expected gains from scaling and root planing but also to what more may be required to maintain any gains or prevent the initiation of disease in new sites or its progression in existing sites.

## References

Apatzidou, D.A. and Kinane, D.F. (2004a). Quadrant root planing versus same-day full-mouth root planing. I. Clinical findings. *J. Clin. Periodontol.* 31 (2): 132–140.

Apatzidou, D.A. and Kinane, D.F. (2004b). Quadrant root planing versus same-day full-mouth root planing. II. Microbiological findings. *J. Clin. Periodontol.* 31 (2): 141–148.

Badersten, A., Nilveus, R., and Egelberg, J. (1984). Effect of nonsurgical periodontal therapy. II. Severely advanced periodontitis. *J. Clin. Periodontol.* 11 (1): 63–76.

Baehni, P., Thilo, B., Chapuis, B., and Pernet, D. (1992). Effects of ultrasonic and sonic scalers on dental plaque microflora in vitro and in vivo. *J. Clin. Periodontol.* 19 (7): 455–459.

Barendregt, D.S., van der Velden, U., Timmerman, M.F., and van der Weijden, F. (2008). Penetration depths with an ultrasonic mini insert compared with a conventional curette in patients with periodontitis and in periodontal maintenance. *J. Clin. Periodontol.* 35 (1): 31–36.

Boretti, G., Zappa, U., Graf, H., and Case, D. (1995). Short-term effects of phase I therapy on crevicular cell populations. *J. Periodontol.* 66 (3): 235–240.

Bower, R.C. (1979). Furcation morphology relative to periodontal treatment. Furcation entrance architecture. *J. Periodontol.* 50 (1): 23–27.

Brayer, W.K., Mellonig, J.T., Dunlap, R.M. et al. (1989). Scaling and root planing effectiveness: the effect of root surface access and operator experience. *J. Periodontol.* 60 (1): 67–72.

Buchanan, S.A. and Robertson, P.B. (1987). Calculus removal by scaling/root planing with and without surgical access. *J. Periodontol.* 58 (3): 159–163.

Caffesse, R.G., Sweeney, P.L., and Smith, B.A. (1986). Scaling and root planing with and without periodontal flap surgery. *J. Clin. Periodontol.* 13 (3): 205–210.

Cheetham, W.A., Wilson, M., and Kieser, J.B. (1988). Root surface debridement— an in vitro assessment. *J. Clin. Periodontol.* 15 (5): 288–292.

Claffey, N., Nylund, K., Kiger, R. et al. (1990). Diagnostic predictability of scores of plaque, bleeding, suppuration and probing depth for probing attachment loss. 3.5 years of observation following initial periodontal therapy. *J. Clin. Periodontol.* 17 (2): 108–114.

Cobb, C.M. (1996). Non-surgical pocket therapy: mechanical. *Ann. Periodontol.* 1: 443–490.

Cobb, C.M. (2002). Clinical significance of non-surgical periodontal therapy: an evidence-based perspective of scaling and root planing. *J. Clin. Periodontol.* 29 (Suppl 2): 6–16.

Copulos, T.A., Low, S.B., Walker, C.B. et al. (1993). Comparative analysis between a modified ultrasonic tip and hand instruments on clinical parameters of periodontal disease. *J. Periodontal.* 64 (8): 694–700.

Cugini, M.A., Haffajee, A.D., Smith, C. et al. (2000). The effect of scaling and root planing on the clinical and microbiological parameters of periodontal diseases: 12-month results. *J. Clin. Periodontal.* 27 (1): 30–36.

De Soete, M., Mongardini, C., Peuwels, M. et al. (2001). One-stage full-mouth disinfection. Long-term microbiological results analyzed by checkerboard DNA-DNA hybridization. *J. Periodontal.* 72 (3): 374–382.

Dragoo, M.R. (1992). A clinical evaluation of hand and ultrasonic instruments on subgingival debridement. Part 1. With unmodified and modified ultrasonic inserts. *Int. J. Periodontics Restorative Dent.* 12 (4): 310–323.

Drisko, C.L. and Lewis, L. (1996). Ultrasonic instruments and antimicrobial agents in supportive periodontal treatment and retreatment of recurrent or refractory periodontitis. *Periodontal. 2000* 12: 90–115.

Fleischer, H.C., Mellonig, J.T., Brayer, W.K. et al. (1989). Scaling and root planing efficacy in multirooted teeth. *J. Periodontol.* 60 (7): 402–409.

Flemmig, T.F., Petersilka, G.J., Mehl, A. et al. (1997). Working parameters of a sonic scaler influencing root substance removal in vitro. *Clin. Oral Invest.* 1 (2): 55–607.

Fowler, C., Garrett, S., Crigger, M., and Egelberg, J. (1982). Histologic probe position in treated and untreated human periodontal tissues. *J. Clin. Periodontal.* 9 (5): 373–385.

Haffajee, A.D., Cugini, M.A., Dibart, S. et al. (1997). The effect of SRP on the clinical and microbiological parameters of periodontal diseases. *J. Clin. Periodontal.* 24 (5): 324–334.

Jervoe-Storm, P.M., Semaan, E., AlAhdab, H. et al. (2006). Clinical outcomes of quadrant root planing versus full-mouth root planing. *J. Clin. Periodontal.* 33 (3): 209–215.

Jespen, S., Ayna, M., Hedderich, J., and Eberhard, J. (2004). Significant influence of scaler tip design on root substance loss resulting from ultrasonic scaling: a laserprofilometric in vitro study. *J. Clin. Periodontal.* 31 (11): 1003–1006.

Kalkwarf, K.L., Kaldahl, W.B., and Patil, K.D. (1988). Evaluation of furcation region response to periodontal therapy. *J. Periodontol.* 59 (12): 794–804.

Khatiblou, F.A. and Ghodossi, A. (1983). Root surface smoothness or roughness in periodontal treatment. A clinical study. *J. Periodontol.* 54: 365–367.

Kocher, T., Rosin, M., Langenbeck, N., and Bernhardt, O. (2001). Subgingival polishing with a teflon-coated sonic scaler insert in comparison to conventional instruments as assessed on extracted teeth (II). Subgingival roughness. *J. Clin. Periodontal.* 28 (8): 723–729.

Kocher, T., Ruehling, A., Momsen, H., and Plagmann, H.C. (1997). Effectiveness of subgingival instrumentation with power-driven instruments in the hands of experienced and inexperienced operators. A study on manikins. *J. Clin. Periodontal.* 24 (7): 498–504.

Lang, N.P., Adler, R., Joss, A., and Nyman, S. (1990). Absence of bleeding on probing. An indicator of periodontal stability. *J. Clin. Periodontal.* 17 (10): 714–721.

Laurell, L. and Pettersson, B. (1988). Periodontal healing after treatment with either the Titan-S sonic scaler or hand instruments. *Swed. Dent. J.* 12 (5): 187–192.

Leknes, K.N., Lie, T., Wikesjö, U.M. et al. (1994). Influence of tooth instrumentation roughness on subgingival microbial colonization. *J. Periodontol.* 65 (4): 303–308.

Leon, L.E. and Vogel, R.I. (1987). A comparison of the effectiveness of hand scaling and ultrasonic debridement in furcations as evaluated by differential dark-field microscopy. *J. Periodontol.* 58 (2): 86–94.

Lindhe, J., Nyman, S., Socransky, S.S. et al. (1982). "Critical probing depth" in periodontal therapy. *J. Clin. Periodontal.* 9: 323–336.

Loe, H., Theilade, E., and Jensen, S. (1965). Experimental gingivitis in man. *J. Periodontol.* 36: 177–187.

Loos, B., Kiger, R., and Egelberg, J. (1987). An evaluation of basic periodontal therapy using sonic and ultrasonic scalers. *J. Clin. Periodontol.* 14 (1): 29–33.

Loos, B., Nylund, K., Claffey, N., and Egelberg, J. (1989). Clinical effects of root debridement in molar and non-molar teeth. A 2-year follow-up. *J. Clin. Periodontol.* 16 (8): 498–504.

Mombelli, A., Schmid, B., Rutar, A., and Lang, N.P. (2000). Persistence patterns of Porphyromonas gingivalis, Prevotella intermedia/nigrescens, and Actinobacillus actinomycetemcomitans after mechanical therapy of periodontal disease. *J. Periodontol.* 71 (1): 14–21.

Mongardini, C., van Steenberghe, D., Dekeyser, C., and Quirynen, M. (1999). One state full-versus partial-mouth disinfection in the treatment of chronic adult or generalized early-onset periodontitis. I. Long -term clinical observations. *J. Periodontol.* 70 (6): 632–645.

Nagata, M.J.H., Anderson, G.B., and Bonaventura, G.T. (2001). Full-mouth disinfection versus standard treatment of periodontitis: a clinical study. *J. Periodontol.* 72 (11): 1636.

Oberholzer, R. and Rateitschak, K.H. (1996). Root cleaning or root smoothing. An in vivo study. *J. Clin. Periodontol.* 23 (4): 326–330.

Oda, S. and Shikawa, I. (1989). In vitro effectiveness of a newly-designed ultrasonic scaler tip for furcation areas. *J. Periodontol.* 60 (11): 634–639.

Oosterwaal, P.J., Matee, M.I., Mikx, F.H. et al. (1987). The effect of subgingival debridement with hand and ultrasonic instruments on the subgingival microflora. *J. Clin. Periodontol.* 14 (9): 528–533.

Quirynen, M. and Bollen, C.M. (1995). The influence of surface roughness and surface-free energy on supra- and subgingival plaque formation in man. A review of the literature. *J. Clin. Periodontol.* 22 (1): 1–14.

Quirynen, M., Mongardini, C., Pauwels, M. et al. (1999). One-stage full-versus partial-mouth disinfection in the treatment of chronic adult or generalized early-onset periodontitis. II. Long-term impact on microbial load. *J. Periodontol.* 70 (6): 646–656.

Rabbani, G.M., Ash, M.M. Jr., and Caffesse, R.G. (1981). The effectiveness of subgingival scaling and root planing in calculus removal. *J. Periodontol.* 52 (3): 119–123.

Ritz, L., Hefti, A.F., and Rateitschak, K.H. (1991). An in vitro investigation on the loss of root substance in scaling with various instruments. *J. Clin. Periodontol.* 18 (9): 643–647.

Rosenberg, R.M. and Ash, M.M. Jr. (1974). The effect of root roughness on plaque accumulation and gingival inflammation. *J. Periodontol.* 45 (3): 146–150.

Sbordone, L., Ramaglia, L., Gulletta, E., and Lacono, V. (1990). Recolonization of the subgingival microflora after scaling and root planing in human periodontitis. *J. Periodontol.* 61 (9): 579–584.

Schlageter, L., Rateitschak-Pluss, E.M., and Schwarz, J.P. (1996). Root surface smoothness or roughness following open debridement. An in vivo study. *J. Clin. Periodontol.* 23 (5): 460–464.

Shiloah, J. and Patters, M.R. (1994). DNA probe analysis of the survival of selected periodontal pathogens following scaling, root planing, and intra-pocket irrigation. *J. Periodontol.* 65 (6): 568–575.

Smart, G.J., Wilson, M., Davies, E.H., and Kieser, J.B. (1990). The assessment of ultrasonic root surface debridement by determination of residual endotoxin levels. *J. Clin. Periodontol.* 17 (3): 174–178.

Stambaugh, R., Dragoo, M., Smith, D., and Carasali, L. (1981). The limits of subgingival scaling. *Int. J. Periodontics Restorative Dent.* 1 (5): 30–41.

Theilade, E., Wright, W.H., Jensen, S.B., and Loe, H. (1966). Experimental gingivitis in man ll. A longitudinal clinical and bacteriological investigation. *J. Periodontal. Res.* 1: 1–13.

Tunkel, J., Helnecke, A., and Flemmlg, T.F. (2002). A systematic review of efficacy of machine-driven and manual subgingival debridement in the treatment of chronic periodontitis. *J. Clin. Periodontol.* 29 (Suppl 3): 72–81.

Van der Weijden, G.A. and Timmerman, M.F. (2002). A systematic review on the clinical efficacy of subgingival debridement in the treatment of chronic periodontitis. *J. Clin. Periodontol.* 29 (Suppl 3): 55–71.

van Winkelhoff, A.J., Van der Velden, U., and de Graaff, J. (1988). Microbial succession in recolonizing deep periodontal pockets after a single course of supra- and subgingival debridement. *J. Clin. Periodontol.* 15 (2): 116–122.

Vastardis, S., Yukna, R.A., Rice, D.A., and Mercante, D. (2005). Root surface removal and resultant surface texture with diamond-coated ultrasonic inserts: an in vitro and SEM study. *J. Clin. Periodontol.* 32 (5): 467–473.

Wylam, J.M., Mealey, B.L., Mills, M.P. et al. (1993). The clinical effectiveness of open versus closed scaling and root planing on multi-rooted teeth. *J. Periodontol.* 64 (11): 1023–1028.

## 5

# Occlusion

*Steven M. Morgano*

## Introduction

Concepts of occlusion in the early twentieth century were based primarily on the rehabilitation of totally edentulous patients with complete dentures. At the time, a relatively large segment of the population was edentulous, in part because of the widespread acceptance of the focal infection theory (Goymerac and Woollard 2004). Complete mouth extraction was commonly prescribed by physicians for patients with systemic diseases in an attempt to eliminate any oral infections that were assumed to act as focal infections and cause the systemic disease.

## Centric Relation and Centric Occlusion

Concepts of centric relation evolved as dentists refined their treatment methods for edentulous patients (Hanau 1929). It was observed by many dentists that the mandible of an edentulous patient could be guided upward and backward to a stable, repeatable position. In this position, the mandible appeared to hinge or rotate about an axis (Figure 5.1). Because these dentists assumed that each condyle was centered in its respective glenoid fossa when the mandible reached this position, the position was referred to as centric relation (Hanau 1929). Many dentists believed that the condyles were in the most retruded position when the mandible was in centric relation (Thompson 1946), and by the latter half of the twentieth century, most definitions of centric relation described it as the most retruded mandibular position. It was also assumed, at the time, that the condyles were in centric relation when a dentate patient brought together the maxillary and mandibular opposing teeth (Niswonger 1934); therefore, the position with the opposing teeth fitting together was referred to as centric occlusion. Posselt's (1952) research on mandibular movements clearly demonstrated that, with

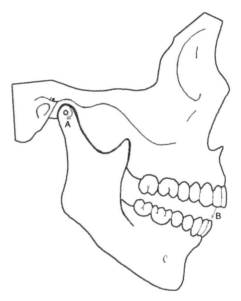

Figure 5.1   When the mandible is in centric relation it rotates about an axis.

most patients, the condyles were not in centric relation when the teeth fit together best. He suggested the term intercuspal position (ICP) to designate the best fit of the teeth, rather than centric occlusion.

American dentists ignored Posselt's suggestion and continued to use the term centric occlusion to designate the ICP. Finally, in 1987, the *Glossary of Prosthodontic Terms*, fifth edition (Academy of Prosthodontics 1987), introduced the term maximum intercuspal position (MIP) (later modified to maximal intercuspal position in a subsequent edition of the *Glossary*) as the designation for the best fit of the teeth.

The term centric occlusion was not abandoned but was redefined as "the occlusion of opposing teeth when the mandible is in centric relation" (Academy of Prosthodontics 1987), a position that may or may not coincide with MIP. In that fifth edition of the *Glossary*, centric relation was also redefined as, "the maxillomandibular relationship in which

*Practical Periodontal Diagnosis and Treatment Planning*, Second Edition. Edited by Serge Dibart and Thomas Dietrich.
© 2024 John Wiley & Sons, Inc. Published 2024 by John Wiley & Sons, Inc.

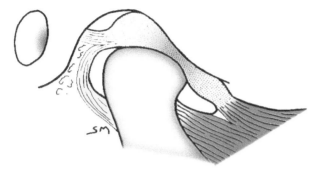

Figure 5.2 The current definition of centric relation describes condyles as articulating with the thinnest avascular portion of their respective disks with the complex in the anterior-superior position against the slopes of the articular eminencies.

the condyles articulate with the thinnest avascular portion of their respective disks with the complex in the anteriorsuperior position against the slopes of the articular eminences. This position is independent of tooth contact. This position is clinically discernible when the mandible is directed superiorly and anteriorly. It is restricted to a purely rotary movement about the transverse horizontal axis." This definition was based on a new understanding of the physiology of the temporomandibular joint (Figure 5.2). Centric relation was not relocated; it was redefined. McDevitt et al. (1995) conducted a magnetic resonance imaging study of a group of patients and confirmed the validity of the new definition.

It has become universally accepted that the MIP for a totally edentulous patient should coincide with centric relation. This concept was later applied to patients with natural teeth. Many dentists believed that a natural MIP that did not coincide with the centric relation position was a malocclusion, while others disagreed.

## Balanced Articulation

Developing an MIP that coincides with centric relation provides denture stability in MIP; however, mastication is not restricted to pure hinge movement. Mastication involves lateral, protrusive, and retrusive three-dimensional movements. Arranging the artificial teeth of complete dentures to allow simultaneous contact of the teeth in eccentric positions can enhance denture stability, uniformly distribute the forces directed to the edentulous ridges, and improve masticatory performance and patient comfort (Khamis et al. 1998; Ohguri et al. 1999; Sutton and McCord 2007) (Figure 5.3). Dentists noticed, empirically, that if the artificial teeth for complete dentures were set to balanced articulation (cross-arch, cross-tooth balance, whereby all teeth contact without interferences in all eccentric

positions), there appeared to be less resorption of the edentulous ridges, and the dentures were more stable during mastication. Balanced articulation became the gold standard for complete denture occlusion.

A modified form of balanced articulation was described by Payne (1941). Payne suggested an arrangement of the artificial teeth with cross-arch balance, but not cross-tooth balance (Figures 5.4, 5.5). The term lingualized occlusion was later used to describe this method of developing an artificial occlusion (Pound 1970). This occlusal concept has become popular and is commonly advocated for implant-supported removable prosthodontics. Clinical and in vitro studies have shown that balanced lingualized occlusion can be as effective as classical balanced articulation (Khamis et al. 1998; Ohguri et al. 1999; Sutton and McCord 2007).

## Occlusal Concepts for Conventional Fixed Prosthodontics

With advances in materials and techniques in the 1930s and 1940s, it became possible to rehabilitate a natural dentition with fixed restorations. Early attempts to provide complete-mouth rehabilitation with fixed prosthodontics used occlusal concepts that were established for complete denture prosthodontics; i.e., balanced articulation was prescribed. It is understandable that dentists would attempt to mimic an occlusal scheme that was highly successful for edentulous patients. It was obvious that balanced articulation resulted in dentures that did not loosen; also, with occlusal balance, there appeared to be less bone resorption beneath the dentures. At the time, the cause of periodontal disease was obscure. The term dental plaque did not exist. Many dentists assumed that bone loss around natural teeth was the result of occlusal overload. Balancing the occlusion was assumed to be a method to uniformly distribute the forces of occlusion and avoid occlusal overload.

Developing balanced articulation with dentate patients required very sophisticated instrumentation. An articulator that could precisely mimic eccentric jaw movements (a fully adjustable instrument) was necessary, and much of the efforts of prosthodontists in the 1930s and 1 940s were directed toward developing tracing devices and articulators that could transfer a patient's 3D jaw movements to an articulator that could be adjusted to reproduce these movements.

In the late 1950s and early 1960s the concept of developing balanced articulation for fixed prosthodontics was challenged. Two primary philosophical approaches were suggested. Unilateral balance, later referred to as group function, was advocated by Schuyler (1963) (Figure 5.6). Stuart (1964) suggested eliminating all posterior tooth contacts in

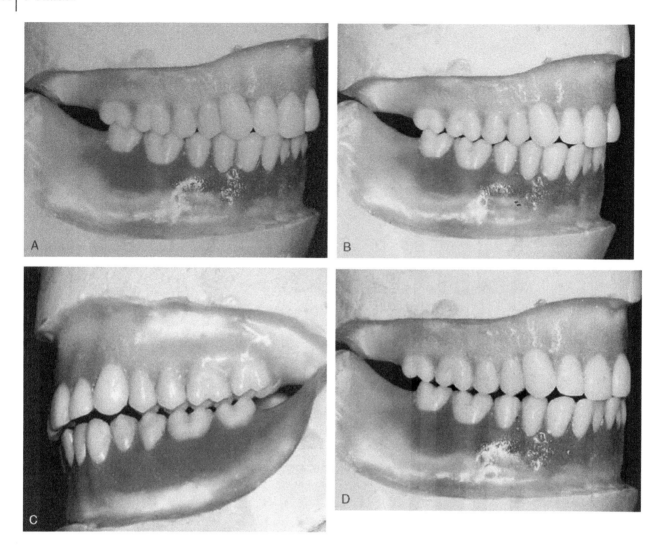

Figure 5.3    Thirty-degree anatomical teeth have been arranged in wax with balanced articulation. A, MIP; B, working side contacts; C, nonworking side (balancing-side) contacts; D, contacts in protrusion.

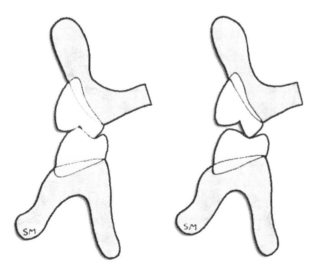

Figure 5.4    Left, classical balanced articulation; right, lingualized occlusion.

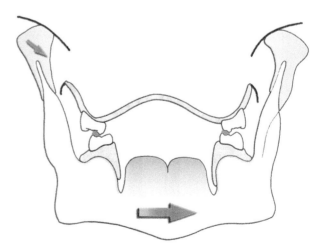

Figure 5.5    With lingualized occlusion, there is cross-arch balance but no cross-tooth balance.

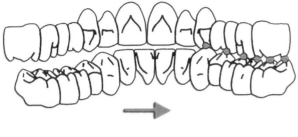

● **Working contacts**

Figure 5.6    Group function or unilateral balance.

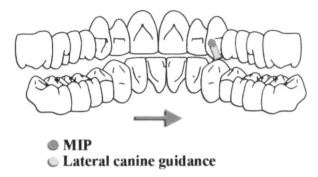

● **MIP**
○ **Lateral canine guidance**

Figure 5.7    Mutually protected occlusion with lateral canine guidance.

eccentric positions. This occlusal scheme has been described as mutually protected occlusion because the posterior teeth act as vertical stops (closure stoppers) and prevent excessive contact of the anterior teeth in MIP, and the anterior teeth disengage the posterior teeth in eccentric positions to protect the posterior teeth from lateral forces (Figure 5.7). Another term that has been used to describe this occlusal scheme is anterior disclusion (anterior teeth discluding the posterior teeth in eccentric positions). If the canine alone (without involvement of the incisors) discludes the posterior teeth in lateral eccentric positions, the mutually protected occlusal scheme is described as canine disclusion.

## Anterior Disclusion (Canine Disclusion) and Group Function

Throughout the 1960s and 1970s there was considerable controversy concerning the best eccentric occlusal scheme for a fixed prosthodontic oral rehabilitation. Group function was considered optimal by some dentists, primarily periodontists, because empirically it appeared that simultaneous contact of all teeth on the working side in a lateral occlusal position would uniformly distribute forces among all teeth. Nevertheless, most prosthodontists were advocating anterior disclusion or canine disclusion. Some periodontists felt that anterior disclusion

or canine disclusion would cause occlusal overload of the anterior teeth, trauma from occlusion, and eventual hypermobility of the anterior teeth; however, prosthodontists were commonly prescribing this occlusal arrangement with good results.

Arguments ensued for at least two decades concerning the optimal eccentric occlusal scheme, but definitive research by Gibbs and Lundeen (1982) shed new light on the physiology of mastication and quelled the arguments. Gibbs and Lundeen reported three distinct adult chewing patterns. They described these as good occlusion, malocclusion, and worn occlusion.

Patients with good occlusion had an arrangement of the dentition whereby the anterior teeth prevented contact of the posterior teeth in eccentric positions. These patients chewed with smooth, repeatable strokes. During mastication, tooth gliding contacts occurred while the mandible was entering MIP. However, these contacts occurred at the very end of the closing stroke, and they were of short duration and low magnitude when compared with the forces generated in MIP. The investigators tracked the envelope of motion or border envelope (Posselt 1952) and the envelope of function with superimposed tracings. It was clear from these tracings (Figure 5.8) that the maxillary

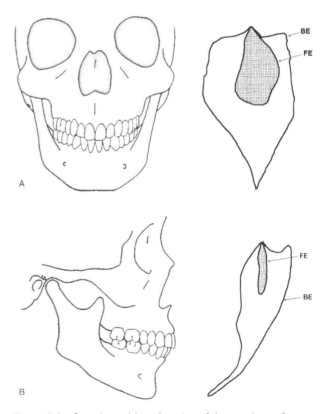

Figure 5.8    Superimposition of tracing of the envelope of motion or border envelope (BE) and functional envelope (FE) clearly demonstrated that maxillary and mandibular anterior teeth passed very close to each other during mastication, without contacting. A, frontal view; B, sagittal view.

and mandibular anterior teeth passed very close to each other during mastication, without contacting. It was the tactile sensation and tactile memory, or proprioception (Crum and Loiselle 1972) of the teeth, as governed by the periodontal ligaments, that appeared to guide the chewing strokes for these patients with good occlusion, always returning to MIP without long gliding contacts on the anterior teeth.

A different chewing stroke was observed with patients whose anterior teeth did not prevent contact of the posterior teeth in eccentric positions. These patients lacked repeatable strokes. Chewing was erratic with long, gliding contacts. This group of patients was designated as having malocclusion.

A third type of chewing stroke was observed in patients with worn occlusal and incisal surfaces. These patients lacked overlap of the anterior teeth and chewed with broad side-to-side strokes. This group was described by the investigators as having a worn occlusion.

The results of these studies by Gibbs and Lundeen confirmed the desirability of anterior disclusion or canine disclusion for the restoration of a dentition with fixed prosthodontics (Figure 5.9.) The results also refuted the contention that a patient's natural MIP must coincide with centric relation. In Gibbs and Lundeen's studies, patients always returned to the MIP during mastication because of the tactile memory and tactile sensation of the teeth. Therefore, when a patient has a normal, healthy MIP and a functional anterior guidance (vertical and horizontal overlap of the anterior teeth), the dentist should preserve this occlusal relationship when placing several crowns or a short-span fixed partial denture (FPD). If the MIP is dysfunctional and cannot be preserved because it will be destroyed with crown preparations (as with complete-mouth oral rehabilitation), or

does not exist (as with a patient edentulous in one or both jaws), centric relation would be the treatment position. It is interesting to note that Gibbs and Lundeen found only a small difference when condylar positions in MIP and centric relation were compared. The mean anterior-posterior difference was 0.13 mm and the mean superior-inferior difference was less than 0.5 mm. These findings suggest that restoring a dentition by developing an MIP coincidental with CR is physiologically sound because this position coincides very closely, but not precisely, with the condylar position of a healthy MIP.

## Splinting

With further improvements in materials and techniques in the 1960s, it became possible to accurately seat castings that were splinted together. Many prosthodontists would routinely splint crowns in series to protect the natural teeth from trauma from occlusion. Often a complete-mouth rehabilitation would be fabricated as maxillary and mandibular one-piece prostheses, each arch completely splinted together. Splinting of natural teeth is no longer advocated. Splinting makes it more difficult to fabricate the prosthesis. An occlusal interference on one splinted crown will be transmitted to all teeth and the interfering tooth cannot move away from the interference (Figure 5.10). A problem with one tooth or one crown can jeopardize the prognosis of the entire prosthesis. Complete-arch splinting is especially undesirable in the mandible because of the phenomenon of mandibular flexure (Fischman 1976) (Figure 5.11). Splinting of implant-supported crowns in series is often advocated and is discussed below.

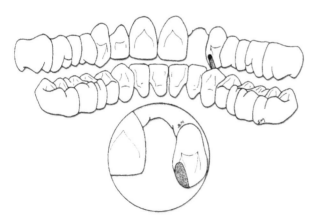

Figure 5.9 The patient will receive three-unit fixed partial denture to replace a missing lateral incisor. The canine relationship of natural teeth should be preserved in the final restoration to ensure canine disclusion.

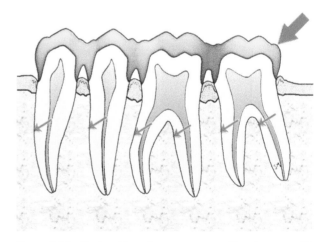

Figure 5.10 Occlusal interference on one splinted crown will be transmitted to all teeth and the interfering tooth cannot move away from the interference.

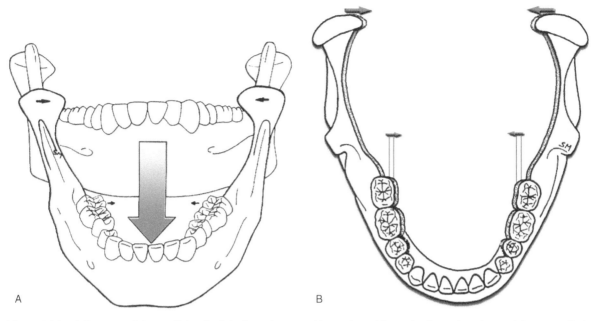

Figure 5.11 A, Because of the medial pull of the lateral pterygoid muscles, with maximal opening, the condyles are pulled medially. B, The result is flexure of the mandible and contraction of the mandibular arch. Splinting teeth from last molar to last molar in the mandible can create unfavorable stresses.

## Implant-supported Artificial Occlusion

Perceptions of occlusion vary with different dental specialties. Orthodontists are interested in moving teeth to develop an Angle Class I occlusal relationship because the maxillary and mandibular teeth tend to fit together best with this arrangement. Prosthodontists are concerned with fabricating dental prostheses in a laboratory on an articulator, and then delivering the prostheses to restore esthetics, phonetics, and function with favorable biomechanics. Traditionally, periodontists were primarily concerned with controlling trauma from occlusion in the natural dentition; however, the contemporary periodontist devotes a considerable amount of time to surgically placing dental implants. Implant dentistry is planned from the crown down; i.e., the prosthodontist or restorative dentist determines the required location and contour of the planned artificial tooth or teeth with a wax trial arrangement of an artificial tooth or teeth, and the implant is then planned to permit this required position of the tooth or teeth (Figure 5.12). To do this effectively, the periodontist must have more background related to occlusal biomechanics.

### Fixed Implant-supported Restorations

Gibbs and Lundeen's research highlighted the importance of proprioceptive input from the periodontal ligaments for fine motor control of the masticatory stroke. Because osseointe-grated implants lack a periodontal ligament, the sensation generated from occlusal contacts is completely different from the sensation experienced with natural teeth (Figure 5.13). A clinical study by Jacobs and van Steenberghe (1993) on passive tactile sensation of natural teeth and implant-supported prostheses reported a threshold that is 50 times greater with implant-supported prostheses when compared with natural teeth. This marked difference in sensation suggests that a patient could easily, and without awareness, overload an implant-supported restoration.

Careful control of biomechanics is essential to the long-term serviceability of implant-supported fixed prostheses. Poor placement can lead to biomechanical overload, which can manifest itself as chronic screw loosening, screw fracture, implant fracture, or loss of osseointegration (Figure 5.14). A retrospective study by Eckert et al. (2000) of fractured implants reported that screw loosening preceded implant fracture for the majority of the implants, suggesting that screw loosening can be a sign of occlusal overload.

When a single missing tooth is replaced with an implant-supported crown, the differences in displaceability of the natural teeth and single implant must be considered. The tooth can be displaced within its socket, but the implant is, for all practical purposes, non-displaceable (Figure 5.15). When the patient occludes lightly on a single implant-supported crown, shim stock (a Mylar strip, 8 μm in thickness) should easily pass through the occlusal surfaces of the implant-supported crown and opposing natural tooth.

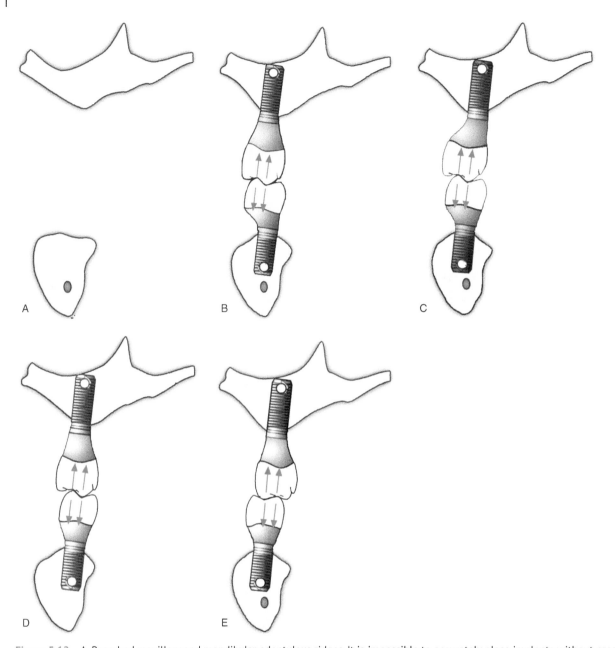

Figure 5.12   A, Resorbed maxillary and mandibular edentulous ridges. It is impossible to accurately place implants without prosthetic planning. B, Forces on the maxillary crown are compressive (favorable), but unfavorable torquing forces exist with the mandibular crown. C, Improved force distribution. D, Optimal force distribution. E, Sometimes optimal forces require a cross-bite occlusal relationship due to the pattern of bone resorption.

When the patient occludes with heavy force, the implant-supported crown should not hold the shim stock any tighter than the adjacent teeth hold a shim stock (Figure 5.16).

The method of implant support will also influence the biomechanics. A finite element analysis (Morgano and Geramy 2004) of a mandibular single molar supported by a 3.75-mm diameter implant, a 5-mm diameter implant, and two implants reported a reduction of approximately 50% in micro-motion of the crown with the 5-mm diameter implant and the double

implant support (Figure 5.17). Micro-motion is an important consideration in implant prosthodontics because it has been reported to produce various clinical problems for implant-supported crowns, including soft tissue complications (Dixon et al. 1995), bone loss (Hermann et al. 2001), and mechanical problems, such as fracture and loosening of screws (Gratton et al. 2001). A strain gauge study (Seong et al. 2000) with a similar design to the study by Morgano and Geramy reported similar results. Also, when implants are in a series, splinting them

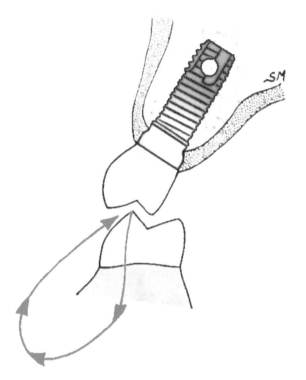

quality of life for totally edentulous patients (Awad et al. 2003). However, it is important to appreciate that implant-supported restorations are not trouble free (Goodacre et al. 2003). One important consideration is occlusal stability (Kohavi 1993). The acrylic resin teeth commonly used with conventional complete dentures tend to wear rapidly with implant-supported overdentures because of the amount of force the patient can generate. The use of porcelain artificial teeth or custom metal occlusal surfaces should be seriously considered, especially for patients with strong musculature.

With implant-supported overdentures, classical balanced articulation or balanced lingualized occlusion should be used to ensure favorable force distribution and masticatory efficiency. Lingualized occlusion has become very popular with implant-supported overdentures because of the improved lever balance. Lever balance was first described by Ortman (1977), and relates to directing the forces of occlusion over the supporting area of a complete denture, thus reducing unfavorable leverage. Because the maxillary palatal cusp is the only intercuspating cusp with lingualized occlusion, it is easier to centralize forces over the supporting implants with lingualized occlusion.

**Figure 5.13** Fine motor control of the envelope of function depends on tactile sensation and tactile memory from receptors within periodontal ligaments of teeth; however, osseointegrated implants lack a periodontal ligament.

together helps distribute forces more uniformly and improve the biomechanics (Guichet et al. 2002) (Figure 5.18).

### Implant-supported Removable Prosthodontics (Overdentures)

The application of osseointegrated implants to support and retain complete dentures has the potential to improve the

## Articulators

An articulator, which has several functions, is used when restoring a dentition. An articulator must serve as a holding instrument for the maxillary and mandibular casts and ensure a positive centric lock. It is desirable for an articulator to accept a face-bow to transfer the patient's opening and closing axis to the instrument. Adjustable condylar guidances are also important features.

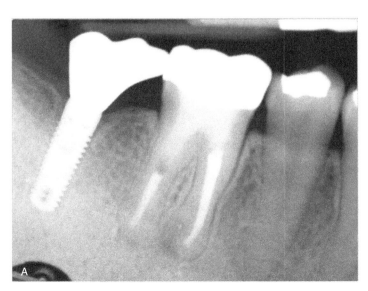
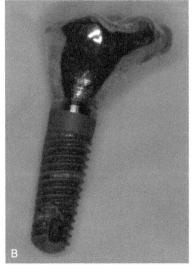

**Figure 5.14** A, The implant was placed too far distally, resulting in an artificial crown with poor biomechanics. B, The result was loss of osseointegration.

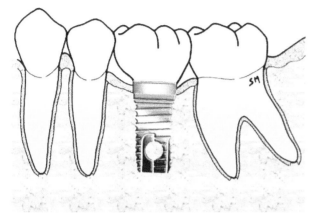

**Figure 5.15** Differences in displaceability of natural teeth, which are surrounded by periodontal ligaments, and a single implant must be considered when adjusting occlusion.

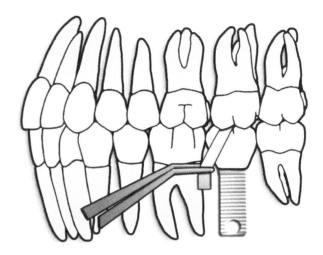

**Figure 5.16** A shim stock is used to adjust occlusion.

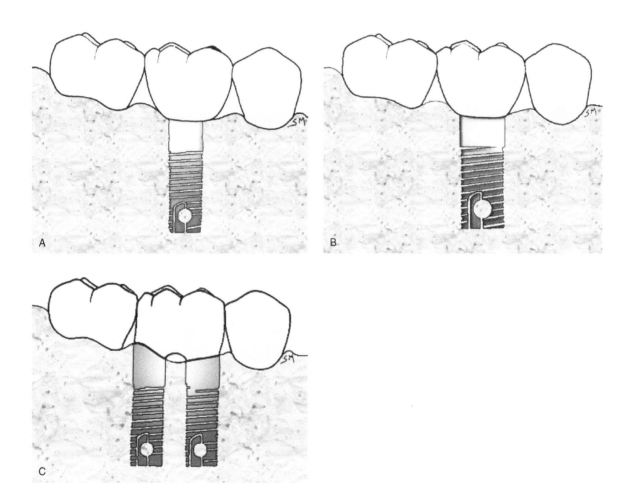

**Figure 5.17** A finite element analysis by Morgano and Geramy (2004) of a mandibular single molar supported by A, a 3.75 mm diameter implant, B, a 5-mm diameter implant, and C, two implants reported approximately 50% reduction in micromotion of the crown with the 5-mm diameter implant and the double implant design. Morgano et al., 2004 / with permission of Elsevier.

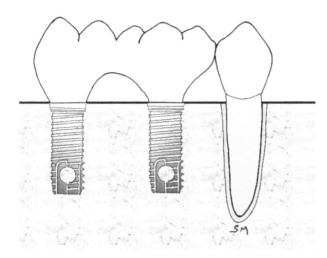

Figure 5.18   In vitro evidence suggests that splinting implants together can distribute forces more uniformly and improve biomechanics.

## Rehabilitation with Fixed Prosthodontics

Mutually protected occlusion is commonly prescribed when rehabilitating a dentition with conventional fixed prosthodontics. Because the goal of mutually protected occlusion is the disclusion of all posterior teeth in eccentric positions, this type of occlusal scheme can be achieved with the use of a semi-adjustable articulator (Lundeen 1979). A semi-adjustable articulator can be programmed for positive or negative error. If an eccentric tooth contact on the articulator is an interference in the mouth, it is described as positive error. If an eccentric tooth contact on the articulator discludes in the mouth, it is negative error (Figure 5.19).

Setting the horizontal condylar guidance below the normal range found in clinical studies will result in negative error in protrusion and in a nonworking (mediotrusive) movement because the separation of the posterior teeth on the articulator will be less than the separation that occurs in the mouth. Therefore, if the posterior teeth disclude in protrusion and nonworking movements in the articulator, they will disclude by more in the mouth.

With a working-side movement, the setting of the Bennett angle (angle of the progressive side shift) on the articulator can be used to produce negative error. The amount of progressive lateral movement is determined by the Bennett angle (the wider the Bennett angle, the greater the progressive lateral movement). Therefore, setting the Bennett angle on the articulator wider than what has been reported in clinical studies will allow the articulator to move laterally a greater amount than can occur in the mouth. As a consequence, posterior teeth on the working side will disclude in the mouth with a separation greater than what occurred on the articulator.

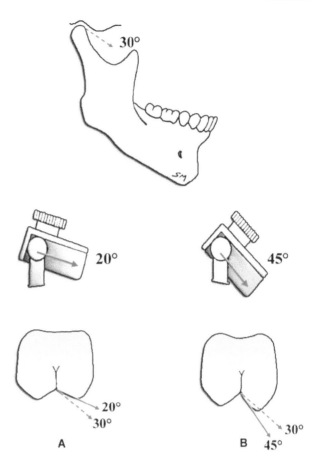

Figure 5.19   An articulator can be programmed for negative or positive error. A patient's natural condylar guidance is 30 degrees (dotted line). A, The articulator has been set with a 20-degree condylar inclination. What contacted on the articulator (solid line) missed in mouth (dotted line) – negative error. B, The articulator has been set with a 45-degree condylar inclination. What contacted on the articulator (solid line) became interference in the mouth (dotted line) – positive error.

The range of the protrusive angle has been reported as 25–65 degrees, and the Bennett angle has been reported as 7–8 degrees (Lundeen 1979; Lundeen and Wirth 1973). If a semi-adjustable articulator is set with a protrusive angle of 20 degrees and a Bennett angle of 1 5 degrees, it will be programmed for negative error (Figure 5.20).

## Rehabilitation with Complete Dentures

With complete denture prosthodontics, balanced articulation is desired, whereby the posterior teeth contact simultaneously in the right and left lateral occlusal positions and in protrusion. Harmonious eccentric occlusal contacts firmly seat the denture(s) and distribute the occlusal load, promoting denture stability and masticatory efficiency (Figure 5.21). Because posterior eccentric contacts are desirable, the concept of negative error cannot be used. A

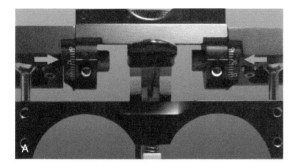

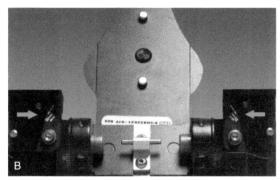

Figure 5.20  If a semi-adjustable articulator is set with A, a protrusive angle of 20 degrees and B, a Bennett angle of 15 degrees, it will be programmed for negative error, ensuring anterior disclusion.

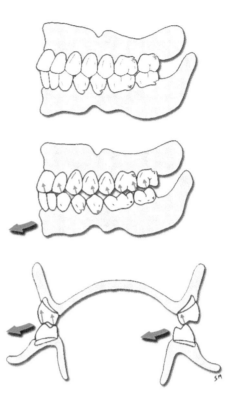

Figure 5.21  Balanced articulation firmly seats the dentures and distributes the occlusal load, promoting denture stability and masticatory efficiency.

protrusive record is made to set the protrusive angle on the articulator. Lateral check records can be made to set the Bennett angles; however, the variability in the Bennett angles of edentulous patients is very small. Langer and Michman (1970) reported that the Bennett angle for edentulous patients was approximately twice the values reported for dentate patients ±2 degrees. Therefore, commonly, the Bennett angle is set arbitrarily at 15 degrees for edentulous patients.

## Authors' Views/Comments

Early principles of occlusion were empiric concepts designed for complete dentures that were almost entirely mechanical. Centric relation was used as the treatment position for the MIP of the dentures, and the occlusion was designed with eccentric balance. This balanced arrangement of the teeth was used to promote denture stability and uniformly distribute forces. Dentists learned that a single interceptive occlusal contact could disturb the position of the denture bases on the mucosa, thus promoting instability, poor retention, tissue trauma, soreness, and accelerated bone resorption. Several clinical studies have reported improved performance with complete dentures when classical balanced articulation or lingualized occlusion was used.

Attempts to apply this mechanical approach to complete mouth rehabilitation with fixed prosthodontics were unsuccessful. The concepts of occlusion for fixed prosthodontics gradually moved from a mechanical approach to a biomechanical approach. Current scientific knowledge suggests that mutually protected occlusion is a biomechanically sound approach to designing the occlusal scheme for a fixed prosthodontic rehabilitation. With a complete-mouth rehabilitation, the MIP will be destroyed because of the tooth preparations, so the treatment position for the newly created MIP would be centric relation.

There is no evidence to suggest that a stable, healthy MIP that does not coincide with centric relation should be altered. Most patients have a slight discrepancy between the condylar positions when the condyle is in centric relation and when the teeth are in MIP. Simple restorations that involve a few teeth should be made to harmonize with the existing MIP.

The masticatory function of natural teeth depends on feedback from the receptors in the periodontal ligaments of the teeth. Because implants are not surrounded by periodontal ligaments, the sensation from implants is different from that of natural teeth. The dentist must be cognizant of this difference in the sensation when designing the occlusal scheme for implants. Steep vertical overlap of natural anterior teeth is considered desirable because the receptors in the periodontal ligaments of the anterior teeth

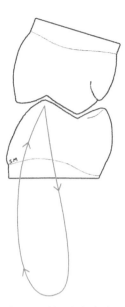

will guide the mandible through the 3D space with a relatively vertical chewing stroke. This vertical stroke helps to protect the posterior teeth from lateral forces (mutually protected occlusion) (Figure 5.22). Because implant-supported anterior crowns lack periodontal ligaments, the sensation is also lacking. Steep anterior vertical overlap is likely to cause chipping of porcelain. An implant-supported fixed rehabilitation should be developed with very shallow anterior guidance, shallow cusps, and narrowed occlusal tables (for improved lever balance). Group function occlusion is also an option. A functionally generated path recording can be used to develop group function with the use of a semi-adjustable articulator (Meyer 1959).

The occlusion for implant-supported overdentures should mimic the occlusion for conventional complete dentures—either classic balanced articulation or balanced lingualized occlusion. Special attention should be directed toward ensuring occlusal stability by preventing excessive wear of the occlusal surfaces of the posterior teeth (Figure 5.23).

**Figure 5.22** Relatively steep overlap of the anterior teeth (anterior guidance) produces a vertical chewing stroke, protecting posterior teeth from lateral forces.

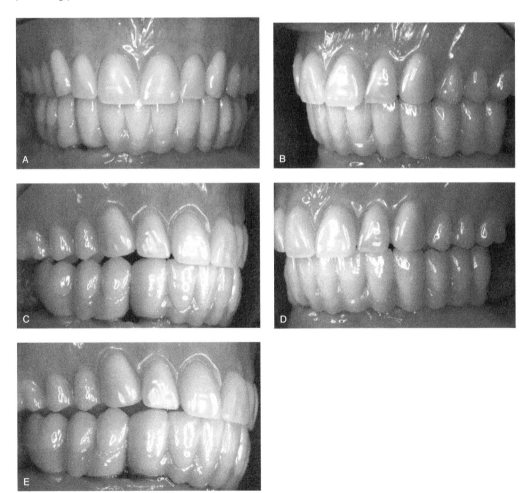

**Figure 5.23** Maxillary implant-supported overdenture that occludes with mandibular implant-supported fixed prostheses. Lingualized occlusion has been used, with porcelain posterior artificial teeth in overdenture and porcelain occlusal surfaces on mandibular metal-ceramic fixed partial dentures. A and B, MIP; C, right nonworking; D, left working (note the lack of contact of buccal cusps); E, protrusion. Courtesy of Dr. Dmitri Svirsky, Toronto, Ontario, Canada.

# References

Academy of Prosthodontics (1987). Glossary of prosthodontic terms, 5th ed. *J. Prosthet. Dent.* 58: 725.

Awad, M.A., Lund, J.P., Shapiro, S.H. et al. (2003). Oral health status and treatment satisfaction with mandibular implant overdentures and conventional dentures: a randomized clinical trial in a senior population. *Int. J. Prosthodont.* 16: 390–396.

Crum, R.J. and Loiselle, R.J. (1972). Oral perception and proprioception: a review of the literature and its significance to prosthodontics. *J. Prosthet. Dent.* 28: 215–230.

Dixon, D.L., Breeding, L.C., Sadler, J.P., and McKay, M.L. (1995). Comparison of screw loosening, rotation, and deflection among three implant designs. *J. Prosthet. Dent.* 74: 270–278.

Eckert, S.E., Meraw, S.J., Cal, E., and Ow, R.K. (2000). Analysis of incidence and associated factors with fractured implants: a retrospective study. *Int. J. Oral Maxillofac. Implants.* 15: 662–667.

Fischman, B.M. (1976). The influence of fixed splints on mandibular flexure. *J. Prosthet. Dent.* 35: 643–647.

Gibbs, C.H. and Lundeen, H.L. (1982). Jaw movements and forces during chewing and swallowing and their clinical significance. In: *Advances in Occlusion*, (ed. C.H. Gibbs and H.L. Lundeen), 2–50. Boston: John Wright PSG, Inc.

Goodacre, C.J., Guillermo, B., Rungcharassaeng, K., and Kan, J.Y.K. (2003). Clinical complications with implants and implant prostheses. *J. Prosthet. Dent.* 90: 121–132.

Goymerac, B. and Woolard, G. (2004). Focal infection: a new perspective on an old theory. *Gen. Dent.* 52: 357–361.

Gratton, D.G., Aquilino, S.A., and Stanford, C.M. (2001). Micro-motion and dynamic fatigue properties of the dental-1 implant interface. *J. Prosthet. Dent.* 85: 47–52.

Guichet, D.L., Yoshinobu, D., and Caputo, A.A. (2002). Effect of splinting and interproximal contact tightness on load transfer by implant restorations. *J. Prosthet. Dent.* 87: 528–535.

Hanau, R.H. (1929). Occlusal changes in centric relation. *J. Am. Dent. Assoc.* 16: 1903–1915.

Hermann, J.S., Schoolfield, J.D., Schenk, R.K. et al. (2001). Influence of the size of the microgap on crestal bone changes around titanium implants. A histometric evaluation of unloaded nonsubmerged implants in the canine mandible. *J. Periodontol.* 72: 1372–1383.

Jacobs, R. and van Steenberghe, D. (1993). Comparison between implant-supported prostheses and teeth regarding passive threshold level. *Int. J. Oral Maxillofac. Implants.* 8: 549–554.

Khamis, M.M., Zaki, H.S., and Rudy, T.E. (1998). A comparison of the effect of different occlusal forms in mandibular implant overdentures. *J. Prosthet. Dent.* 79: 422–429.

Kohavi, D. (1993). Complications in the tissue integrated prostheses components: clinical and mechanical evaluation. *J. Oral. Rehabil.* 20: 413–422.

Langer, A. and Michman, J. (1970). Evaluation of lateral tracings of edentulous subjects. *J. Prosthet. Dent.* 23: 381–386.

Lundeen, H.C. (1979). Mandibular movement recordings and articulator adjustments simplified. *Dent. Clin. North Am.* 23: 231–241.

Lundeen, H.C. and Wirth, C.G. (1973). Condylar movement patterns engraved in plastic blocks. *J. Prosthet. Dent.* 30: 866–875.

McDevitt, W.E., Brady, A.P., Stack, J.P., and Hobdell, M.H. (1995). A magnetic resonance imaging study of centric maxillomandibular relation. *Int. J. Prosthodont.* 8: 377–391.

Meyer, F.S. (1959). The generated path technique in reconstruction dentistry. Part II. Fixed partial dentures. *J. Prosthet. Dent.* 9: 432–440.

Morgano, S.M. and Geramy, A. (2004). Finite element analysis of three designs of an implant-supported molar crown. *J. Prosthet. Dent.* 92: 434–440.

Niswonger, M.F. (1934). The rest position of the mandible and centric relation. *J. Am. Dent. Assoc.* 21: 1572–1582.

Ohguri, T., Kawano, F., Chikawa, T., and Matsumoto, N. (1999). Influence of occlusal scheme on the pressure distribution under a complete denture. *Int. J. Prosthodont.* 12: 353–358.

Ortman, H.R. (1977). Complete denture occlusion. *Dent. Clin. North. Am.* 21: 299–320.

Payne, S.H. (1941). A posterior set-up to meet individual requirements. *Dent. Digest.* 47: 20–22.

Posselt, U. (1952). Studies in the mobility of the human mandible. *Acta Odont. Scandinav.* 10 (19–160, Suppl. 10).

Pound, E. (1970). Utilizing speech to simplify a personalized denture service. *J. Prosthet. Dent.* 24: 586–600.

Schuyler, C.H. (1963). The function and importance of incisal guidance in oral rehabilitation. *J. Prosthet. Dent.* 13: 1011–1029.

Seong, W.J., Korioth, T.W., and Hodges, J.S. (2000). Experimentally induced abutment strains in three types of single-molar implant restorations. *J. Prosthet. Dent.* 84: 318–326.

Stuart, C.E. (1964). Good occlusion for natural teeth. *J. Prosthet. Dent.* 14: 716–724.

Sutton, A.F. and McCord, J.F. (2007). A randomized clinical trial comparing anatomic, lingualized, and zero-degree posterior occlusal forms for complete dentures. *J. Prosthet. Dent.* 97: 292–298.

Thompson, J.R. (1946). The rest position of the mandible and its significance to dental science. *J. Am. Dent. Assoc.* 33: 151–180.

6

# Systemic and Local Drug Delivery of Antimicrobials

*Dimitra Sakellari*

## Introduction

The recognition of the importance of bacteria as etiologic agents of periodontal disease and the seminal studies of previous decades which identified key pathogens have led to numerous investigations into the role of antibiotics in periodontal treatment. Unfortunately, due to differences of these studies in design, duration, antibiotic class and dosage, concomitant mechanical treatment, and disease classification, the extrapolation of concise conclusions is not easy, as several authors in the field have noted. In addition, during the last two decades, advances in laboratory technology have provided new insight about the structure and properties of the subgingival biofilm and its resistance to antimicrobials and raised questions about their efficacy. The abovementioned parameters combined with the emerging global threat of antimicrobial resistance and the well-known side effects or adverse reactions during antibiotic administration have developed a trend among clinicians for more cautious prescription of this class of drugs.

Knowledge of the disadvantages of systematic administration of antibiotics and difficulties in patient compliance (especially in long-term regimens) have also prompted researchers to develop several local delivery systems in periodontology, i.e., antimicrobial agents embodied in excipients for direct placement and action in periodontal pockets. Due to advanced material technology, a number of such products are available for clinicians and several studies have evaluated their effects on periodontal conditions.

This chapter focuses on evidence-based systemic and local administration of antibiotics in periodontology and provides guidelines for their indications, according to current evidence and documentation.

## Evidence-based Outcomes

Historically, clinical studies regarding the benefits of the systematic administration of antimicrobials in periodontology began in the late 1970s and initially referred to patients with localized juvenile periodontitis (LJP), a disease which partially coincides with localized aggressive periodontitis. In the classical studies of the 1980s and 1990s, both in the US and Scandinavia, it has been shown that in LJP patients, systemic administration of antibiotics such as the tetracyclines can improve clinical parameters and decrease the pathogenic subgingival microflora, especially *Aggregatibacter (Actinobacillus) actinomycetemcomitans* (Saxen and Asikainen 1993; Saxen et al. 1990; Slots and Rosling 1983). The efficiency of the combined systemic administration of metronidazole and amoxicillin in LJP patients was investigated by Van Winkelhoff et al. (1989), who have shown an improvement of clinical parameters and elimination of *A. actinomycetemcomitans* for at least nine months and therefore introduced this regimen in other classes of periodontal diseases.

After years of including antimicrobials in clinical practice, current major issues of concern among clinicians include the following: Can antibiotics be considered as a sole therapy for periodontal diseases? Are there adjunctive benefits to conventional mechanical treatment or periodontal surgery? Can antibiotics enhance periodontal regeneration or treat acute periodontal conditions and peri-implantitis? In this section, we review current evidence which should guide clinicians to indications and methods of delivery.

The issue of using antibiotics as monotherapy to treat periodontal disease has been addressed in several studies. Current data regarding biofilm structure and resistance to antimicrobials show that subgingival biofilms can be more effectively controlled when they are mechanically disrupted. When their dense structure has been altered and the huge number of bacteria diminished, the antimicrobials have the potential to better diffuse and eliminate the microbial target (Socransky and Haffajee 2002). In addition, antimicrobial activity has been shown to be more effective in "young" and not well-organized biofilms. In the Sixth European Workshop on Periodontology, in 2008, Herrera and coworkers addressed the question of whether systemic antimicrobials can be efficacious if the biofilm is not disrupted. The authors reviewed the existing literature and concluded, in agreement with previous position papers and systematic reviews (AAP 1996; Haffajee et al. 2003; Herrera et al. 2002), that clinicians should not consider antibiotics as a sole therapy for periodontal diseases and that antibiotics should be combined with mechanical means of disrupting or removing biofilms in gingival sulci and pockets. Therefore, currently, clinicians should act based on good medical practice and administer systemic antibiotics as adjuncts rather than as the main and sole therapy. The cornerstone of effective periodontal therapy should include meticulous mechanical therapy by a highly skilled operator, patient compliance (oral hygiene and smoking cessation), and effective control of systemic diseases such as diabetes.

As mentioned above, although numerous studies have tested the role of systematic administration of antimicrobials in patients with periodontitis, several discrepancies among them preclude the comparison and classification of their results and the extrapolation of guidelines. Today, scientifically sound clinical studies should be designed as randomized clinical trials (RCTs) with the inclusion of controls, a duration of at least six months, and in accordance with strictly defined criteria and statistical analysis as described in the Consolidated Standards for Reporting Trials (CONSORT) statement (Altman et al. 2001). Therefore, clinicians are encouraged to thoroughly examine the design of scientific trials on antibiotics before considering their conclusions. The most recent relevant report of the European Federation of Periodontology (Teughels et al. 2020) has addressed the following question: which is the efficacy of adjunctive systemic antimicrobials, in patients with periodontitis, compared to subgingival debridement plus a placebo, regarding probing pocket depth (PPD) reduction in RCTs with at least 6 months duration? In this report, data from 34 articles which strictly fulfilled criteria for inclusion were pooled and analyzed. According to the most recent classification of periodontal diseases (2018), the clinical entities chronic and aggressive periodontitis are no longer valid. However, a number of previous conducted studies are based on the previous classification. Data referring to aggressive periodontitis cases correspond to Stages III/IV and Grade C periodontitis and have been incorporated to the meta-analysis accordingly.

For PPD, statistically significant benefits ($p < 0.001$) from adjunctive systemic antibiotics were observed in short-term studies (Weighted Mean Differences = 0.448 mm, 95% Confidence Intervals [0.324; 0.573], Prediction Intervals [−0.10 to 0.99]) and long-term studies (WMD = 0.485 mm, 95% CI [0.322; 0.648], PI [−0.11 to 1.08]). Additionally, statistically significant benefits were also found for clinical attachment level, bleeding on probing, pocket closure, and frequency of residual pockets (Teughels et al. 2020).

In specific, the administration of the combination of amoxicillin plus metronidazole as an adjunct to scaling and root planing (SRP) results in statistically significant greater reduction of PPD, reduction in frequency of pockets of > 4, 5, 6, and 7 mm and bleeding on probing, higher percentage of pocket closure and higher CAL gain. The additional PPD reduction and CAL gain elicited by the combination of metronidazole and amoxicillin and to a lesser extent by metronidazole alone and azithromycin are more pronounced in initially deep than in initially moderately deep pockets and these clinical effects are maintained up to 12 months after their administration. Currently, there is no evidence for the benefits of systemic antimicrobials as adjuncts to SRP, above 2 years of follow-up and no indications that these effects are different between the former aggressive and chronic periodontitis. Metronidazole alone and azithromycin result in clinical benefits but of a smaller magnitude compared to the combination of metronidazole and amoxicillin (Teughels et al. 2020).

It should be noted that although statistically significant clinical benefits were observed in patients who received systemic antimicrobials, adverse events were more frequently reported in these groups, with the group administered the combination of metronidazole and amoxicillin exhibiting the largest frequency of side effects.

During the last years, the tetracyclines are no longer popular as adjuncts of periodontal therapy. One of the main reasons is that bactericidal and not bacteriostatic antimicrobials have been proven to be effective against periodontal pathogens, especially in the biofilm structure and density of microbial populations. In addition, the phenomenon of antimicrobial resistance to this class of antimicrobials is widespread due to overuse or misuse not only for medical purposes in humans, but also in veterinary medicine, agriculture, livestock, and fishing farms.

In fact, the global emergence of specific-drug resistant and multidrug-resistant species (among them periodontal pathogens) and the possible contribution of clinical dentistry to this serious health and socioeconomic problem should be taken into consideration before prescribing systemic antimicrobials for periodontal therapy. It has been noted that populations with higher consumption of antimicrobials in Europe exhibit higher percentages of resistant periodontal pathogens or carriage of antimicrobial resistance genes in the oral cavity (Koukos et al. 2016; Van Winkelhoff et al. 2005). The 2020 report of the EFP highlights the issue of contribution to antimicrobial resistance among the possible adverse effects from excessive prescribing of systemic antimicrobials for periodontal therapy, despite favorable clinical outcomes and encourages clinicians for antibiotic stewardship (Teughels et al. 2020).

The results of clinical studies concerning the systematic administration of antimicrobials in combination with periodontal surgery to eliminate the pockets or to achieve periodontal regeneration are contradictory. It is known that antimicrobials can be useful for preventing postsurgical complications. In this case, antibiotic coverage usually targets bacteria that can cause transfections, although for periodontal surgery there are no studies confirming the necessity of antimicrobial administration. It is suggested that sterile conditions and antiseptic mouthwashes can be efficient in preventing complications (Newman and van Winkelhoff 2001).

Findings concerning the clinical benefits of the combined use of antimicrobials with surgical periodontal treatment are controversial. Based on the limited data in the literature, both the Haffajee et al. (2003) and Herrera et al. (2008) reports suggest marginal or insufficient evidence for additional clinical benefits from periodontal surgery when combined with systemic antimicrobials.

The combination of guided tissue regeneration (GTR) with the administration of several antimicrobial regimens also does not appear to uniformly offer stable beneficial clinical outcomes, neither to efficiently prevent bacterial colonization nor to prevent complications (Demolon et al. 1993; Loos et al. 2002; Vest et al. 1999; Zucchelli et al., 1999). The relevant report of the Sixth European Workshop states that there is no sufficient evidence to support the administration of antibiotics during regenerative procedures.

At this point, it should be emphasized, the microflora of patients with deep periodontal pockets, especially after the repeated administration of antimicrobials, can include nonoral Gram-negative species such as enteric rods and *Pseudomonas* spp., where the administration of other classes of antimicrobials such as the quinolones are indicated (Rams et al. 1992; Slots et al. 1990). In this group of patients the administration of a combination of metronidazole and ciprofloxacin appears to provide additional clinical improvement.

Antimicrobials also have been administrated for acute inflammatory conditions of the periodontal tissues, such as periodontal abscess, necrotizing gingivitis (NG) or periodontitis (NP), and peri-implantitis.

In the previous century, antiseptics were used for the treatment of NG, while in the 1960s it was confirmed that the systematic administration of penicillin or metronidazole could contribute to the management of the acute phase of inflammation, especially when systemic manifestations such as fever, malaise, and lymphadenitis are present (Collins 1970; Fletcher and Plant 1966). Clinical cases without these symptoms can be adequately managed with no antimicrobials (Holmstrup and Westergaard 2003).

The frequent occurrence of NG in patients who are HIV positive raised the question about the necessity of administration of antimicrobials in this patient category. According to the latest findings there is no need for antimicrobial coverage of this group if generalized symptoms are absent. In addition, the possibility of *Candida* spp. infection as a side effect of systemic antimicrobial administration suggests that antibiotics should be prescribed with caution and after consulting the physician.

There is insufficient or contradictory evidence in the literature to document the necessity of antimicrobial administration for treatment of acute periodontal abscess. Existing studies are usually case reports and there are no comparative studies that demonstrate adjunctive benefits from systemic antimicrobials. Generally, in the case of acute periodontal abscess, antimicrobials are considered necessary when the abscess is very extended, diffused, and accompanied by intense pain and/or coexisting compromising medical conditions and systemic manifestations. The combination of drainage with systemic administration of penicillin, hydrochloric tetracycline, or metronidazole was found efficient for the management of the acute conditions, while the combination of amoxicillin/clavulanic and the newer macrolide azithromycin resulted in recovery from acute symptoms without the simultaneous initial drainage of the abscess (Genco 1991; Herrera et al. 2000a; Palmer 1984; Smith and Davies 1986). In any event, according to good medical practice, the initial drainage or surgical fission of the periodontal abscess is considered the necessary first step for managing its acute phase (AAP 2000; Herrera et al. 2000b).

Limited documentation also exists about the effectiveness of antimicrobials in peri-implantitis, an infection in which there are no established treatment protocols. Existing data from animal and human studies are suggestive of a positive contribution of the systemic or local administration of antimicrobials, especially nitroimidazoles or the combination of amoxicillin and metronidazole, but the effectiveness of adjunctive antimicrobial therapy remains debatable (Javed et al. 2013; Mombelli 2002; Mombelli and Lang 1998; Renvert et al. 2008).

In addition, there is insufficient scientific documentation about administering antimicrobials to prevent complications during dental implant surgery. Two relative studies present controversial results. The Swedish study questions the need for antimicrobial use to prevent postsurgical complications (Gynther et al. 1998), while the American study indicates that the administration of antimicrobials is related to lower percentages of implant failures (Laskin et al. 2000). Nevertheless, because there are no RCTs on this issue, in everyday practice, clinicians usually prescribe antibiotics for implant placement based on the possibility of a complication and less on scientific documentation.

It should be pointed out that the abovementioned data refer to systemically healthy individuals, whereas the approach for medically compromised subjects is modified. In addition, certain medical conditions require antimicrobial prophylaxis for all periodontal procedures, as will be described in the indications and protocols section below.

Data in the literature regarding evidence-based outcomes of local delivery systems in periodontology are more limited and include several studies and a few systematic reviews. Most of the existing systems (fibers, chips, gels, and microspheres) were originally tested in split-mouth models as monotherapy and compared to scaling and root-planing or no treatment and then as adjuncts to mechanical treatment, mainly in "chronic" periodontitis patients. These systems were usually applied at the initial treatment phase or in treated sites with poor response or recurrent disease activity during supportive treatment (Bonito et al. 2005; Hanes and Purvis 2003; Matesanz-Pérez et al. 2013; Smiley et al. 2015).

The most recent systematic review and meta-analysis for the European Federation of Periodontology (Herrera et al. 2020) has addressed the following question: which is the efficacy of adjunctive locally delivered antimicrobials, in adult patients with periodontitis, in comparison with subgingival debridement alone or plus a placebo, regarding probing pocket depth (PPD) reduction, in RCTs with at least 6 months

duration ? In this report, data from 59 articles which fulfilled criteria for inclusion were included. For PPD, statistically significant differences were observed in 6–9 month studies (Weighted Mean Differences = 0.365 mm, 95% Confidence Intervals [0.262; 0.468], Prediction Intervals [−0.29 to 1.01]). Significant differences for PPD but not for CAL were also observed in long-term studies. No increase in adverse side effects was reported.

Albeit the statistical differences regarding PPD reduction reported from the use of locally delivered subgingival antimicrobials, as pointed out by the authors, significant heterogeneity was observed in most of the studies, since they combined different products with different active agents, and results may also be influenced by the study design (for example split-mouth studies or partial-mouth assessments). Therefore, the clinical value of these effects and the cost–benefit of local delivery systems and the precise indications of their applications have not yet been clearly established (Herrera et al. 2020).

## Indications and Protocols

The indications for prescribing systemic antibiotics in periodontology are listed in Table 6.1 and are guided by combining current data and evidence in the literature and the current trend in the medical community to limit antibiotic use under the global threat of antimicrobial resistance. Clinicians are encouraged to constantly review the literature for updated information on this important aspect of periodontal therapy.

For all periodontal procedures in medically compromised individuals, clinicians should carefully review the subject's medical history and consult with the physician. Specific medical conditions require antibiotic prophylaxis and practitioners should comply with revised, periodically issued guidelines from scientific societies. The British Society for Antimicrobial Chemotherapy (2006) and the American Heart Association (2007) and the European Society of Cardiology (2009) have revised their guidelines for antimicrobial chemoprophylaxis during dental procedures after carefully reviewing evidence

Table 6.1 Evidence-based indications for systemic antibiotics in periodontology.

| | |
|---|---|
| Periodontitis | The adjunctive use of systemic antibiotics may be considered for specific patient groups (e.g., generalized periodontitis Stage III in young adults) |
| Acute periodontal abscess | When generalized symptoms are present |
| Necrotizing gingivitis | When generalized symptoms are present |
| Necrotizing periodontitis | Yes |
| Peri-implantitis | Documentation not clear |

about the correlation of dental procedures with infective endocarditis (Gould et al. 2006; Habib et al.,2009; Wilson et al. 2007). These scientific societies have limited the cardiological conditions requiring chemoprophylaxis and emphasize the need for oral hygiene and healthy periodontal tissues in order to minimize the risk for infective endocarditis-causing bacteremia from daily routine activities such as tooth brushing and chewing. These indications, the dental procedures, and the recommended regimens are presented in Tables 6.2 and 6.3.

The antibiotic regimens usually prescribed in periodontology for indications listed above are presented in Table 6.4.

**Table 6.2** Dental procedures and cardiac conditions for which antibiotic prophylaxis is required. Wilson et al., 2007 / American Heart Association.

| Dental procedures for which endocarditis prophylaxis is recommended for patients | Cardiac conditions associated with the highest risk of adverse outcome from endocarditis for which prophylaxis with dental procedures is recommended |
| --- | --- |
| All dental procedures that involve manipulation of gingival tissue or the periapical region of teeth or perforation of the oral mucosa.[*] | • Prosthetic cardiac valve<br>• Previous infective endocarditis<br>• Congenital heart disease (CHD)[†]<br>• Unrepaired cyanotic CHD, including palliative shunts and conduits<br>• Completely repaired congenital heart defect with prosthetic material or device, whether placed by surgery or by catheter intervention, during the first six months after the procedure[‡]<br>• Repaired CHD with residual defects at the site or adjacent to the site of a prosthetic patch or prosthetic device (which inhibits endothelialization)<br>• Cardiac transplantation recipients who develop cardiac valvulopathy |

[*] The following procedures and events do not need prophylaxis: routine anaesthetic injections through noninfected tissue, taking dental radiographs, placement of removable prosthodontic or orthodontic appliances, adjustment of orthodontic appliances, placement of orthodontic brackets, shedding of primary teeth, and bleeding from trauma to the lips or oral mucosa.

[†] Except for the conditions listed above, antibiotic prophylaxis is no longer recommended for any other form of CHD.

[‡] Prophylaxis is recommended because endothelialization of prosthetic material occurs within six months after the procedure. Wilson W, Taubert KA, Gewitz M, and colleagues. Prevention of infective endocarditis: Guidelines from the American Heart Association. *JADA* 2007; 138 (6): 739–60.

**Table 6.3** Regimens for a dental procedure. Wilson et al., 2007 / American Heart Association.

| Situation | Agent | Regimen: Single dose 30 to 60 minutes before procedure | |
| --- | --- | --- | --- |
| | | Adults | Children |
| Oral | Amoxicillin | 2 g | 50 mg/kg |
| Unable to take oral medication | Ampicillin<br>OR | 2 g IM[*] or IV[†] | 50 mg/kg IM or IV |
| | cefazolin or ceftriaxone | 1 g IM or IV | 50 mg/kg IM or IV |
| Allergic to penicillins or ampicillin oral | Cephalexin[‡§]<br>OR | 2 g | 50 mg/kg |
| | clindamycin<br>OR | 600 mg | 20 mg/kg |
| | azithromycin or clarithromycin | 500 mg | 15 mg/kg |
| Allergic to penicillins or ampicillin and unable to take | Cefazolin or ceftriaxone OR | 1 g IM or IV | 50 mg/kg IM or IV |
| oral medication | Cephalexin[‡§] | 600 mg IM or IV | 20 mg/kg IM or IV |

[*] IM: Intramuscular.

[†] IV: Intravenous.

[‡] Or other first- or second-generation oral cephalosporin in equivalent adult or pediatric dosage.

[§] Cephalosporins should not be used in a person with a history of anaphylaxis, angioedema, or urticaria with penicillins or ampicillin.
Wilson W, Taubert KA, Gewitz M, and colleagues. Prevention of infective endocarditis: Guidelines from the American Heart Association. *JADA* 2007; 138 (6): 739–60.

Table 6.4 Antibiotic regimens for periodontal conditions (when indicated).

**A. Periodontitis**

| Antimicrobial | Dosage |
| --- | --- |
| Metronidazole | 500 mgr/8 hours for 7 days |
| Tetracycline | 250 mgr/6 hours for 21 days |
| Doxycycline | 200 mgr the first day 100 mgr/24 hours for 21 days |
| Minocycline | 200 mgr the first day 100 mgr/24 hours for 21 days |
| Clindamycin | 100 mgr/12 hours for 21 days |
| Azithromycin | 500 mgr 1–3 /day, for 3–5 days |
| Metronidazole and amoxicillin | 500 mgr each/8 hours for 7 days |

**B. Periodontal abscess (a), necrotic gingivitis (b), peri-implantitis (c)**

| Antimicrobial | Dosage |
| --- | --- |
| Metronidazole (a, b, c) | 500 mgr/8 hours for 7 days |
| Amoxicillin (a) | 500 mgr/6 hours for 7 days |
| Amoxicillin and clavulanic acid (a) | 625 mgr/12 hours for 7 days |
| Clarithromycin (a) | 250 mgr/12 hours for 7 days |
| Metronidazole and amoxicillin (c) | 500 mgr each/8 hours for 7 days |

It should be noted that differences exist between various countries, according to the manufacturing company. Regarding local delivery systems, the main indication currently remains residual or recurrent pockets during supportive periodontal therapy, according to existing data in the literature and clinicians should be aware of advantages of their use as presented in Table 6.5.

Other factors to be considered by clinicians when choosing a local delivery system include the antimicrobial agent that it contains, the initial concentration and pharmacokinetics of this agent in the periodontal pocket environment, and the form, structure, and chemical properties of the excipient which regulate the time and rate of delivery of the antimicrobial (Goodson 1996). It must be remembered that the initial efforts to deliver antimicrobials by subgingival irrigations (Rams and Slots 1996) had limited clinical results, while the incorporation of antimicrobial substances in polymers ensured a more stable rate of diffusion and release and therefore a more predictable presence of active concentration of the antimicrobials for efficient time in the subgingival environment. The anatomy of the pocket region and the restriction of antimicrobial activity in a confined

Table 6.5 Advantages of local delivery antimicrobial systems.

Release rate of antimicrobials that ensures therapeutic results

Reduction of toxicity and side effects of systematic delivery

Difficulty in antimicrobial agent decomposition

Patient compliance

(Possibly) lower cost and lower waste of antimicrobials

area of the body are favorable for these systems but the continuous flow of the gingival crevicular fluid is a major challenge to be overcome by the biomaterials technology and, more recently, nanotechnology (Goodson 2003).

The most widely known local delivery systems are presented in Table 6.6. Tetracycline fibers, the only system with zero order kinetics and thus with stable concentration of the antibiotic for the 10 days that they remain in the pocket environment, are not currently available on the market and they are the only system that requires physical removal of the system, since they are nondegradable. All of the other systems listed in the table are degradable and user-friendly because they are applied subgingivally either with a blunt needle that is provided or with a blunt instrument in the case of chips.

## Author's Views/Comments

Therapeutic planning in contemporary periodontology should be driven by scientific evidence. The use of antibiotics, especially systemic ones, has been a matter of debate and contradictory findings for several years. Clinicians should be aware that currently only results from well-organized randomized clinical trials should be taken into consideration. Periodically issued systematic reviews and meta-analyses provide data and guidelines useful for clinical practice. The current trend in the medical and dental community to confine the use of antimicrobial agents should also apply to contemporary periodontology

Table 6.6 Local delivery systems in periodontology.

| System | Antimicrobial | Form | Initial concentration in GCF | Biodegradability |
|--------|---------------|------|------------------------------|------------------|
| Actisite | Chlortetracycline | Fiber | 1,300 µgr/ml | – |
| Elyzol | Metronidazole | Gel | 461 µgr/ml | + |
| Periochip | Chlorhexidine | Chip | 500 ppm | + |
| Atridox | Doxycycline | Gel | 148 µgr/ml | + |
| Arestin | Minocycline | Microspheres | 340 µgr/ml | + |

and therefore, they should be considered as adjuncts and not substitutes for proper mechanical treatment. Because specific clinical situations or certain microbiological profiles appear to benefit from adjunctive antimicrobials, in the future, a personalized antibiotic regimen, preferably after microbial analysis, could be a desirable target.

## References

Altman, D.G., Schulz, K.F., Moher, D. et al. (2001). The revised CONSORT statement for reporting randomized trials: explanation and elaboration. *Ann. Int. Med.* 13: 663–694.

American Academy of Periodontology (1996). Systemic antibiotics in periodontics. *J. Periodontol.* 67: 831–866.

American Academy of Periodontology (2000). Parameters on acute periodontal diseases. *J. Periodontol.* 71: 863–866.

Bonito, A.J., Lux, L., and Lohr, K.N. (2005). Impact of local adjuncts to scaling and root planing in periodontal disease therapy: a systematic review. *J. Periodontol.* 76: 1227–1236.

Collins, J.F. (1970). Antibiotic therapy in the treatment of acute necrotizing ulcerative gingivitis. *J. Oral Med.* 25: 3–6.

Demolon, I.A., Persson, G.R., Moncla, B.J. et al. (1993). Effects of antibiotic treatment on clinical conditions and bacterial growth with guided tissue regeneration. *J. Periodontol.* 64: 609–616.

Fletcher, J.P. and Plant, C.G. (1966). An assessment of metronidazole In the treatment of acute ulcerative pseudomembranous gingivitis (Vincent's disease). *Oral Surg. Oral Med. Oral Pathol.* 22: 729–736.

Genco, R.J. (1991). Using antimicrobial agents to manage periodontal diseases. *J. Am. Dent. Assoc.* 122: 30–38.

Goodson, J.M. (1996). Principles of pharmacologic intervention. *J. Clin. Periodontol.* 23: 268–272.

Goodson, J.M. (2003). Gingival crevice fluid flow. *Periodontol. 2000* 31: 43–54.

Gould, F.K., Elliott, T.S., Foweraker, J. et al. (2006). Guidelines for the prevention of endocarditis report of the working party of the British Society for Antimicrobial Chemotherapy. *J. Antimicrob. Chemother.* 57: 1035–1042.

Gynther, G.W., Kondell, P.A., Moberg, L.E., and Heimdahl, A. (1998). Dental implant installation without antibiotic prophylaxis. *Oral Surg. Oral Med. Oral Pathol. Oral Radiol. Endod.* 85: 509–511.

Habib, G., Hoen, B., Tornos, P., and Thuny, F. ESC Committee for Practice Guidelines. (2009). Guidelines on the prevention, diagnosis, and treatment of infective endocarditis. *Eur. Heart J.* 30: 2369–2413.

Haffajee, A.D., Socransky, S.S., and Gunsolley, J.C. (2003). Systemic anti-infective periodontal therapy. A systematic review. *Ann. Periodontol.* 8: 115–181.

Hanes, P.J. and Purvis, J.P. (2003). Local anti-infective therapy: pharmacological agents. A systematic review. *Ann. Periodontol.* 8: 79–98.

Herrera, D., Alonso, B., León, R. et al. (2008). Antimicrobial therapy in periodontitis: the use of systemic antimicrobials against the subgingival biofilm. *J. Clin. Periodontol.* 35 (S. 8): 45–66.

Herrera, D., Matesanz, P., Martín, C. et al. (2020). Adjunctive effect of locally delivered antimicrobials in periodontitis therapy: a systematic review and meta-analysis. *J. Clin. Periodontol.* 47: 239–256.

Herrera, D., Roldan, S., Connor, A., and Sanz, M. (2000a). The periodontal abscess (II). Short-term clinical and microbiological efficacy of 2 systemic antibiotic regimes. *J. Clin. Periodontol.* 27: 395–404.

Herrera, D., Roldan, S., and Sanz, M. (2000b). The periodontal abscess: a review. *J. Clin. Periodontol.* 27: 377–386.

Herrera, D., Sanz, M., Jepsen, S. et al. (2002). A systematic review on the effect of systemic antimicrobials as an adjunct to scaling and root planing in periodontitis patients. *J. Clin. Periodontol.* 29: 136–159.

Holmstrup, P. and Westergaard, J. (2003). Necrotizing periodontal disease. In: *Clinical Periodontology and Implant Dentistry*, 4e (ed. J. Lindhe, T. Carring, and N. Lang), 243–259. Blackwell-Munksgaard.

Javed, F., Alghamdi, A., Ahmed, A. et al. (2013). Clinical efficacy of antibiotics in the treatment of peri-implantitis. *Int. Dent. J.* 63: 169–176.

Koukos, G., Konstantinidis, A., Tsalikis, L. et al. (2016). Prevalence of β-lactam (*bla*$_{TEM}$) and Metronidazole (*nim*) Resistance genes in the oral cavity of Greek subjects. *Open Dent. J.* 10: 89–98.

Laskin, D.M., Dent, C.D., Morris, H.F. et al. (2000). The influence of preoperative antibiotics on success of endosseous implants at 36 months. *Ann. Periodontol.* 5: 166–174.

Loos, B.G., Louwerse, P.H.G., Van Winkelhoff, A.J. et al. (2002). Use of barrier membranes and systemic antibiotics In the treatment of Intraosseous defects. *J. Clin. Periodontol.* 29: 910–921.

Matesanz-Pérez, P., García-Gargallo, M., Figuero, E. et al. (2013). A systematic review on the effects of local antimicrobials as adjuncts to subgingival debridement, compared with subgingival debridement alone, in the treatment of chronic periodontitis. *J. Clin. Periodontol.* 40: 227–241.

Mombelli, A. (2002). Microbiology and antimicrobial therapy of peri-implantitis. *Periodontol. 2000* 28: 177–189.

Mombelli, A. and Lang, N.P. (1998). The diagnosis and treatment of peri-implantitis. *Periodontol. 2000* 17: 63–76.

Newman, M.G. and van Winkelhoff, A.J. (2001). *Antibiotic and Antimicrobial Use in Dental Practice*, 2e. Quintessence Publishing.

Palmer, R.M. (1984). Acute lateral periodontal abscess. *Br. Dent. J.* 157: 311–312.

Papapanou, P.N. and Sanz, M. et al. (2018). Periodontitis: consensus report of workgroup 2 of the 2017 World Workshop on the Classification of Periodontal and Peri-Implant Diseases and Conditions. *J. Clin. Periodontol.* 45 (Suppl 20): S162–S170. https://doi.org/10.1111/jcpe.12946.

Rams, T.E., Feik, D., Young, V. et al. (1992). *Enterococci* in human periodontitis. *Oral Microbiol. Immunol.* 7: 249–252.

Rams, T.E. and Slots, J. (1996). Local delivery of antimicrobial agents in the periodontal pocket. *Periodontol. 2000* 10: 139–159.

Renvert, S., Roos-Jansaker, A.M., and Claffey, N. (2008). Non-surgical treatment of peri-implant mucositis and peri-implantitis: a literature review. *J. Clin. Periodontol.* 35 (8 Suppl): 305–315.

Saxen, L. and Asikainen, S. (1993). Metronidazole in the treatment of localized juvenile periodontitis. *J. Clin. Periodontol.* 20: 166–171.

Saxen, L., Asikainen, S., Kanervo, A. et al. (1990). The long-term efficacy of systemic doxycycline medication in the treatment of localized juvenile periodontitis. *Arch. Oral Biol.* 35: 227S–229S.

Slots, J., Feik, D., and Rams, T.E. (1990). Prevalence and antimicrobial susceptibility of *Enterobacteriaceae, Pseudomonadaceae* and *Acinetobacter* in human periodontitis. *Oral Microbiol. Immunol.* 5: 149–154.

Slots, J. and Rosling, B.G. (1983). Suppression of the periodontopathic microflora in localized juvenile periodontitis by systemic tetracycline. *J. Clin. Periodontol.* 10: 465–486.

Smiley, C.J., Tracy, S.L., Abt, E. et al. (2015). Systematic review and meta-analysis on the nonsurgical treatment of chronic periodontitis by means of scaling and root planing with or without adjuncts. *J. Am. Dent. Assoc.* 146: 508–524.

Smith, R.G. and Davies, R.M. (1986). Acute lateral periodontal abscesses. *Br. Dent. J.* 161: 176–178.

Socransky, S.S. and Haffajee, A.D. (2002). Dental biofilms: difficult therapeutic targets. *Periodontol. 2000* 28: 12–55.

Teughels, W., Feres, M., Oud, V. et al. (2020). Adjunctive effect of systemic antimicrobials in periodontitis therapy: a systematic review and meta-analysis. *J. Clin. Periodontol.* 47: 212–281.

Van Winkelhoff, A.J., Herrera, D., Oteo, A., and Sanz, M. (2005). Antimicrobial profiles of periodontal pathogens isolated from periodontitis patients in the Netherlands and Spain. *J. Clin. Periodontol.* 32: 893–898.

Van Winkelhoff, A.J., Rodenburg, J.P., Goene, R.J. et al. (1989). Metronidazole plus amoxicillin in the treatment of *Actinobacillus actinomycetemcomitans* associated periodontitis. *J. Clin. Periodontol.* 16: 128–131.

Vest, T.M., Greenwell, H., Drisko, C. et al. (1999). The effect of postsurgical antibiotics and a bioabsorbable membrane on regenerative healing in Class II furcation defects. *J. Periodontol.* 70: 878–887.

Wilson, W., Taubert, K., Gewitz, M. et al. (2007). Prevention of infective endocarditis. Guidelines from the American Heart Association. *J. Am. Dent. Assoc.* 138: 739–760.

Zucchelli, G., Sforza, N.M., Clauser, C. et al. (1999). Topical and systemic antimicrobial therapy in guided tissue regeneration. *J. Periodontol.* 70: 239–247.

# 7

# Periodontal Osseous Resective Surgery

*Luca Landi*

## Introduction

Successful treatment of periodontal disease can be achieved today through a number of surgical and nonsurgical procedures, each aiming to control infection and inflammation and reduce pocket depth. Periodontal surgery can still be considered a keystone in the treatment of periodontitis. Osseous resective surgery is defined as a means of changing the diseased tissue contour to reproduce a more physiologic anatomy. Knowledge of the pathogenetic mechanisms of the disease process and identification of the defect characteristics enable the clinician to select the appropriate surgical therapy to correct the deformity and establish a healthy environment.

The degree of destruction of periodontal tissues involving bone, periodontal ligament, cementum, and connective tissue depends on several factors such as type of bacteria, host response, teeth anatomy, hard and soft tissue biotypes, and so forth. Once the lesion has progressed apically, a discrepancy between the gingival margin and bone contour is established, resulting in a pocket. The characteristics of this pocket are determined by gingival biotype, morphology of the osseous crest, and teeth anatomy and location. As the inflammation caused by the periodonto-pathogens moves apically in the periodontal apparatus, a change in the anatomy of the zone takes place. If the bone is thick enough, a funnel-shaped defect is created while the surrounding bone not involved in the demineralization process maintains the gingival tissue in the same position. In the case of thin bone, such as buccal bone or interproximal bone between mandibular incisors, a horizontal pattern of resorption usually takes place, and depending on the soft tissue thickness, a recession or a suprabony pocket is formed.

## Indications and Endpoints

The goal of osseous resective surgery is to establish minimal or physiologic probing depth and create a gingival contour compatible with good self-performed oral hygiene (Barrington 1981). Even if regeneration of the lost periodontal apparatus is considered to be the ideal form of treatment, this can be successfully applied only to a limited number of defects according to their infra-osseous depth and morphology. There is a clear indication in the literature that regenerative principles should be applied to those defects with an intra-osseous component greater than or equal to 4 mm. Therefore, osseous resection is indicated in a number of clinical situations whenever the infra-osseous defect depth is in the 3-mm range or whenever a one-wall defect is present (Ochsenbein 1986).

Bone recontouring should be carried out to achieve the so-called positive architecture. This term refers to the physiologic morphology of the alveolar bone that is located in a more coronal position interproximally compared to the radicular buccal and palatal/lingual aspect of the teeth (Figure 7.1). The bone contour follows the cementoenamel junction of the teeth and may be more or less concave, according to the tooth type and genetic biotype (Becker et al. 1997). Therefore, the alveolar crest architecture would have a more pronounced scalloping around incisors and canines, while that toward the molar region would progress in a more flat profile (Figure 7.2).

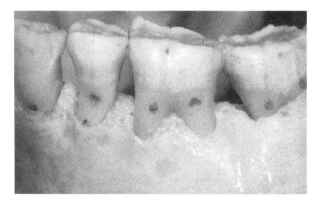

Figure 7.1 An example of positive architecture is shown in this human dry mandible. The buccal alveolar bone is apical to the interproximal crest. Courtesy of Dr. Hyman Smukler, Brookline, MA, USA.

*Practical Periodontal Diagnosis and Treatment Planning*, Second Edition. Edited by Serge Dibart and Thomas Dietrich.
© 2024 John Wiley & Sons, Inc. Published 2024 by John Wiley & Sons, Inc.

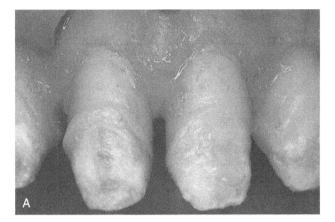 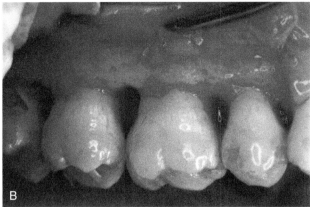

Figure 7.2 A, Surgical exposure of the alveolar crest around maxillary incisors during a crown lengthening procedure. Note how the bone architecture follows the CEJ outline, creating a scalloped morphology. B, A full-thickness flap of a maxillary posterior sextant for pocket elimination. The alveolar crest at the molar area runs with minimal scalloping according to the CEJ morphology.

In a healthy condition, the gingival margin follows the bone architecture so that a consistency between the two entities can be recorded (Matherson 1988). This is considered during surgical correction of osseous defects to avoid excessive or inappropriate remodeling of the osseous crest. Another field of application for osseous resective surgery is in the case of pre-prosthetic applications. Exposing sound tooth structure, reestablishing a biologic space between alveolar bone and the restoration margin, or correcting an unesthetic gingival contour can be achieved through osseous resective surgery. In those instances the surgical approach is best known as a crown lengthening procedure (Ingber et al. 1977).

## Physiologic and Pathologic Alveolar Bone Anatomy

Unaltered alveolar bone morphology is characterized by the following conditions:

- The interproximal bone peaks are located at a more coronal position compared to the buccal or palatal bone. This is identified as a positive architecture. A negative architecture is considered whenever, due to the effect of periodontal disease, the position of the interdental bone is apical to the one of the buccal or palatal/lingual side. A flat type of architecture is identified whenever interproximal and buccal or palatal bone contour lie on the same line. This can be an effect of periodontal disease or the result of a surgical treatment if an ideal osseous recontouring cannot be achieved.
- The buccal or palatal/lingual bone architecture follows the cementoenamel junction (CEJ) of the related tooth. Therefore, the concavity may be more or less accentuated according to the tooth anatomy. The bone crest appears

to be more scalloped at the single-rooted teeth compared to the molars, which present a more flat contour.
- The interproximal bone anatomy reflects the position and root anatomy of the proximal teeth. In the anterior areas, because of the reduced interproximal embrasure and the more or less conical anatomy of the root of the adjacent teeth, this morphology has a knife-edge contour. On the contrary, in the molar area the embrasure is wider and the roots have a more complex anatomy with concavity and convexity leading to a flatter morphology.

These differences also have an impact from a histologic point of view. A thin knife edge interproximal area usually includes only cortical bone with minimal or no cancellous component (Figure 7.3). This is true, as demonstrated by Tal (1984), any time the distance between two adjacent roots is less than 3 mm. In this case, around 1 mm on each tooth side of the interradicular space is occupied by the periodontal ligament and only about 1 mm is left for the alveolar crest that would be made of only cortical bone. In a molar area the embrasure is usually wider and therefore the interradicular bone may include both cortical and cancellous bone compartments (Figure 7.4). These abovementioned anatomical features play a significant role in the pathogenesis of an infra-osseous defect. The inflammatory process, in the case of a narrow interproximal space with a mainly cortical interdental bone, usually determines a horizontal pattern of resorption. Conversely, in the case of a wider embrasure, with thicker cortical and cancellous bone, an infra-osseous defect is more likely to occur (Figure 7.5).

- The buccal bone is usually thinner than the corresponding palatal or lingual bone according to the biotype. Root prominence, such as in the case of canines or the mesiobuccal root of the first maxillary molars, may determine a further reduction of the bone thickness predisposing to buccal bone

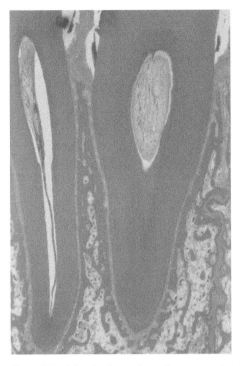

Figure 7.3 Histologic specimen from a monkey (*Macaca fascicularis*) showing the interproximal bone septum between the canine and incisor. The coronal part of the crest consists of only cortical bone, while cancellous bone becomes evident toward the middle third of the septum. Courtesy of Dr. Morris Ruben, Boston, MA, USA.

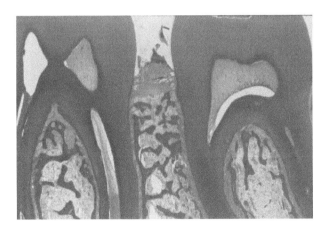

Figure 7.4 Histologic view of a block section taken from a nonhuman primate at the molar area. The interproximal distance is greater than 3 mm and cortical and cancellous bone are well represented. Courtesy of Dr. Morris Ruben, Boston, MA, USA

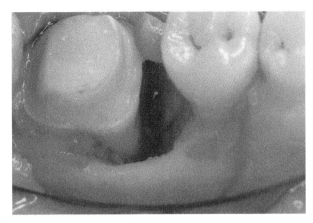

Figure 7.5 A large semi-circumferential three-wall defect around the mesiolingual aspect of a mandibular first molar is exposed during surgery. The thickness of the lingual cortex and the interradicular distance account for the defect morphology.

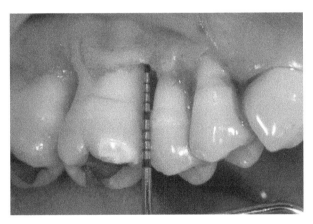

Figure 7.6 After flap elevation for pocket elimination, a dehiscence at the distobuccal roots of the first molar has occurred. This finding greatly affects treatment strategy and approach. Courtesy of Dr. Alessandro Crea, Viterbo, Italy.

## Principles

The principles of osseous resective surgery, as it is conceived today, date back to Schluger (1949) and Friedman (1955). Those authors reported the need for eliminating osseous defects so that a consistency between osseous topography and gingival tissue could be reestablished, but at a more apical level. According to the *Glossary of Periodontal Terms*, osseous resective surgery includes two different steps: (1) osteoplasty, the reshaping of the alveolar process to achieve a more physiologic form without removing supporting bone, and (2) ostectomy, the excision of bone or portion of a bone that is part of a periodontal defect and includes removal of supporting bone.

According to Friedman (1955), osteoplasty is indicated in the case of buccal and/or interproximal thick bony ledges (Figure 7.7), whereas ostectomy should be used to

dehiscences and fenestrations. Eliot and Bowers (1963), studying human skulls, reported an incidence of bone defects of about 20%. Fenestrations were more frequent in the maxilla, whereas dehiscences occurred at a higher rate in the mandible. The occurrence of one of these defects during periodontal surgery may complicate the osseous recontouring or may determine a significant change in the treatment goals (Figure 7.6).

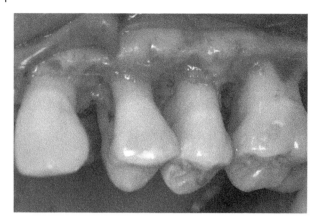

**Figure 7.7** A thick buccal bony ledge can be observed after a full-thickness flap is raised. Bony ledges are often accompanied by infra-osseous defects and craters. Their elimination includes a generous osteoplasty to achieve a physiologic osseous anatomy.

correct shallow interproximal defects such as craters and hemisepti. This resective approach has several limitations and side effects, and often the application of these principles may determine extraction of involved teeth or an unacceptable esthetic result for the patient. Those limitations have been discussed by Siebert (1976), who reported that the main side effect was the loss of attachment induced by the surgery. He also listed a series of factors that should be taken into account before selecting ostectomy as the surgical treatment modality. Those factors include the length and shape of the roots, location and dimension of the defect, width of investing bone, root prominence, and relationship between the intrabony defects and the adjacent teeth or anatomic structures (maxillary sinus, alveolar nerve, etc.). For these reasons, osseous resection underwent a series of modifications through the years, aiming to reduce the amount of bone removal during surgery and thus decreasing the resulting attachment loss.

It should be stressed that osseous resective surgery must be used cautiously whenever an area with esthetic concern is involved in the surgical plan. To simplify the surgical approach to esthetic areas, the key to deciding whether or not to use resective surgery is related to the presence of or a need for a prosthetic involvement. In those cases, osseous resection may be ideal. When there is no prosthetic commitment, only limited and selected cases, including patients with a low smile line and with low esthetic expectations, may be appropriate for this technique (Figure 7.8; Tables 7.1, 7.2).

## Technique

If osseous resective surgery is selected as a treatment option, several steps should be followed to correctly apply the technique.

### Flap Design

Osseous resective surgery is usually coupled with an apical position of the flap. A para-marginal or submarginal incision using a 15 or 15C blade is carried out according to the soft tissue characteristics. A split or combined full-split flap may be used to expose the underlying alveolar bone. Releasing incisions may be necessary to gain better surgical visibility or to easily position the flap at the end of the surgery. Vertical incisions should always be carried out beyond the muco-gingival line buccally and lingually, while the palatal aspect should be extended far enough to allow flap mobilization. The main concern in designing the flap is to provide an adequate vascular supply to the margin of the mobilized flap. Therefore, the apical portion of the flap must be wider than the coronal one and should include the major vessel of the area. For this reason vertical releasing incisions should go by the following general principles: (a) must be beveled, (b) must be divergent toward the apex, (c) should be placed at the mesial and/or distal line angle of the last tooth included in the surgical area, and (d) radicular and interproximal areas must be avoided due to the major blood supply.

### Degranulation and Root Debridement

Once the flap is reflected, degranulation of the soft tissue must be done with surgical curettes (Goldman-Fox n.2, n.3; Barnhardt n. 1/2, etc.) and with sonic/ultrasonic and hand scalers. Once the degranulation is completed and the defect can be identified thoroughly, the root surfaces should be cleaned and planed. Root preparation must be carried out with great care because it greatly influences the type of healing that will take place at the end of the surgical procedures. Polson and Caton described the factors influencing periodontal repair in a primate model (Polson and Caton 1982). They showed that root surface alterations and contamination inhibit new connective tissue attachment and they stressed the importance of a complete root surface debridement for periodontal healing.

### Identification and Measurement of the Defect

Once the surgical field is cleaned, the defect is measured and identified. This is critical in determining the amount of ostectomy and osteoplasty that is indicated. In addition, location of the furcation entrance, root trunk length, or anatomical characteristics of the surgical area must be identified.

### Osteoplasty/Ostectomy

The first step is reducing the interproximal bone thickness. This procedure, called grooving, determines the amount of

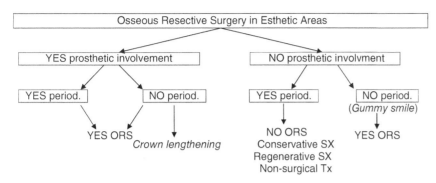

**Figure 7.8** Strategic use of resective surgery according to the presence of prosthetic involvement and the diagnosis of periodontal disease.

**Table 7.1** Indications and contraindications to the surgical therapy in the case of anterior areas with no prosthetic involvement.

| Therapy | Indications | Notes |
|---|---|---|
| Nonsurgical therapy (SRP) | √ PPD > 4 mm<br>√ Horizontal defects | Attention to thin biotypes for recessions |
| Access surgery<br>1. Labial curtain<br>2. Papilla preservation | √ PPD > 6 mm<br>√ Vertical defects<br>√ Palatal defects | Attention to the high smile |
| Osseous resective surgery | √ Rarely<br>√ Low lip line<br>√ Low esthetic expectation | Attention to the post-op teeth sensitivity |

**Table 7.2** Indications and contraindications to the surgical therapy in the case of anterior areas with prosthetic involvement.

| Therapy | Indications | Notes |
|---|---|---|
| Nonsurgical therapy (SRP) | √ PPD 4–5 mm<br>√ Horizontal defects | Attention to thin biotypes for recessions |
| Access surgery<br>1. Labial curtain<br>2. Papilla preservation | √ Palatal defects<br>√ Severe buccal recessions and extremely long crowns | No if infrabony defect > 4 mm<br>Attention to the high smile |
| Osseous resective surgery | √ PPD > 4 mm<br>√ Medium and shallow intrabony defects | Att.: Crown-to-root ratio<br>Att.: Clinical crown length |

osteoplasty that is needed at the radicular bone. In the case of a very thin buccal or palatal/lingual bone, a minimal or no osteoplasty is required. In other instances, a thick bony ledge may be present, requiring aggressive bone re-contouring. This is usually done with diamond coarse or carbide round burs mounted on a hand piece or a high speed hand piece under abundant water cooling irrigation (Figure 7.9). In the case of a bony ledge, a thin cortical layer may be encountered and if care is not taken during the osteoplasty a deep groove into the ledge may be produced as the bur drops into the cancellous bone once the resistance offered by the cortical bone is gone.

As soon as the grooving is accomplished, a radicular blending must be done to produce a smooth and blended surface (also known as a sluice-way profile) to enhance flap adaptation. During this step a careful evaluation of root position and anatomy will reduce the risk of causing any fenestration or dehiscence. At this point ostectomy comes into play. One wall, craters, or other defects should be removed and interproximal and radicular bone

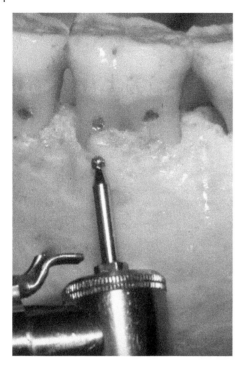

Figure 7.9   A diamond coarse round bur (Brassler, USA) can be used to perform osteoplasty. Due to its moderate cutting ability, compared to the carbide bur, it may be indicated whenever minimal osteoplasty must be done.

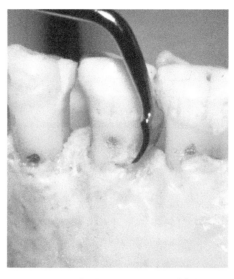

Figure 7.10   A back action (Rhodes 36–37 Hu-friedy, USA) is used in a dry mandible to demonstrate how to perform fine ostectomy. The blade of the instrument is placed on the radicular bone and moved backward toward the root to eliminate the supporting bone involved in the defect.

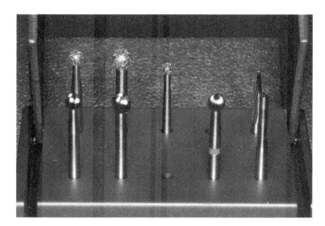

Figure 7.11   An osseous resective surgery bur kit (Brassier, USA), including different sized round burs made of diamond coarse and carbide. The end-cutting bur 957c-H207C is used to remove supporting bone around the tooth without damaging the root surface.

designed to achieve a positive architecture. Radicular bone removal is usually carried out with hand instruments. The Ochsenbain chisel (n.1 and 2) and back action chisel (Rhodes 36–37) (Figure 7.10) are the most popular instruments used for this purpose. Rotary instruments also may be used, but great care must be taken so as to not damage the root while carrying out the ostectomy. Special burs with only an end-cutting head have been designed for this purpose and may be very useful in the interproximal areas (Figure 7.11).

The more bone that is removed from the radicular or interproximal areas, the thicker the alveolar margin; this phenomenon is known as ledging. The desired newly established alveolar bone morphology should have a knife-edged profile to allow better flap adaptation and reduce the chance of pocket re-formation. However, there are instances, such as during crown lengthening, in which a certain degree of margin thickness (ledge) is desirable to support soft tissue stability (Figure 7.12).

The last surgical step is the correction of the interdental area. The presence of a crater or a one-wall defect may be managed according to the location and anatomy of the tooth, either by a complete flattening of the crest or by a palatal/lingual approach. This can be done initially with a round bur and completed with bone files (Sugerman file, Kramer and Nevins, etc.). In addition, the removal of the so-called widow's peak is critical. These peaks consist of residual bone left at the facial and palatal/lingual line angles of the teeth. During the healing process, the persistence of these formations may lead to a soft tissue bridging with a re-pocketing of the area. Their elimination is achieved with hand chisels (Wiedelstadt n.1 and n.2) that are run into the interdental area against the radicular surfaces.

Another important factor that influences the ability to achieve a positive architecture is the amount of the residual attachment apparatus. Performing osseous resection to eliminate pockets and defects should not jeopardize tooth

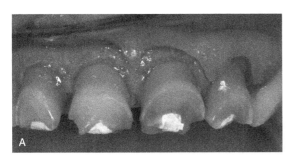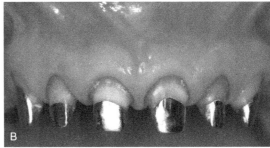

Figure 7.12  A, It may be useful to create a bone ledge in the esthetic area. In this case a crown lengthening has been done and a certain degree of crestal thickness has been intentionally achieved. B, Six months after surgery and before final prosthetic delivery. It is observable that the thickness of crest contributed to the creation of a thick and firm gingival unit.

stability. The length and anatomy of the roots and evaluation of the residual periodontal support help determine whether osseous resection may be the treatment of choice. The amount of bone that is removed during osseous surgery may vary according to the defect characteristics, the bone architecture, and the teeth morphology. Selipsky (1976) showed that an average of 0.6 mm of support per tooth may be removed with osseous resective surgery. He concluded that although a significant amount of the total bone had to be removed, only a minimal amount of the removed portion would be the supporting apparatus. The increase of mobility following the surgical therapy is transitory and returns to the preoperative level in about 12 months.

## Suturing

Once the osseous recontour is completed the flap is placed apical to the preoperative margin. Its position may be apical to or at the osseous crest. In the first case, a small portion of exposed bone, with or without its periosteum, is left exposed. A vertical or horizontal periosteal mattress suture may be used to hold the flap in position; the sutures may be interrupted or continuous. The use of sling sutures is also recommended any time the lingual/palatal or buccal flap must be placed at a different level. A periodontal dressing may or may not be used according to the operator's preference. In the authors' experience it seems that periodontal eugenol-free dressing (Coe-pack) may be indicated any time the flap is positioned apical to the osseous crest to improve patient comfort during healing and reduce the risk for flap displacement during healing. However, it is important to remember that the use of a periodontal dressing may delay the healing process and therefore routine use is no longer justified.

## Modifications to the Original Surgical Approach

### Palatal Approach

Ochsenbein and Bohannan (1963) were the first to introduce a modification of the original protocols, by describing the palatal approach. This approach was based on the observation that, due to teeth location and alveolar bone anatomy, infra-osseous defects in the maxillary arch were located mainly interproximally and palatally. The palatal approach has several advantages: (a) the presence of an abundant amount of keratinized tissue on the palatal side, (b) an increased thickness of the alveolar bone compared to the buccal aspect, (c) a wider embrasure area between the molars, facilitating the surgical access, and (d) the cleansing effect of the tongue in the postoperative period.

By using this approach a palatally inclined ramp is created with minimal ostectomy. The majority of the osteoplasty and ostectomy are carried out from the palatal aspect and only minimal osseous contour is done buccally, preserving furcation entrance integrity in the molars and reducing the amount of root exposure in esthetically sensitive areas. In 1964, the same authors classified the interproximal defects (craters) in four different entities. Class I defect was characterized by a 2–3-mm deep component with thick facial and palatal walls; Class II was 4–5 mm deep with thin facial and palatal walls; Class III more than 6 mm deep with a sharp drop from the walls to a flat base, and Class IV, the least common situation, was characterized by a crater with a variable depth but extremely thin buccal and palatal walls. The authors associated a treatment option with each defect so that Class I could be managed only with palatal ramping, while Class II and III should be approached with both buccal and palatal ramping, and treatment of Class IV, although very unfavorable, included the elimination of buccal and palatal walls.

## Lingual Approach

The same concept used in the maxilla was later introduced for the mandible. Tibbets et al. (1976) reported on how the mandibular molars and premolars should be approached from the lingual aspect. The rationale for this lies in the observation that molars and premolars have a lingual inclination (Wilson's curve around 29 degrees for the molars and 9 degrees for the premolars) so that the entrance of the lingual furcation is located at a more apical position compared to the buccal one. Furthermore, the lingual bone is thicker compared to the buccal (Figure 7.13) and there is always an adequate amount of keratinized tissue on this side. As for the palatal approach, this technique should be used to minimize the amount of ostectomy carried out in the buccal area, preserving the furcation integrity and reducing the total amount of attachment loss (Figure 7.14).

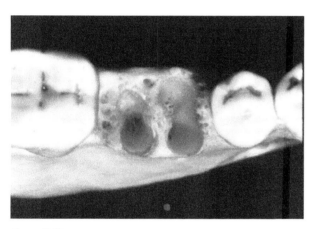

**Figure 7.13** Photograph of a dry human mandible showing the alveolar crest after removal of a first molar. The buccal bone is a very thin lamina compared to the lingual crest. Removal of lingual bone to correct a periodontal defect is preferred to prevent furcation exposure and severe buccal dehiscence.

## Fiber Retention Osseous Resective Surgery

Another and more recent modification of the osseous resective surgical technique has been presented by Carnevale (2007). This technique is based on the concept that supracrestal fibers inserted into the root cementum are always present coronal to the alveolar crest, both in diseased and healthy situations (Carnevale et al. 1985; Gargiulo et al. 1961). Therefore, it seems reasonable from a biological and clinical standpoint that preservation of those fibers during surgery may have two effects: (a) relocating the deepest portion of the defect at a more coronal position, and (b) reducing the amount of ostectomy required to eliminate the defect. In other words, the presence of a connective tissue attachment coronal to the crest determines a coronal shift of the apical component of the osseous defect.

The technique includes a split thinned flap and the careful removal of the soft tissue using a blade or an interproximal knife (Goldman-Fox n.11, Orban 5/6, Buck 1/2). This sharp dissection is followed by the identification of the residual attachment apparatus within the bone defect using a periodontal probe. The nonattached soft tissue is then removed and resection of the osseous crest is carried out. At the end of the alveolar bone recontouring, only bone with attached fibers should be left around the tooth. This technique has been proven to be effective in reducing and maintaining probing depth within the normal range. Carnevale et al. (1991) reported on 304 periodontally compromised patients treated with the fiber retention osseous resective surgery who were followed for 3–17 years. The majority of the patients (86%) belonged to ADA case types 3 and 4. Patients were further divided into three groups according to the length of the follow-up period. Ninety-two patients were followed for 11.3 years. At the end of the study only 147 out of 8,572 sites were deeper than 4 mm (1.72% of the total sites), demonstrating a remarkable

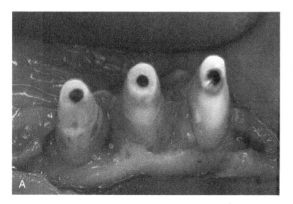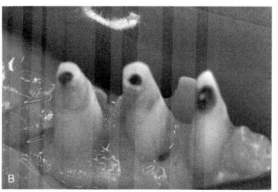

**Figure 7.14** A, Craters and combined infrabony defect less than 3 mm deep lingually to prosthetic abutments. Lingual osteoplasty and minimal ostectomy are indicated to manage this defect. B, The result after osseous recontouring and tooth preparation. No defects remain.

long-term stability of the results achieved at the completion of active therapy.

Data on teeth extraction also have been reported by the authors. It is significant that the majority of the teeth (576, that is, 7.5% of the total sample) were extracted during active treatment. Most of these teeth (63.7%) belonged to patients falling in the ADA case type 4 category, and the main reason for their loss was advance periodontal breakdown. During supportive therapy, however, the incidence of teeth extraction was dramatically reduced (67 teeth; 0.9% of the total sample) and limited to a subgroup of 50 patients. These results confirmed the effectiveness of this technique in treating and controlling advanced periodontal disease.

Furthermore, this technique should be considered a very reliable option in the case of complex perio-prosthetic case involvement.

## Soft Tissue Management

The soft tissue component must be managed during the osseous surgery. Positioning the gingival margin apical to the preoperative level is recommended any time elimination of the defect is indicated. This can be done in several ways according to the soft tissue biotype and osseous determinants.

### Buccal/Facial Flap

Whenever an adequate band of keratinized tissue is present a submarginal scalloped incision may be outlined about 1–2 mm apical to the gingival margin or as deep as the required probing depth (Figure 7.15). A full-thickness thinned flap up the mucogingival line followed by a partial dissection or a complete partial-thickness flap

may be elevated to gain access to the underlying bone. In the case of inadequate or minimal keratinized gingiva an intra-sulcular incision is preferred to preserve as much attached gingiva as possible. In the case of a very thin biotype a mucoperiosteal flap is preferred because the chance of flap perforation and necrosis may increase (Wood et al. 1972). Once the flap is elevated and osseous recontouring is performed, the mobility of the flap should be tested so that a passive positioning is obtained at or apical to the newly recontoured alveolar crest. As previously described, if vertical releasing incisions are indicated to freely move the flap, these should be extended into the alveolar mucosa.

### Palatal Flap

A different approach is required on the palatal side because the gingiva in this area is completely keratinized and cannot be moved in an apico-coronal position. This approach, best known as palatal thinned flap, is used any time pocket reduction or elimination is required. The primary scalloped incision should be outlined according to the probing depth and following the anatomy of the teeth involved in the surgical area. For instance, the primary incision around a second premolar is more concave compared to that around a first molar. Another factor that influences flap design is root anatomy and morphology. As the defect moves apically, the size of the roots narrows. So in the case of a deep probing around the palatal root of a maxillary first molar, the scalloping should be calibrated to the root morphology rather than the mesiodistal dimension of the clinical crown. It is therefore root morphology that dictates the incision outline, rather than clinical crown anatomy. In addition, tooth position and consequently root direction must be considered in the

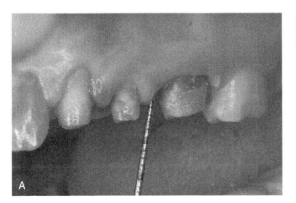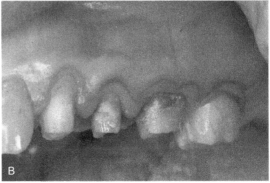

**Figure 7.15**    A, Presurgical probing for crown lengthening. Surgical incisions are planned according to probing depth, tooth and root anatomy, and amount of keratinized tissue. B, In this case the abundance of keratinized tissue allows the outline of a submarginal scalloped full-thickness flap. Surgical papillae are created interproximally and facial to the furcation entrance to protect this area during healing.

surgical planning. Most of the time palatal roots of maxillary first and second molars have a disto-palatal direction. This must be considered in the flap design.

The palatal vault is another important anatomic issue for the thinned palatal flap. In the case of a high vault palate the incision may correspond to the probing depth, while in the case of a flat vault it should be outlined close to the gingival margin. This is mainly due to the presence of the greater palatal artery that runs into the soft tissue at a distance from the CEJ of the molars that varies according to the vault extension (Reiser et al. 1996).

A thinned flap is indicated to reduce the soft tissue component and achieve a pocket reduction with a better flap adaptation. The final crest morphology should be estimated during flap incisions so that minimal trimming of the flap is needed at the end of the surgery (Figure 7.16). A bone sounding under anesthesia is required to determine the preoperative bone contour. The periodontal probe is run into the palatal tissue until it stops, so that the thickness of the gingiva may be estimated.

The presence of an exostosis or osseous defect also may be recorded. This information will help the operator to create an evenly thinned flap along its entire extension. An interproximal thickening of the flap may determine poor tissue adaptation at the radicular aspect of the bone, thus creating an anatomical dead space that may result in a sloughing of the marginal tissue.

Remember that flap design and osseous anatomy are by far more crucial than the suturing technique in achieving passive flap adaptation. However, care must be taken during suturing to hold the flap in the proper position.

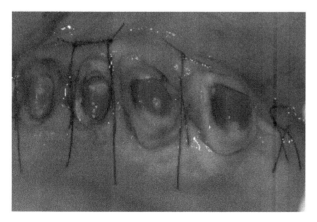

Figure 7.16 If properly outlined, a palatal thinned flap will drop on the recontoured alveolar crest following the root anatomy. Minimal or no trimming should be required if proper tissue incisions are made. The picture shows a passive adaptation of a thinned flap. Note how the primary incisions have been designed according to the root position and anatomy.

## Effect of Surgery on the Alveolar Bone

Flap elevation with or without bone reshaping determines a certain degree of crestal bone remodeling, leading to a loss of bone ranging from 0 mm to 0.8 mm (Donnenfeld et al. 1964). Studying the amount of postsurgical bone remodeling in a human model, Moghaddas and Stahl (1980) reported that the net bone loss at six months after osseous surgery combined with a full-thickness flap varied according to the location. Crestal bone loss averaged 0.23 mm in the interproximal space, 0.55 mm at the radicular aspect, and 0.88 mm in the furcation region of a molar. In their study the three months' data did not reach any statistically significant difference from the six months' data.

Another interesting finding of this work was that no correlation could be made between the amount of resection and the degree of remodeling. During a reentry procedure, Donnenfeld and coworkers (1970) measured the amount of bone remodeling that took place in three patients undergoing osseous resective procedures both immediately after surgery and at six months. They reported an average of 0.6 mm of bone loss interproximally and 1 mm at the radicular location. Another study (Smith et al. 1980) described the bone loss after osseous resective surgery only through a bone sounding procedure at six months. They found 0.2 mm of radicular bone loss and 0.3 mm of interproximal bone loss. Pennell and coworkers (1967) described in a landmark paper the pattern of wound healing obtained from 34 teeth from 20 patients treated with a full-thickness flap followed by osteoplasty on 5 mm of marginal bone and ostectomy at the first mm of crestal bone. The postsurgical observation period ranged from 14 to 545 days and they reported an average bone crest resorption of 0.54 mm. The majority of the teeth (82%) showed less than 1 mm of resorption, while severe bone loss (more than 3 mm) was recorded in only two cases.

### Histologic Effect of Osseous Surgery

The best histologic evidence on the effect of resective procedures on the alveolar crest is reported by Wilderman et al. (1970). The sample included 23 block sections of teeth that underwent a mucoperiosteal flap followed by osteoplasty in the first 5 mm of alveolar bone and 1 mm of crestal bone reduction. The effect of bone surgery varies according to the nature of the alveolar bone. Superficial bone necrosis with intense osteoclastic activity was a common finding. In the case of a thin alveolar bone, resorption took place at the periodontal ligament side, while when a thick bone was found, the osteoclastic activity started within the marrow spaces toward the periosteal side. Osteoblastic activity reached its peak after 21 days, and after six months very little additional bone remodeling could be detected.

Interestingly, the mean loss of bone was 0.8 mm in the case of a thick alveolar crest, while it reached 3.1 mm in the case of a thin crest. This may be due to the different intrinsic healing potential of different bone anatomy. Thick cancellous bone holds better healing potential compared to thin cortical bone. Therefore, great attention must be paid to the quality of the bone during osseous surgery because the knowledge of these characteristics may be of great importance in determining the final surgical result.

## Evidence-based Outcomes

In the past 50 years a number of studies comparing different treatment approaches to periodontal pockets have been published. It is worth noticing that different conclusions may be drawn from the results presented with a certain degree of discrepancy. Evidence-based dentistry, as it is established today, is a very important tool for gaining a better understanding of the limitations and benefits of different treatment options. However, ideal studies fulfilling all of the requisites for the highest scientific evidence have yet to be performed. This chapter attempts to summarize the results of some of the most representative studies to give the reader some indications that may be useful in a clinical setting. A more in-depth and precise examination of the literature on this topic is suggested to gain a broader understanding of each of the studies quoted.

Osseous resective surgery has been studied alone and compared with other surgical and nonsurgical techniques in several longitudinal studies. Most of the studies reported on short-term results, while only a few extended to a five-year follow-up. Here we discuss only those studies with at least five years of follow-up. Although there are some differences, the layout of these studies is somewhat similar as different modalities of treatment have been tested in a split mouth design. The treatments rendered were osseous resective surgery with apical positioning of the flap, modified Widman flap surgery, and scaling and root planing. The results have been analyzed according to the initial probing depth. Three depth categories have been identified: 1–3 mm, 4–6 mm, and greater than 7 mm.

Knowles and coworkers (1979) treated 72 patients and found that while in a 1–3-mm depth there was a slight loss of attachment with all of the treatment modalities (thus demonstrating that there is no indication for any kind of treatment in a shallow pocket), for the 4–6 mm category osseous resective surgery achieved greater pocket depth reduction compared to scaling and root planing but similar results compared to Widman flap surgery. Interestingly, in

this depth category all three modalities determined the same amount of attachment level gain. For the greater than 7 mm pockets, all of the treatments reduced the probing depth, but the Widman flap achieved a more significant reduction and a greater gain of attachment compared to the other two.

Ramfjord et al., in 1987, published a second study with a five-year follow-up. The general conclusions were similar to those previously reported except for the greater than 7 mm pockets. In this category the probing depth reduction, although greater compared to the other probing categories, did not show any significant difference in any of the three therapies (ORS 3.53 mm, MWF 3.13 mm, SRP 2.92 mm). This finding was also true for the attachment level gain; none of the treatments was superior to the others. Comparing the results of the one year of maintenance with the final examination at five years, it is notable that some periodontal deterioration took place in most of the patients. Although no statistically significant differences could be reported between the treatments in terms of probing depth reduction and gain of attachment, the incidence of loosing sites was twice in the Widman flap and scaling-treated quadrants compared to the resective surgery quadrants. It is also noteworthy that no molar furcations were included in this study.

In a similar study, Kaldahl and coworkers (1996) reported on 72 patients who were followed for more than five years. Osseous resective surgery was able to produce a greater probing depth reduction compared to Widman flap surgery and scaling and root planing during the entire study in the 5–6 mm pocket category (–1.85 mm for ORS, –1.48 for MWF, –1.52 for SRP). In terms of attachment level gain, osseous resective surgery had the least gain, 0.44 mm, while modified Widman flap surgery (0.60 mm) and scaling and root planing (0.90 mm) showed the greatest performance. In the greater than 7 mm pocket category, osseous resection was the most efficacious treatment in probing reduction (3.38 mm) compared to the other two (MWF 3.09 mm, SRP 2.88 mm). No statistically significant difference could be found in terms of clinical attachment gain between the three therapies at five years (ORS 1.83 mm, MWF 2.07 mm, SRP 1.88 mm).

Several considerations should be made before drawing a definitive conclusion from these studies. Probing depth alone does not reflect the anatomy and morphology of the underlying bony defect, so a deeper or shallower intrabony defect associated with the same probing depth may respond differently to the same treatment modality. The split mouth design may carry an innate bias related to the effect that one treatment may have on the others over the long term. Also, clear endpoints in the performance of osseous surgery have not been stated in any of the studies except those from the Nebraska group (Kaldahl et al. 1996). In this study the achievement of a positive architecture led to the extraction of several teeth and roots during surgery. This is clearly in contrast to other studies in which no mention of root resection or extraction was reported (Knowles et al. 1979; Ramfjord et al. 1987). This may be considered a major limitation in defining the effect of a specific treatment modality.

Another interesting point is the fact that attachment loosing sites appeared to have a higher incidence in those quadrants not treated with osseous resection. Usually the statistical comparison between treatments that has been reported has been based on the mean changes. Now if the number of attachment loosing sites is relatively small, it may be overshadowed by the majority of the stable sites. However, a site analysis may bring up differences that may be significant in the clinical setting. Therefore, the fact that patients treated with osseous resective procedures have a low incidence of attachment loosing sites (Carnevale et al. 2007; Kaldhal et al. 1996; Kalkwarf et al. 1988) may be very important in the case of perio-prosthetic rehabilitation in which disease recurrence may determine prosthetic failure.

A possible explanation for this stability of the apical positioning of the flap has been reported as a major contributor. Several studies (Levy et al. 2002; Mombelli et al. 1995) have shown that the apical displacement of the gingival margin exposing the previously contaminated root determines the formation of a new dento-gingival unit apical to the diseased cementum. This may also determine a positive shift of the microflora by modifying the existing habitat (Levy et al. 2002) and reduce the chance for microorganisms (that have been dormant in the dentinal tubuli) to inhabit the newly formed shallow sulcus (Adriaens et al. 1988).

## Treatment of Furcated Molars with Resective Techniques

Furcation lesions traditionally have been seen as a major challenge for periodontists and restorative dentists. Complicated root anatomy combined with limited access to the area due to teeth location has been cited for the poor prognosis of those areas. Furcation anatomy presents several characteristics that must be known before continuing with their treatment. Furcation entrance size, root trunk length, root concavities, and dome morphology all contribute to make treatment of furcation involvement a difficult task.

## Classification of Furcation Involvement

Once a furcation is periodontally involved different treatment options may be contemplated in relation to the degree of involvement. A furcation lesion may be detected using a dedicated curved probe (Nabers probe) with color marking every 3 mm. Hamp et al. (1975) categorized furcation defects according to the degree of horizontal probing. Three different classes of severity were identified: Class I, when the probing was in the 3 mm range; Class II, if the probing was greater than 3 mm but not passing through the furcation; and Class III, if a through and through lesion was detectable. Tarnow and Fletcher (1984) added to the Hamp classification the evaluation of the vertical probing, identifying three different categories: Subclass A, 1–3 mm; Subclass B, 4–6 mm; and Subclass C, greater than 6 mm. According to the authors, this may help clinicians to improve treatment choices and predictability.

## Ability to Remove Calculus

Furcation is a critical area for cleaning. Caffesse and coworkers (1986) showed that even with an open approach it was very difficult to achieve complete removal of the calculus from an involved furcation area. Matia et al. (1987), using a surgical approach, was able to remove calculus from only seven out of the 26 treated furcation surfaces. These difficulties in achieving a satisfactory result are determined mainly by the complicated anatomy of the area.

## Molar Root Anatomy

Bower (1979a, b) and Gher and Vernino (1980), analyzing extracted maxillary and mandibular molars, reported that the furcation aspect of mandibular molars presents a concavity up to 1 mm deep 100% of the time for the mesial root and 99% of the time for the distal root. In the maxillary molars 100% of the mesiobuccal roots have a 1 mm deep concavity while the distal has this concavity 97% of the time and the palatal has this 17% of the time. Furthermore, 75% of the time the furcation entrance is less than 1 mm, limiting the accessibility to scalers and sonic devices. For these reasons new designs and miniaturized hand and sonic instruments have been introduced in the market and have become very popular. In spite of these technological advancements, each clinician should bear in mind that the result in treating a furcation depends on the strategic value of the tooth.

## Enamel Pearl Projections

Other anatomical determinants may complicate the furcation area. Enamel pearl projections have been reported in the literature as cofactors for furcation lesion formation. Masters and Hoskins (1964) found that cervical enamel projections were present at 29% of the buccal surfaces of mandibular molars, while only 17% of the observed maxillary molars had the same anatomical feature. Moskow and

Canut (1990) found a lower incidence of the enamel pearl projections, with a range from 1.1% to 9.7%. The teeth with the highest frequency were the maxillary third and second molars. Two different papers (Bissada and Abdelmalek 1973; Swan and Hurt 1976) reported a 50% correlation between furcation involvement and enamel pearl projections. In 1987 Hou and Tsai were able to correlate furcation involvement with the presence of cervical enamel projections based on a study of 87 furcated molars that showed cervical enamel projections in 63% of the cases.

### Intermediate Bifurcational Ridge

These formations can be found on the mandibular molars; they consist of cementum formation originating from the mesial surface of the distal root, extending to the mesial root. Everett et al. (1958) found that 73% of the observed extracted mandibular molars were affected by these anatomical aberrations.

### Accessory Pulp Canals

Since Bender and Seltzer (1972) reported on the presence of a great number of accessory pulp canals in the furcation area of molars, many other authors have investigated the incidence of these canals and their role in the establishment of periodontal lesions. While there is enough evidence to support the fact that accessory pulp canals open in the furcation area with a great deal of frequency (with a range of 27.4–76%) (Burch and Hulen 1974; Gutman 1978; Lowman et al. 1973; Vertucci and Williams 1974), there is still some controversy regarding their role in the pathogenesis of a periodontal lesion.

### Resective Options

According to the 1992 *Glossary of Periodontal Terms* we can define the following treatment modalities:

**Root amputation:** The surgical removal of a root without the related crown portion (this can be done before or after the endodontic treatment).

**Root resection:** The removal of a root and the related crown portion from a multi-rooted tooth.

**Root separation:** The surgical sectioning of the root complex and the maintenance of all roots.

**Hemisection:** The surgical separation of a multi-rooted tooth with the extraction of one root with the overhanging crown. Usually refers to mandibular molars.

**Tunnelization:** Conservative treatment by creating a space between the roots that can be cleaned by the patient. (Usually refers to mandibular molars.)

The modalities are described in detail below.

### Root Amputation

This treatment may be considered a conservative treatment modality; it may not include the prosthetic restoration of the involved tooth. This may be indicated whenever one of the roots is involved periodontally or endodontically and the overhanging crown is sound (Figure 7.17 a, b). In this case, after a flap is raised the root is cut right at its emergence from the root trunk. A fissure bur is used to bevel the amputation. A minimal ostectomy should be performed on the buccal aspect of the root (or palatal aspect in the case of a palatal maxillary molar) to allow the extraction of the root without the risk of buccal bony plate fracture (Figure 7.17 c, d). Once the root is extracted the orifice on the crown should be filled and the flap sutured back. Smukler and Tagger (1976) showed in a clinical and histological study that this procedure may be carried out as an emergency procedure before endodontic treatment has been performed. The pulp of the amputated molars remains vital for up to two weeks without symptoms. However, all efforts should be made to treat the tooth endodontically before the amputation is performed.

**Evidence:** There is scarce evidence regarding the long-term effect of this modality of treatment.

### Root Resection/Separation/Hemisection

In the case of Class II and III furcation involvement, a root resection or separation may be considered. Several factors should be evaluated before considering this option: root anatomy, root length, amount of attachment loss and attachment apparatus left on the residual roots, tooth mobility before resection, restorability of the crown, strategic importance, and alternative treatment. This treatment includes endodontic therapy, tooth reconstruction, and prosthetic coverage. All of the operators involved in the treatment must be acquainted with the objectives of the treatment so that appropriate minimally invasive root canal shaping and conservative root preparation is done.

Once the tooth has been judged appropriate for this treatment, it must undergo endodontic therapy first and then must be prepared for a complete crown coverage (Figure 7.18). After raising a flap, the furcation entrance must be clearly identified and the anatomy of the root selected for resection carefully evaluated (Figure 7.19). Using a carbide or diamond fissure bur, a trough will be outlined connecting the entrances of the two furcations. The extraction can be done once the root and the related portion of the crown are isolated (Figure 7.20). Some crestal bone may be removed to facilitate root mobilization and minimize the chance of fracture of the buccal bony plate during root extraction. At this point the residual tooth should be checked for any further furcation involvement; if this is the case a separation of the residual roots may be considered.

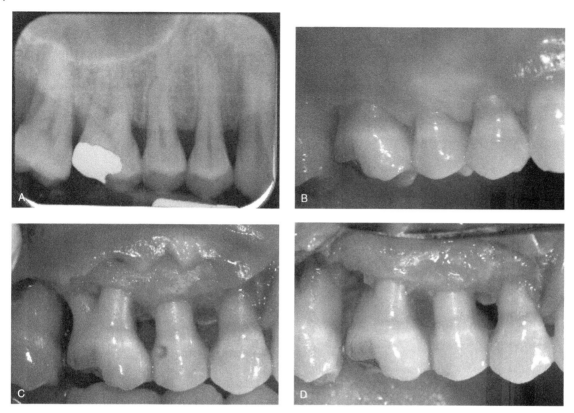

Figure 7.17 A, Radiograph of a maxillary first molar with a root proximity and a Class II defect of the buccal furcation. B, Clinical view, preoperative. C, After mucoperiosteal flap elevation, the buccal furcation is clearly visible. D, The root amputation is performed by cutting the base of the distobuccal root with a fissure bur to create a sluiceway to allow proper cleaning.

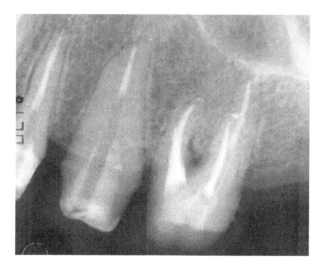

Figure 7.18 Radiographic view of a Class II furcation.

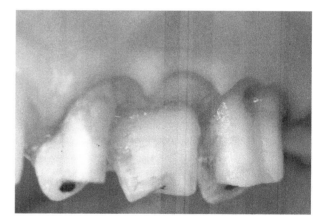

Figure 7.19 The furcation is identified and measured at flap elevation.

It is very important in this procedure to consider each separated root as an individual unit and the furcation space as an interdental area. Osseous surgery around each of the resected roots should therefore follow the same basic principles of creating a positive architecture. The amount of the attachment apparatus left on each root combined with root morphology and length determines the degree of stability of the root. It should be remembered that the majority of the attachment apparatus of a maxillary molar is in the root trunk area and that the mesiobuccal root has a greater attachment area followed by the palatal and distobuccal roots. A maxillary molar with a short root trunk will be affected by a furcation lesion earlier, but may have a better prognosis if resective procedures are used as most of the attachment is still present.

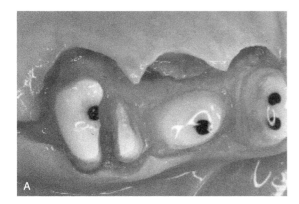

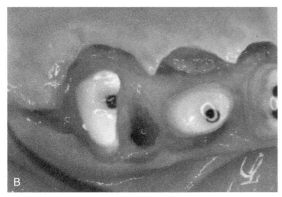

Figure 7.20   The mesiobuccal root is isolated (A) and extracted (B).

On the contrary, a long root trunk, once involved, has a lesser chance to be treated with resective means because the amount of residual attachment on the remaining root is reduced. Therefore, the root to be resected should be carefully selected both pre- and intraoperatively, particularly when mesiobuccal or palatal roots are indicated for extraction.

After root extraction and/or separation, the tooth must be reshaped and prepared to ensure physiologic soft tissue adaptation and allow patient cleansing maneuvers.

Osteoplasty of the residual alveolus also may be indicated to allow better flap adaptation.

Temporary restorations play a significant role in this treatment technique because they ensure stability and protection of the residual tooth during the healing period. At the end of the surgery the temporary restorations should be relined and adapted, leaving the margin at least 3 mm away from the osseous crest to allow tissue maturation and establishment of physiologic supra-crestal gingival tissue (Figure 7.21). Kon and Majzoub (1992) reported that the distance between the pulp floor and the furcation entrance in maxillary resected first molars was, on average, less than 3 mm (Figure 7.22). The significance of this finding may have a major restorative impact because it may imply that all of the restorations in those areas may violate the supra-crestal gingival tissue dimension.

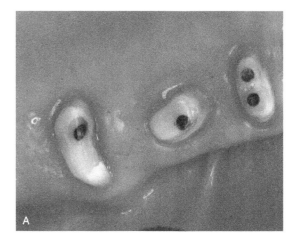

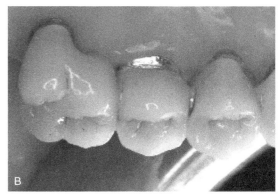

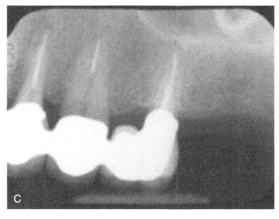

Figure 7.21   A, Two months healing demonstrates good tissue quality and adequate plaque control by the patient. B, Clinical view two years after crown delivery. C, Two-year radiographic control. Courtesy of Dr. Paolo Manicone, Rome, Italy.

Root resection for mandibular molars deserves some additional considerations. Mesial root anatomy is far more complex compared to the distal root anatomy because it contains two canals and in 100% of the cases has a curvature and a deep concavity on the furcation aspect (Bower 1979a, b). Removal of the mesial root is therefore preferable because the distal root may be easier to restore and manage periodontally. Fracture of the resected mandibular molar is

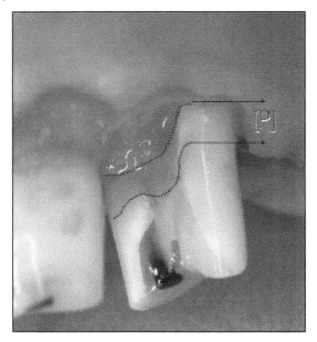

Figure 7.22 Maxillary first molar with a resected mesiobuccal root. The distance between the pulp chamber and the furcation entrance (P) is on average less than 3 mm, as in this case.

more frequent when the mesial root is retained (Langer et al. 1981). In the author's experience resection of the mandibular molar may be indicated when the adjacent teeth are involved in the prosthetic plan (Figure 7.23).

The restoration of a resected mandibular molar with an individual crown is the least advantageous because a mesial or distal cantilever is created, along with a great chance of fracture. On the contrary, once the resected molar is involved in a more extended bridgework, the mechanical loading is distributed along the entire bridge span, reducing the risk for fracture. Prosthetic management of resected teeth is beyond the scope of this chapter, but usually requires conservative preparations to spare as much tooth structure as possible to avoid weakening the abutments.

Mandibular furcated molars, and to a lesser extent maxillary molars, may also be treated by root separation, better known as hemisection. In this instance the roots are separated and maintained. This procedure may be indicated whenever each of the roots has an adequate periodontal apparatus and is judged to be able to be maintained from a prosthetic and endodontic standpoint. The surgical principles are the same as for root resection; however, prosthetic

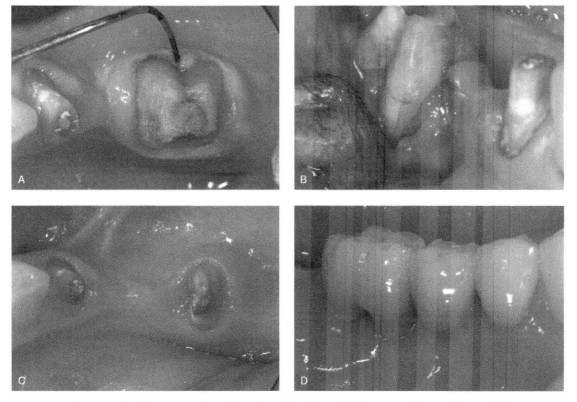

Figure 7.23 A, Lower right first molar with a Class I furcation. B, A vertical fracture of the mesial root is found and the tooth is resected with the extraction of the mesial root. C, Three months after the extraction the distal root is checked for stability and a final fixed partial denture is delivered. D, The pontic design should be adequate to allow good home care. Courtesy of Dr. Paolo Manicone, Rome, Italy.

management may differ because a tunneled molar crown must be fabricated to ensure good access for home care (Figure 7.24). The interproximal distance between the roots must be adequate to allow space for the crown margin (that should only be made of metal) and for interproximal space. Therefore, molars with a narrow interradicular space or with roots that connect or converge toward the apex may not be candidates for this treatment modality. The use of an orthodontic device to increase the interradicular space has also been advocated, even though it may increase the complexity and length of the therapy.

**Evidence:** Gathering a general consensus on the effectiveness of root resection therapy on a long-term basis may not be so easy. Conflicting data can be found in the scientific literature regarding this subject. Poor treatment outcomes on a long-term basis have been reported by Langer et al. (1981), who in a 10-year study found that 38 of 100 resected molars had to be extracted. The main reasons for failure were root fracture (18%), periodontal breakdown (10%), and endodontic lesion (7%). Only three teeth failed because of cemental leakage and recurrent decay. Buhler (1988) reported a 32% failure rate at 10 years on 34 resected

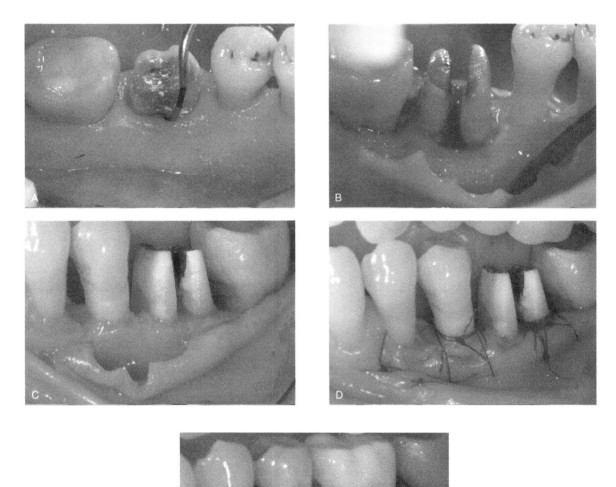

Figure 7.24   A, A Class II lingual furcation is detected at the lower left first molar. B, A root resection is performed and an osteoplasty is also carried out to reduce the infrabony defect around the roots on the lingual side. C, A buccally minimal ostectomy is necessary. D, The buccal flap is apically repositioned using continuous sling vertical mattress sutures. E, Three weeks' healing after surgery. Courtesy of Dr. Antonello Pavone, Rome, Italy.

molars. Again, the main causes of failure were endodontic pathology and root fracture, while only one tooth was extracted due to periodontal breakdown. The same failure rate was found by Blomlof et al. (1997) in a follow-up 3–10 years later. The results of this study should be interpreted with caution because the authors compared the survival of 146 root-resected molars with 100 endodontically treated single-rooted teeth. Interestingly, at five years the survival rate between the two groups did not differ significantly (82% vs. 83%), while at 10 years the survival rate for multi-rooted teeth dropped to 68% compared to 77% of single-rooted teeth. These differences, however, did not provide statistical significance. In this study the primary reason for failure was recurrence of periodontitis, and smoking was identified as a strong risk factor in this group of patients.

On the other hand, several studies report favorable results with the use of root resection. Taken together, the failure rate described in those studies ranged from zero to 8%, at 2–23 years of follow-up. Hamp et al. (1975) reported on the effect of various treatment modalities in the case of furcation involvement of 310 molars. Eighty-seven of these teeth received root resection. After five years no teeth were lost and periodontal conditions were stable; only two teeth had a probing depth greater than 6 mm. This would indicate that a change in the supra- and sub-gingival environment, allowing good self-performed home care, may be critical for periodontal stability. The same periodontal success has been reported by Erpenstein (1983), treating 34 molars with root resection. During the average follow-up time of 2.9 years (range one to seven years) only four teeth were lost, three of which had endodontic failure.

The main study dealing with root resection therapy is the one from Carnevale and coworkers (1998), who treated 194 patients for a total of 488 resected molars. All of the teeth were prosthetically restored. The follow-up time ranged from 3–11 years. At the end of the study all of the patients were included in a strict regimen of supportive therapy. The success rate was 94% (28 teeth failed) and the reasons for failure included endodontic recurrence (four teeth), caries (nine teeth), abutment fracture (three teeth), and root fracture (nine teeth). Three teeth with a probing depth of greater than 5 mm were also included as failures. The conclusion of this study was that resective therapy may be considered to be a viable option in the treatment of advanced periodontal disease on a long-term basis.

**Comments:** Root resection therapy is a highly demanding procedure that can still be considered an option in the armamentarium of a periodontist. The introduction of implant therapy has greatly affected the application of this technique in the daily practice. Nevertheless, any time the decision whether to treat and maintain a multi-rooted tooth or extract and replace it with an implant has to be made, there are several considerations. These considerations must be made by every single member of the restorative team because a team effort is required to achieve a predictable result:

- The endodontist should perform the least invasive therapy possible, sparing as much root structure as possible.
- A fiber post or post and core reconstruction with a temporary crown should be done before resective surgery is initiated.
- A positive architecture must be achieved during surgery and the tooth profile must be reshaped to ensure good access for maintenance and easy prosthetic finalization.
- The precision of the final crown is a critical step and the lab technician should be instructed to create space for cleaning.
- A strict periodontal support program is critical to achieve long-term success, as has been widely demonstrated by several authors (Axelsson et al. 1981).

Although all of these steps may seem overwhelming, the extraction of a periodontally compromised maxillary molar and its replacement with an implant may not be as hard as it seems. One should note that most of the time the sinus in that area is highly pneumatized and drops into the inter-radicular space. Once the tooth is extracted, an alveolar bone remodeling takes place, further reducing the amount of remaining crestal bone. Furthermore, posterior maxillary sextants are physiologically associated with poor bone quality, which is directly correlated with a higher implant failure rate (Jaffin and Berman 1991). Therefore, the alternative to root resection therapy may be tooth extraction followed by sinus elevation surgery and implant placement. Although this procedure is now considered to be routine, with good results (Del Fabbro et al. 2004), the data are rarely higher than those reported by Carnevale et al. (1998). A careful evaluation of each individual case, considering patient risk profile, local determinants, and possible alternatives, is always recommended.

### Tunnelization

This conservative technique has been employed in the treatment of advanced furcation lesions that mainly affect mandibular molars. The primary indication for this approach is the case of an existing Class III furcation with no or a minimal vertical component (Figure 7.25). The anatomy of the affected molar is critical to determining the possibility of performing this procedure. Usually a short or medium root trunk with divergent and long roots may be considered as an ideal candidate for this treatment. The technique includes a certain degree of osteoplasty/ostectomy to widen the furcation entrance and achieve a flat bone crest anatomy.

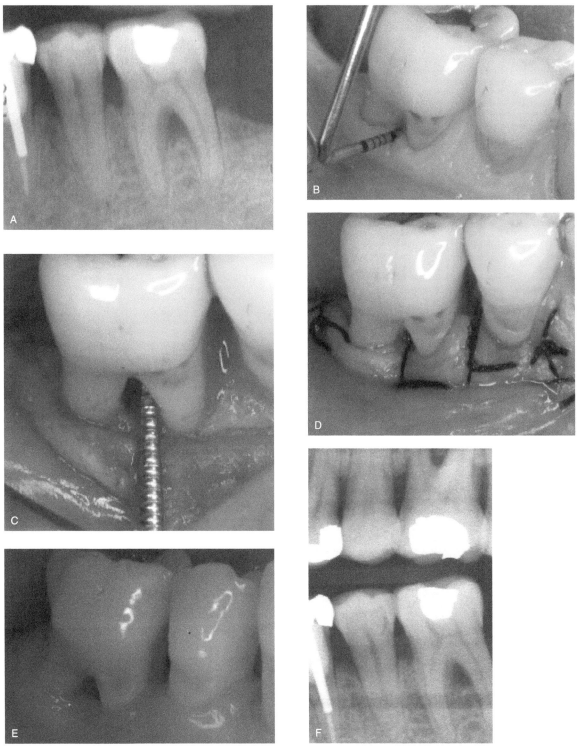

**Figure 7.25** A, A Class III furcation defect is documented radiographically, and B, clinically. C, Tunnelization is performed, and using a Sugerman bone file, the interradicular space is widened and the bone crest flattened. D, Silk sutures provide apical displacement of the tissue. E, Six months' healing shows an adequate opening of the furcation area for cleaning. F, Radiograph at one year, suggesting corticalization of the interradicular bone crest at the first molar with no sign of further loss of support.

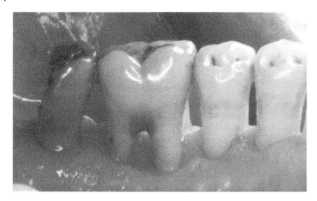

**Figure 7.26** Caries at the furcation of a tunnelized lower left first molar. The unrestored mesial root of a resected second molar is also present. The lack of an adequate prosthetic plan may well be considered a major drawback in this case.

Some odontoplasty has also been proposed to obtain better access to the furcation area. This should be done with great care because it may cause tooth hypersensitivity. Therefore, it is suggested that odontoplasty of the furcation entrance only be performed in the case of an endodontic-treated tooth or when the distance between the dome of the furcation and the floor of the pulp chamber is adequate. Once the osseous resection is accomplished the flap is apically positioned and a mattress suture is passed through the furcation to hold down the flap. As soon as the sutures are removed the patient must be instructed to use an interproximal brush or a superfloss to ensure good cleaning of the area.

**Evidence:** No large studies reporting on this technique have been published in the literature. Relative periodontal stability has been reported using this technique (Little et al. 1995; Muller et al. 1995). According to several authors, the major complication is related to the development of caries in the furcation area (Figure 7.26), with an incidence that ranged from 10% to 57% up to five years. (Hamp et al. 1975; Hellden et al. 1989; Ravald and Hamp 1981). Other authors were unable to report the same cario-susceptibility and described more favorable long-term results. A recent publication by Feres and coworkers (2006) reported on 30 tunnelized teeth in 18 subjects who were followed for a mean period of 3.6 years. Four teeth (13.4%) showed active caries, while there was no difference in the carious lesion between the inner and outer furcation area. Probing depth was, however, higher inside of the furcation compared to the radicular and interproximal sites.

## Author's Views/Comments

This treatment should be reserved for those cases in which a compromised treatment option is selected for strategic or financial reasons. In addition, careful analysis of the tooth anatomy and morphology (root length, interradicular space, root curvatures, etc.) must be reviewed before performing the procedure.

## References

Adriaens, P.A., DeBoever, J.A., and Loesche, W.J. (1988). Bacterial invasion in root cementum and radicular dentin of periodontally diseased teeth in humans—A reservoir of periodontopathic bacteria. *J. Periodontol.* 59: 222–230.

Axelsson, P. and Lindhe, J. (1981). Effect of controlled oral hygiene procedures on caries and periodontal disease in adults. *J. Clin. Periodontol.* 8 (3): 239–248.

Barrington, E.P. (1981). An overview of periodontal surgical procedures. *J. Periodontol.* 52: 518–528.

Becker W., Ochsenbein, C., Tibbetts, L., and Becker, B.E. (1997). Alveolar bone anatomic profiles as measured from dry skulls. Clinical ramification. *J. Clin. Perio.* 24: 727–780.

Bender, I.B. and Seltzer, S. (1972). The effect of periodontal disease on the pulp. *Oral Surg. Oral Med. Oral Pathol.* 33: 458–474.

Bissada, N.F. and Abdelmalek, R.G. (1973). Incidence of cervical enamel projections and its relationship to furcation involvement in Egyptian skulls. *J. Periodontol.* 44: 583–585.

Blomlof, L., Jansson, L., Applegren, R. et al. (1997). Prognosis and mortality of root resected molars. *Int. J. Period. Rest. Dent.* 17: 191–201.

Bower, R.C. (1979a). Furcation morphology relative to periodontal treatment—furcation entrance architecture. *J. Periodontol.* 50: 23.

Bower, R.C. (1979b). Furcation morphology relative to periodontal treatment—furcation root surface anatomy. *J. Periodontol.* 50: 366.

Buhler, H. (1988). Evaluation of root-resected teeth. *J. Peridontol.* 59: 805–810.

Burch, J.C. and Hulen, S. (1974). A study of the presence of accessory foramina and the topography of lower molar furcations. *Oral Surg. Oral Med. Oral Pathol.* 38: 451–454.

Caffesse, R., Sweeney, P.L. and Smith, B.A. (1986). Scaling and root planing with and without periodontal flap surgery. *J. Clin. Periodontol.* 13: 205.

Carnevale, G. (2007). Fibre retention osseous resective surgery: a novel conservative approach for pocket elimination. *J. Clin. Periodontol.* 34: 182–187.

Carnevale, G., Cordioli, G., Mazzocco, C., and Brugnolo, C. (1985). La tecnica della conservazione delle fibre gengivali. *Dent. Cadmos* 19: 15–40.

Carnevale, G., Di Febo, G., Tonelli, M.P. et al. (1991). A retrospective analysis of the periodontal-prosthetic treatment of molars with interradicular lesions. *Int. J. Perio. Rest. Dent.* 11 (3): 189–204.

Carnevale, G., Pontoriero, R., and Di Febo, G. (1998). Long term effects of root resective therapy in furcation involved molars. *J. Clin. Periodontol.* 25: 209–214.

Del Fabbro, M., Testori, T., Francetti, L., and Weinstein, R. (2004). Systematic review of survival rates for implants placed in the grafted maxillary sinus. *Int. J. Period. Rest. Dent.* 24: 565–577.

Donnenfeld, O., Hoag, P.M., and Weissman, D.P. (1970). A clinical study on the effects of osteoplasty. *J. Periodontol.* 41: 131–141.

Donnenfeld, O.W., Marks, R.M., and Glickman, I. (1964). The apically repositioned flap: a clinical study. *J. Periodontol.* 35: 381–387.

Elliott, G.M. and Bowers, G.M. (1963). Alveolar dehiscences and fenestrations. *Periodontics* 1: 245–248.

Erpenstein, H. (1983). A three-year study of hemisectioned molars. *J. Clin. Periodontol.* 10: 1–10.

Everett, F.G., Jump, E.B., Holder, T.D., and Williams, G.C. (1958). The intermediate bifurcational ridge: a study of the morphology of the bifurcation of the lower first molar. *J. Dent. Res.* 17: 62.

Feres, M., Araujo, M.W., Figueiredo, L.C., and Opperman, R.V. (2006). Clinical evaluation of tunneled molars: a retrospective study. *J. Int. Acad. Periodontol.* 8: 96–103.

Friedman, N. (1955). Periodontal osseous surgery: Osteoplasty and ostectomy. *J. Periodontol.* 26: 257–269.

Gargiulo, A., Wantz, F., and Orban, B. (1961). Dimensions of the dentogingival junction in humans. *J. Periodontol.* 32: 261.

Gher, M.E. and Vernino, A.R. (1980). Root morphology— Clinical significance in pathogenesis and treatment of periodontal disease. *J. Am. Dent. Assoc.* 101: 627–633.

Gutman, J.L. (1978). Prevalence, location and patency of accessory canals in the furcation region of permanent molars. *J. Periodontol.* 49: 21–26.

Hamp, S.E., Nyman, S., and Lindhe, J. (1975). Periodontal treatment of multi-rooted teeth. Results after 5 years. *J. Clin. Periodontol.* 2: 126–132.

Hellden, L.B., Elliot, A., Steffensen, B., and Steffensen, J. (1989). The prognosis of tunnel preparations in treatment of class III furcations. A follow-up study. *J. Periodontol.* 60: 182.

Ingber, J.S., Rose, L.F., and Coslet, J.G. (1977). The biologic width: A concept in periodontics and restorative dentistry. *Alpha Omegan* 10: 62–65.

Jaffin, C.L. and Berman, B.A. (1991). The excessive loss of Branemark fixtures in type IV bone. A 5-year study. *J. Periodontol.* 6: 2–5.

Kaldahl, W., Kalkwarf, K., Patil, K.I. et al. (1996). Long-term evaluation of periodontal therapy: I. Response to 4 therapeutic modalities. *J. Periodontol.* 67: 93–102.

Kalkwarf, K.L., Kaldahl, W.B., and Patil, K.D. (1988). Evaluation of furcation region response to periodontal therapy. *J. Periodontol.* 59 (12): 794–804.

Knowles, J., Burgett, F.G., Nissle, R.R. et al. (1979). Results of periodontal treatment related to pocket depth and attachment level—Eight years. *J. Periodontol.* 50: 225.

Langer, B., Stein, S.D., and Wagenberg, B. (1981). An evaluation of root resections. A ten-year study. *J. Periodontol.* 52 (12): 719.

Levy, R.M., Giannobile, W.V., Magda, F. et al. (2002). The effect of apically positioned flap surgery on the clinical parameters and the composition of subgingival microbiota. A 12-month study. *Int. J. Period. Rest. Dent.* 22: 209–219.

Little, L., Beck, B., Bagci, B., and Horton, J. (1995). Lack of furcal bone loss following the tunneling procedure. *J. Clin. Periodontol.* 22: 637–641.

Lowman, J.V., Burke, R.S., and Pelleu, G.B. (1973). Patent accessory canals: incidence in the molar furcation region. *Oral Surg. Oral Med. Oral Pathol.* 36: 580–584.

Majzoub, Z. and Kon, S. (1992). Root Resection of Maxillary First Molars. *J. Periodontal.* 63: 290–296.

Masters, D.H. and Hoskins, S.W. (1964). Projections of cervical enamel in molar furcations. *J. Periodontal.* 35: 49–53.

Matherson, D.G. (1988). An evaluation of healing following periodontal osseous surgery in monkeys. *Int. J. Period. Rest. Dent.* 8: 9–39.

Matia, J.I., Bissada, N.F., Maybury, J.E., and Ricchetti, P. (1987). Efficiency of scaling of the molar furcation area with and without surgical access. *Int. J. Perio. Rest. Dent.* 6: 25.

Moghaddas, H. and Stahl, S.S. (1980 July). Alveolar bone remodeling following osseous surgery. A clinical study. *J. Periodontal.* 51 (7): 376–381.

Mombelli, A., Nyman, S., Bragger, U. et al. (1995). Clinical and microbiological changes associated with an altered subgingival environment induced by periodontal pocket reduction. *J. Clin. Periodontal.* 22: 780–787.

Moskow, B.S. and Canut, P.M. (1990). Studies on root enamel (II). Enamel pearls. A review of their morphology, localization, nomenclature, occurrence, classification, histogenesis and incidence. *J. Clin. Periodontal.* 17: 275–281.

Muller, H.P., Eger, T., and Lange, D.E. (1995). Management of furcation-involved teeth. A retrospective analysis. *J. Clin. Periodontal.* 22: 911–917.

Ochsenbein, C. (1986). A primer for osseous surgery. *Int. J. Perio. Rest. Dent.* 6 (1): 8–47.

Ochsenbein, C. and Bohannan, H.M. (1963). The palatal approach to osseous surgery. I. Rationale. *J. Periodontal.* 34: 60–68.

Pennell, B., King, K.O., Wilderman, M.N., and Barron, J.M. (1967). Repair of the alveolar process following osseous surgery. *J. Periodontal.* 38: 426–431.

Polson, A.M. and Catou, J. (1982). Factors influencing periodontal repair and regenerization. *J Periodontal* 53 (7): 420–424.

Ramfjord, S.P, Caffessee, R.G., Morrison, E.C. et al. (1987). Four modalities of periodontal treatment compared over five years. *J. Clin. Periodontal.* 14: 445.

Ravald, N. and Hamp, S.E. (1981). Prediction of root surface caries in patients treated for advance periodontal disease. *J. Clin. Periodontal.* 8: 400–414.

Reiser, G.M., Bruno, J.F., Mahan, P.E., and Larkin, P.E. (1996). The subepithelial connective tissue graft palatal donor site: anatomic considerations for surgeons. *Int. J. Perio. Rest. Dent.* 16: 130–137.

Schluger, S. (1949). Osseous resection—A basic principle in periodontal surgery. *Oral Surg.* 2: 316–325.

Selipsky, H. (1976). Osseous surgery. How much need we compromise? *Dent. Clin. North Am.* 20: 79–106.

Siebert, J. (1976). Treatment of infrabony lesions by surgical resection procedures. In: *Periodontal Surgery: Biologic Basis and Technique* (ed. S.S. Stahl). Springfield, IL: Charles C. Thomas.

Smith, D.H., Ammons, W.F., and Van Belle, G. (1980). A longitudinal study of periodontal status comparing osseous recontouring with flap curettage. I. Results after 6 months. *J. Periodontol.* 51: 367.

Smukler, H. and Tagger, M. (1976). Vital root amputation: A clinical and histological study. *J. Periodontol.* 47: 324–330.

Swan, R.H. and Hurt, W.C. (1976). Cervical enamel projections as an etiologic factor in furcation involvement. *J. Am. Dent. Assoc.* 93: 342–345.

Tal, H. (1984). Relationship between the interproximal distance of roots and the prevalence of intrabony pockets. *J. Periodontol.* 55: 604–607.

Tarnow, D. and Fletcher, P. (1984). Classification of the vertical component of furcation involvement. *J. Periodontol.* 55: 283–284.

Tibbets, L., Ochsenbein, C., and Loughlin, D.M. (1976). Rationale for the lingual approach to mandibular osseous surgery. *Dent. Clin. North Am.* 20: 61–78.

Vertucci, F.J. and Williams, R.G. (1974). Furcation canals in the human mandibular first molar. *Oral Surg. Oral Med. Oral Pathol.* 38: 308–314.

Wilderman, M.N., Pennell, B., King, K.O., and Barron, J.M. (1970). Histogenesis of repair following osseous surgery. *J. Periodontol.* 41: 551–565.

Wood, D.L., Hoag, P.M., Donnenfeld, O., and Rosenfeld, L.D. (1972). Alveolar crest reduction following full and partial thickness flaps. *J. Periodontol.* 43: 141–144.

# 8

# Contemporary Periodontal Regenerative Treatment

*Ronaldo Barcellos de Santana, Mehmet Ilhan Uzel, and Carolina Miller Mattos de Santana*

Despite the successful clinical results, conventional therapeutic procedures present significant variability depending on the intrinsic healing potential of the patient, which are typically observed as long junctional epithelium and limited regeneration of the periodontal attachment apparatus due to minimal cementogenesis and limited bone formation (Listgarten and Rosenberg 1979; Steiner et al. 1981; Waerhaug 1978). Ideally, the healing process should reestablish the original tissue architecture and function of the support tissues previously destroyed, including the regeneration of alveolar bone, radicular cementum, and periodontal ligament (Caton and Greenstein 1993; Listgarten and Rosenberg 1979; Mellonig 1999). Therefore, several procedures have been employed to optimize the regenerative potential of periodontal lesions, including bone grafts and substitutes, barrier membranes for guided tissue regeneration, bioactive substances such as growth factors and enamel matrix derivatives and combination of these techniques and materials (Pretzl et al. 2009; Sanz et al. 2004, Siciliano et al. 2011; Thakare and Deo 2012; Yukna et al. 2002).

In conjunction with, and irrespective of, the selection of an adequate regenerative approach, the use of a sound treatment protocol and surgical technique is mandatory to optimize the clinical results including the flap design, treatment of the root surface, treatment of the bone defect, maintenance and control and timing of reevaluation.

## Flap Design

Adequate flap design is an important element in periodontal regenerative therapy in order to provide adequate access for root instrumentation, bone defect debridement, placement of regenerative materials in the periodontal defect, and attaining primary coverage of the surgical site. Several types of flaps have been used, including the modified Widman flap (Cortellini et al. 1995; de Miranda et al 2013; Santana et al 1999), the papilla preservation flap (Takei et al. 1989),

modified papilla preservation flap (Cortellini et al. 1995; Santana and de Santana 2015), simplified papilla preservation flap (Cortellini et al 1999), interproximal tissue maintenance (Murphy 1996), and single flap approaches (Trombelli et al. 2012). Traditionally, conventional flap designs such as the modified Widman flap were employed for the treatment of intrabony (Cortellini et al. 1999) and furcation defects (de Miranda et al. 2013; Santana and Van Dyke 1999); however, conventional surgical approaches performed with vertical releasing incisions and without interdental papilla preservation may result in deficient flap closure, limited blood clot stability and, possibly, negatively impacting periodontal wound healing. Thus, the necessity to obtain and maintain adequate levels of soft tissue coverage post-surgery led to the increased test and development of alternative approaches.

The coronally positioned flap was proposed as a method to obtain coverage of regenerative materials and primary closure of the surgical site; however, limited additional benefit in probing depth reduction and attachment level gain was provided after the use of this flap design in the treatment of human furcation defects, in comparison with the modified Widman flap, except for significantly reduced postsurgical gingival recession (Santana and Van Dyke 1999). However, positive outcomes were reported for this procedure when used in conjunction with guided tissue regeneration and bone substitutes (Santana and Van Dyke 1999, Santana et al. 2009).

In order to optimize the healing potential of human intrabony defects, several technical modifications were proposed in order to favor the maintenance of the interproximal soft tissue coverage flap closure (Cortellini et al. 1995; 1999; Murphy 1996; Takei et al. 1989; Trombelli et al. 2012). The preservation of the interproximal soft tissues may result in higher blood clot stability within the periodontal defect and faster vascular stability in the papillary area (Retzepi et al. 2007), promoting primary wound healing, improved wound instability and, ultimately, enhanced clinical results in the treatment of human

*Practical Periodontal Diagnosis and Treatment Planning*, Second Edition. Edited By Serge Dibart and Thomas Dietrich.

intrabony defects (Cortellini and Tonetti 2007a, 2007b; Cortellini et al. 2008; Retzepi et al. 2007). Increased reduction in probing depth and attachment levels with minimal gingival recession and less postoperative discomfort has been reported (Graziani et al. 2012).

## Bone Grafts and Bone Substitutes

Bone grafts and bone substitutes are biocompatible particulate biomaterials that are placed directly into periodontal bone defects to serve as scaffolds for cell attachment, migration, and differentiation.

Several bone grafts/substitutes have been used in the regenerative treatment of periodontal defects, including autografts, allografts, xenografts, and alloplastic materials (Sculean et al. 2015). For many years, bone autografts were considered the gold standard for bone regeneration due to its potential osteogenic, osteoconductive, and osteoinductive potentials. Clinical evidence, however, did not demonstrate significantly enhanced clinical results in comparison to periodontal open flap debridement procedures without the use of bone grafting (Froum et al. 1976; Renvert et al. 1985). Histological evidence in humans is controversial, with some studies demonstrating periodontal regeneration (Dragoo & Sullivan 1973a, 1973b; Hiatt et al. 1978; Stahl et al. 1983), while others demonstrated the formation of a long junctional epithelium (Listgarten and Rosenberg 1979), particularly for bone grafts harvested from intraoral sources. Moreover, complications such as ankylosis and root resorption were also reported, particularly following the use of bone allografts from extra-oral sites, such as medullary bone from the iliac crest (Dragoo and Sullivan 1973a, 1973b). Taken together, the current evidence may limit the indication of bone autografts for the treatment of periodontal bone defects.

Bone allografts may contain bone morphogenetic proteins, providing these materials with osteoinductive activities (Miron et al. 2016; Schwartz et al. 1996, 1998). However, the osteoinductive activity of bone allografts such as DFDBA varies significantly depending on the manufacturer or the gender of the donor (Schwartz et al. 1996, 1998). Thus, adequate donor selection and manufacturing processes that preserve the bioactivity of the material appear to be critical for the production and clinical use of these materials (Schwartz et al. 1996, 1998). In conjunction with adequate clinical (Barnett et al. 1989; Flemmig et al. 1998; Meadows et al. 1993; Rummelhart et al. 1989) and histologic results (Bowers et al. 1989a, 1989b), robust histologic evidence of periodontal regeneration in humans were reported (Bowers et al. 1989a, 1989b) following the use of these materials.

Several xenogeneic materials, derived from bovine, swine, or equine sources, have also been employed, and act as an inert bone scaffold of tridimensional structure like the mineralized bone matrix. It has been hypothesized that these materials could present the risk of antigenicity, being derived from other species (Oliveira et al. 2008) and, despite controversial, the risk for prion infection has also being considered (Kim et al. 2013, 2016). Adequate clinical (Figures 8.10 to 8.17) results were reported for these materials in the treatment of periodontal defects (Camargo et al. 2000; Cosyn et al. 2012; De Bruyckere et al. 2018; Pietruska 2001; Richardson et al 1999; Scheyer et al. 2002; Sculean et al. 2002b).

Systematic analysis of histologic preclinical essays, in which regenerative therapies were used for the treatment of periodontal defects (Ivanovic et al. 2014), demonstrated that most of the biomaterials, used alone or combined, promoted more extensive periodontal regeneration than conventional open flap procedures without the use of biomaterials (Ivanovic et al. 2014). Systematic reviews also concluded that the use of bone grafts/substitutes resulted in significant enhancement in attachment levels, probing depth reduction, increased bone fill, and reduced crestal resorption in comparison with open flap debridement (Reynolds 2003). However, attachment level gains varied significantly among the several individual biomaterials (Trombelli 2002). Similar clinical results were obtained for allografts and alloplastic materials (Barnett et al. 1989; Bowen et al. 1989; Oreamuno et al. 1990). The combined use of bone grafts and membranes can result in increased gains of attachment, bigger probing depth reduction and more defect filling than membranes used alone (Murphy and Gunsolley 2003; Needleman et al. 2006). It has been reported that the use of alloplastic materials may reduce postsurgical gingival recession (Leknes et al. 2009), possibly by avoiding the collapse of the soft tissues into the bone defects. Histologically, DFDBA, autografts, and some xenografts result in the formation of new attachment and periodontal regeneration (Sculean et al. 2003a; Sculean et al. 2003b; Sculean et al. 2005b; Sculean et al. 2015), while the results for alloplastic materials are more limited, specially, when employed in monotherapy (Sculean et al. 2015). However, some alloplastic materials can result in periodontal regeneration when employed in conjunction with enamel matrix derivatives (Sculean et al. 2008c).

## Guided Tissue Regeneration

Guided tissue regeneration is a treatment concept based on the use of membranes or barriers interposed between the surgical flap and the periodontal defect to mechanically exclude non-regenerative cells from the gingival epithelium and connective tissue from the regenerative events at the defect area (Figures 8.1 to 8.9). The modern biological concepts of guided tissue regeneration (GTR) is based in the establishment of a protected environment for the blood clot and competent regenerative cells via the interposition of a physical barrier between the soft tissues of the gingival flap and the osseous defect/root surfaces in order to isolate a secluded space, thus, allowing cells from the periodontal ligament and bone to recolonize the defect area and regenerate the periodontal attachment apparatus (Caffesse et al. 1988; 1990; Gottlow et al. 1986; Magnusson et al. 1988; Nyman et al. 1982; Pitaru et al. 1987; Pfeifer et al. 1989). These concepts have been used clinically for the treatment of several periodontal and bone deformities such as periodontal intrabony (Cortellini and Tonetti 2000), furcation (Santana and Van Dyke 1999; Santana et al. 2009) (Figures 8.6 to 8.10), and recession defects (Trombelli and Calura G 1993); closure of oro-antral communications (Waldrop and Semba 1993); surgical treatment of periodontal defects associated with palato-gingival developmental grooves (Rankow and Kassner 1996); reconstruction of bone defects following surgical removal of oral cysts or tumors (Vitkus and Meltzer 1996); autogenous tooth transplantation (Hurzeler and

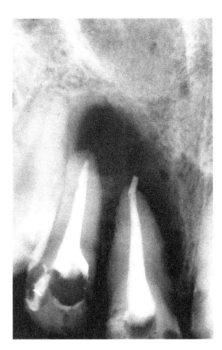

Figure 8.2 Radiographic view at baseline. Santana et al., 2013 / Reproduced with permission from John Wiley & Sons.

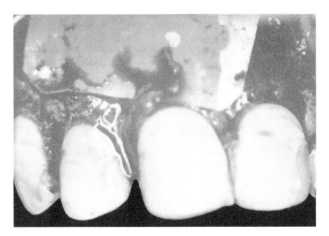

Figure 8.3 Area was grafted with microparticulate hydroxyapaptite and the surgical site was covered with PTFE membranes after root management and apical retrofilling. The flap was coronally advanced and stabilized with interrupted sutures. Santana et al., 2013 / Reproduced with permission from John Wiley & Sons.

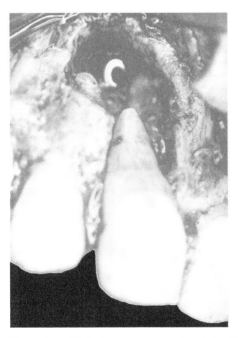

Figure 8.1 Clinical trans-surgical view. A significant bucco-palatal through-and-through maxillary bone defect can be observed extending apically up to the nasal floor. Santana et al., 2013 / Reproduced with permission from John Wiley & Sons.

Quinones 1993); surgical treatment of advanced apical or combined apical-marginal lesions associated with absence of buccal alveolar bone wall (Rankow and Kassner 1996, Santana and Santana 2013) (Figures 8.1 to 8.5); maintenance or enhancement of the osseous ridge, following root amputation of multi-rooted teeth (Conner 1996); and prevention or treatment of distal

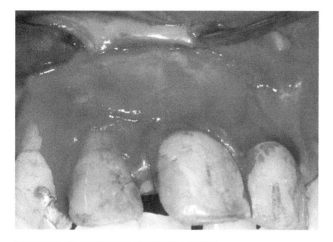

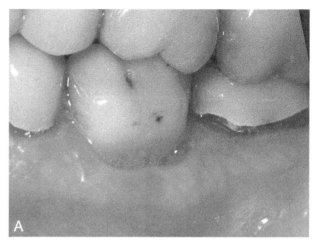

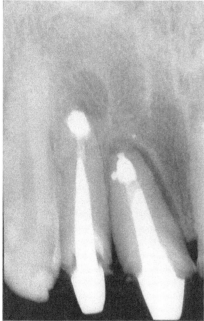

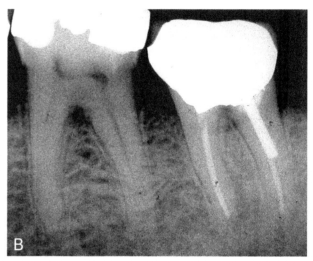

Figure 8.5 Baseline clinical (A) and radiographic view (B). A buccal class II furcation involvement was detected on the mandibular left first molar.

Figure 8.4 Trans-surgical view at the time of membrane removal nine months after the surgical procedure (A) and radiographic view after 15 years of healing demonstrates significant and stable periodontal healing and bone fill. Santana et al., 2013 / Reproduced with permission from John Wiley & Sons.

osseous defects following the removal of impacted third molars (Oxford et al. 1997).

Several materials have been tested as barrier membranes for GTR. These materials exhibit differences in chemical composition, physical properties, and macroscopic and microscopic structure. Criteria for the design of GTR membranes have been proposed (Scanttlebury 1993), and include tissue integration capacity, cell occlusivity properties, clinical manageability, space making ability, and biocompatibility. The biological response to implanted biomaterials is a critical element in reconstructive biology. Significant differences have been described for the response of living tissues to implanted barrier membranes, possibly related to the surface topography and porosity of the device (Buchmann et al. 2001; Lu et al. 2004; Lundgren et al. 1995; Scanttlebury et al 1993; Santana et al. 2010; Wikesjo et al. 2003).

## Nonabsorbable Devices

Polytetrafluorethilene (PTFE) is an inert and biocompatible material. Due to a unique molecular composition and configuration PTFE presents with low chemical reactivity, great stability, and low superficial energy of the polymer. There is no solvent that can dissolve PTFE in temperatures lower than 3,000°C. PTFE can be utilized as barrier devices in porous, dense, and expanded forms (Crump et al. 1996; Scattlebury 1993). Other materials tested as nonabsorbable

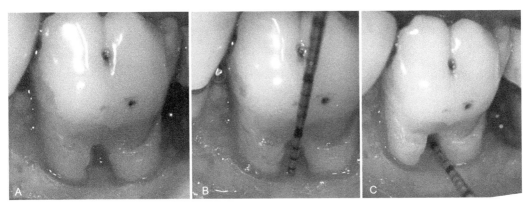

Figure 8.6 Trans surgical view after full-thickness flap reflection and mechanical root treatment (A) revealed 3.5 mm vertical (B) and 7 mm horizontal (C) buccal interradicular bone loss.

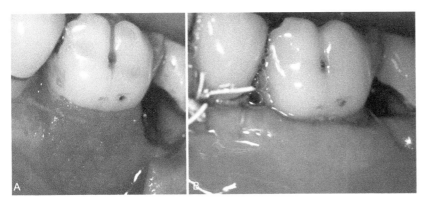

Figure 8.7 A synthetic polylactic acid barrier membrane was adjusted and sutured over the defect (A) and the gingival flap was released, coronally advanced, and sutured with suspensory sutures (B).

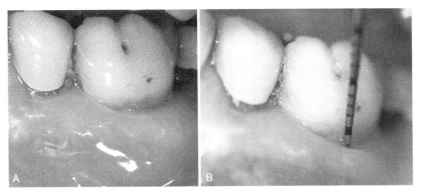

Figure 8.8 Clinical view one year after treatment demonstrated clinically health gingival tissues (A), absence of bleeding on probing, and 2.5 mm probing depth (B).

barriers include microfibrillar alkali-cellulose, aluminum, and titanium. Microfibrillar alkali-cellulose is a safe and biocompatible material, primarily used as a skin substitute for burned people (Novaes Jr. et al 1990a, 1990b, 1992). A core of commercially-pure aluminum (minimum 99.35% of Al), superficially coated with aluminum oxide (minimum of 99.48% of $Al_2O_3$), in a laminated form, $Al_2O_3$ is a ceramic material which has biocompatibility characteristics similar to titanium and tantalus oxides ($TiO_2$, $Ta_2O_5$) that has been used as constituents of endosseous dental implants, both in single-crystal and polycrystalline forms (Babbush et al. 1987; Kawahara and Hirabayashi 1980). Biocompatibility of this material appears to be derived from its high dielectric constant, biomolecule adsorption

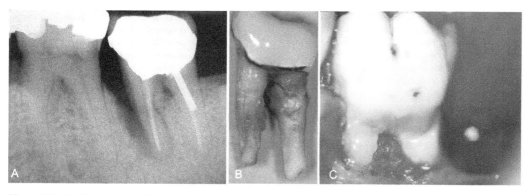

**Figure 8.9** Radiographic evaluation performed five years after treatment revealed significantly increased radiopacity on the furcation of the treated first molar, however, the second molar exhibited clinical and radiographic signs of vertical mesial root fracture (A), which could be confirmed after the tooth was extracted (B) during surgical bone reconstructive approach for implant placement (C). The furcation area of the treated first molar, however, was completely closed with new bone (C).

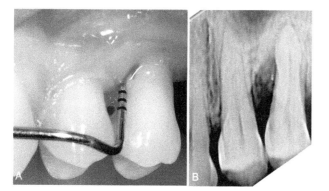

**Figure 8.10** Baseline clinical (A) and radiographic view (B). Deep probing depths, bleeding on probing (A), and vertical radiographic bone radiolucency (B) were noted on the mesial aspect of the maxillary second premolar.

capacity, chemical inertness to corrosion, low dielectric potential difference, and catalyst activity (Kawahara and Hirabayashi 1980; Yamagami et al. 1988). Among the several alternatives for nonabsorbable devices, PTFE is the most studied and well characterized.

## Synthetic Absorbable Devices

Several synthetic materials have been tested as resorbable GTR membranes. Calcium sulfate is one of the materials that have been tested as a barrier for GTR applications (Conner 1996; Sottosanti 1992, 1993, 1995). Although reintroduced in the 90s, similar materials have been used for more than 100 years in medicine and dentistry as adjuncts for bone regeneration (Peltier 1959; Shaffer and App 1971). At present, it is composed of absorbable medical grade calcium sulfate monohydrate ($CaSO_4$), plaster of Paris, mixed with a premeasured accelerator solution. It is used as a barrier over autogenous or allogenous bone grafts, in order to maintain the graft in place. Spagnuolo and Bissada (1995) proposed a new resorbable composite barrier for the

treatment of adult periodontitis membrane composed of calcium sulfate monohydrate ($CaSO_4$) combined to DFDBA and doxycycline in a 4:1:1 ratio by volume.

Polyglactin 910 is a lactide-glicolide copolymer which has been long used as a resorbable suture material (Conn et al. 1974). Such material seemed to be inert, non-antigenic, and non-pyogenic, presenting only a mild tissue reaction during absorption (Conn et al. 1974). It has been manufactured as a mesh for use in neurosurgery (Maurer and McDonald 1985) and is composed of undyed fiber, identical in composition to that of the absorbable sutures. This mesh has also been tested for GTR procedures (Cristgau et al. 1998; Eikholtz and Hausman 1998; Fleisher et al 1988).

A synthetic, liquid polymer of lactic acid, poly(DL-lactide), dissolved in N-methyl-2-pyrrolidone(NMP), has been developed for GTR purposes (Polson et al. 1994, 1995).This material exists as a fluid which transforms to a solid on contact with water or other aqueous solutions. This property is used to form an adaptable partially set barrier extraorally, which is rigid enough to provide GTR function but flexible enough to be easily adapted to the surgical site. The barrier continues to solidify in situ and subsequently bioabsorbs via hydrolysis (Garrett et al 1997). It has a similar composition, rate of absorption, and safety performance as that of Polyglactin 910. It has been shown to be safe, nontoxic, resorbable, and efficacious for GTR attempts in animals and humans (Garrett et al. 1997; Polson et al. 1994, 1995).

Various other polylactic acid-based products have been evaluated for their potential use in GTR surgeries, such as (a) polylactic acid dissolved in chloroform (Magnusson et al. 1988), (b) polylactic acid blended to a citric acid ester (Gottlow 1993), and (c) a polylactic acid porous sheet (Vernino et al. 1995). Such materials are absorbed by hydrolysis and seem to break down with minimal inflammatory reaction (Vernino et al. 1995), which seems to be consistent with a material that was biologically acceptable in the wound healing environment (Vernino et al. 1995). A hydrophilic, biodegradable membrane fabricated from D,L-polylactic acid was introduced (Vernino et al. 1998, 1999). The thickness of this membrane measures from 175 to 250 μm, and the polymer of the membrane is organized in an architecture of randomly sized, randomly positioned, intercommunicating interstices ranging in size from 10 to 15 μm. One surface of the membrane, constituting approximately 10% of the total thickness, is considerably denser than the remainder of the device (Vernino et al. 1998). Another of these polylactic acid-based products is a bioabsorbable material consisting of polylactic acid comprising L-and D-lactic acid enantiomers, and acetyl-tributyl citrate, a citric acid ester. It has a multilayered matrix designed for ingrowth of gingival connective tissue. Periodontal ligament and alveolar bone can also migrate into the matrix and merge with the gingiva. Thus, the matrix barrier would allow for simultaneous regeneration and integration following a single surgical procedure (Gottlow 1993). Clinical results were reported for the treatment of human gingival recession, furcation, and intraosseous lesions with this material (Cristgau et al. 1998; Luepke et al. 1997; Pini Prato et al. 1995).

## Organic Absorbable Devices

Among the products of organic or natural sources, collagen-based devices of different types and origins are probably the most commonly used as barrier membranes due to its weak immunogenic capacity and long-term experimental use in animals and humans (Pitaru et al. 1988). Several characteristics of collagen seem to support its use as barrier membranes for GTR purposes (Pitaru et al. 1988). Collagen is the major extracellular macromolecule of the periodontal connective tissues (Posthlethwaite et al 1978) that can act as a barrier for migrating gingival epithelial cells (Pitaru et al. 1987) by providing a thrombogenic surface (Blumenthal 1993) that inhibits the mitotic function of the basal epithelial cells during the initial phases of wound healing (Numabe et al. 1993), thus limiting the apical migration of epithelium. Simultaneously, the hemostatic properties of collagen (Pitaru et al. 1988) may enhance blood clot stability in the bony defect, while exhibiting a chemotactic activity for fibroblasts (Posthlewaite et al. 1978). Despite the past controversies regarding the safety of using collagenous membranes in human clinical trials, due to localized hypersensitivity reactions developed in sites where collagen was injected (Kammer and Chukurian 1984), collagenous membranes did not elicit any abnormal immunologic responses when implanted as a barrier membrane during GTR attempts in humans (Black et al. 1994; Blumenthal 1993; Mattson et al. 1995; Numabe et al. 1993).

Autogenous "periosteum" grafts were proposed by Lekovic et al. (1991) as an alternative for GTR barriers. In this technique, a partial thickness connective tissue graft is obtained from the palate of the patient, then trimmed and adjusted as a barrier to cover the periodontal defect to be treated according to the principles of GTR. In controlled studies, this technique demonstrated significantly better results than the controls treated by a modified Widman flap procedure (Lekovic et al. 1991), and similar results to those obtained by ePTFE barriers (Bouchard et al. 1993) in the treatment of human mandibular furcation lesions. However, the necessity of a second surgical site to obtain the graft, the limited and great variability of the results obtained with this technique diminished its applicability in routine regenerative periodontal therapy.

Particulate decalcified freeze-dried bone allografts (DFDBA) have been used for many years as a periodontal grafting material (Gouldin et al. 1996; Mellado et al. 1995; Mellonig 1984; Pearson et al. 1981; Quintero et al. 1982; Wallace et al. 1994) due to the safety, biocompatibility, and very weak immunogenic properties of these materials (Friedlaeder et al 1984; Quattlebaum et al. 1988; Turner and Mellonig 1981). Moreover, possible osteoinductive capacity, due to the presence of bone morphogenetic proteins (BMPs), may be retained in the material following its processing (Urist 1965; Urist and Dowell 1968; Urist et al. 1967), promoting bone inductive abilities in vivo (Mellonig et al. 1981a, 1982, 1981b, 1983). Despite the demonstration of biological activity of DFDBA (Shigeyama et al. 1995), such activity could be variable, depending on the source of the product, donor characteristics, and the processing of the material (Schwartz et al. 1996). Thus, the effectiveness of particulate DFDBA on periodontal regeneration has been questioned (Becker et al. 1994, 1995). Laminar sheets of DFDBA are available and have been successfully employed as barriers for GTR (Rankow and

Kassner 1996; Scott et al. 1997; Yamaoka et al. 1996). Positive results were reported in the treatment of human furcation defects (Scott et al. 1997; Yamaoka et al. 1996).

Bioabsorbable composite matrixes were also tested as a barrier for clinical use in GTR applications (Costa-Noble et al 1996). The basic components of this material are elastin and fibrin monomers that are combined under specific physicochemical conditions. The crude product obtained is then further processed with fibronectin, type I collagen, and other aggregating agents as sulfur derivatives and gamma-rays to obtain optimum cohesivity. The derived material is also associated with polyglactic networks to obtain good saturability and treated with aprotinin to control the degradation rate.

Histologic preclinical studies demonstrated that barrier membranes used alone or combined with bone grafts/substitutes result in bone (Santana et al. 2010) and periodontal regeneration (Sculean et al. 2008c). Enhanced results were observed for the combined therapies employing membranes and bone grafts/substitutes in comparison to the use of membranes alone in noncontained two-wall defects and supra-alveolar defects, while no additional benefit was observed for the combined therapy for three-wall defects (Sculean et al. 2008c). Results from histological studies in humans are partially divergent than these results obtained in animals.

The results of clinical studies and systematic reviews demonstrated that regenerative therapies with barrier membranes provide significant clinical benefits, in comparison with open flap procedures alone, as evaluated by reduced gingival recession, probing depth reduction, attachment level gain, and bone fill (Cortellini and Tonetti 2000; Murphy and Gunsolley 2003; Needleman et al. 2005). Clinical results may be maintained for several years in most patients enrolled in frequent periodontal supportive therapy, even with severe intrabony defects (Cortellini et al 2004). Positive outcomes have also been reported for the combined use of membranes and synthetic graft materials in the treatment of human furcation defects (Santana and Van Dyke 1999; Santana et al. 2009). No significant difference was reported for the several types of membranes evaluated; however, the use of different types of membranes may explain the significant variability of clinical results reported in different studies (Murphy and Gunsolley 2003; Needleman 2006).

## Bioactive Substances

The use of bioactive substances offers a new paradigm in periodontal reconstructive therapy as a resource to amplify or accelerate the endogenous healing potential with new therapies that act at the cellular and molecular levels to enhance the periodontal wound healing and regeneration of the attachment apparatus.

### Autogenous Platelet Concentrates

Autogenous platelet concentrates preparations have been widely tested as regenerative biomaterials in periodontics. The main goal of these preparations is to obtain concentrate supraphysiological doses of autologous growth factors from centrifugated blood (Kobayashi et al. 2016). Several types of platelet concentrates have been described, depending on the centrifugation protocol employed (Castro et al. 2019; Choukroun 2015; Choukroun et al. 2001; Cortellini et al. 2018; Miron et al. 2019a, 2019b, 2017; Wend et al. 2017). Platelet rich plasma (PRP) is a platelet concentrate produced using anticoagulants and high g-forces to selectively separate blood cells based on density, under the centrifugation cycles ranging from 15 min to 1 h, depending on the specific harvesting kits employed. PRP protocols traditionally result in the production of three layers: the upper or platelet-poor (acellular) layer, the middle platelet-rich (buffy coat) layer, and a bottom red blood cell (RBC corpuscle) layer. Since anticoagulants are utilized, the cell layers are separated without coagulating; however, it has been also reported that anticoagulant incorporation in formulations may negatively impact tissue regeneration (Anfossi et al. 1989; Fijnheer et al. 1990; Marx 2004).

Platelet-rich fibrin (PRF) was developed as a second-generation platelet concentrate with the aim of eliminating the need for anticoagulants (Choukroun et al. 2001). In this protocol, the centrifugation times were significantly reduced to only 8–12 min. An important modification of the PRF protocol, denominated advanced PRF (A-PRF), was the decreased centrifugation speeds from 2,700 rpm to 1,300 rpm, resulting in a PRF formulation with a higher number of leukocytes which were also more evenly distributed throughout the blood clot (Choukroun 2015; Miron et al. 2019a). This preparation demonstrated higher growth factor release and increased fibroblast migration, proliferation, and collagen mRNA levels than the traditional PRF (Fujioka-Kobayashi et al. 2017; Kobayashi et al. 2016).

The injectable PRF (iPRF) is a variation of the protocol that was developed by further reducing centrifugation speed and time and by using centrifugation tubes with more hydrophobic materials to reduce clotting times (Miron et al. 2017). Comparatively to PRP protocols, the iPRF protocol results in a low yield of isolated platelets and leukocytes (Miron et al. 2019b; Varela et al 2019), which demonstrate significantly increased cellular activity (Abd El Raouf et al. 2017; Miron et al. 2017; Wang et al. 2017, 2018). However, the total platelet yield and growth factor release is higher on PRP preparations (Miron et al. 2017). More recently, in order to improve the platelet and leukocyte yields of i-PRF, a novel protocol, termed concentrated PRF (C-PRF), has been developed (Castro et al. 2019; Cortellini et al. 2018; Miron et al. 2019b; Wend et al. 2017). In this novel protocol, centrifugation times are increased to 4–8 min, centrifugation speeds are increased to 2,700–3,000 rpm, and a horizontal centrifugation (as opposed to conventional fixed angle centrifugation) is employed (Castro et al. 2019; Cortellini et al. 2018; Miron et al. 2019b; Wend et al. 2017). These modifications resulted in increased platelets accumulation in the upper i-PRF layer (Wend et al. 2017), and higher platelet and leukocyte yields and concentrations (Castro et al. 2019; Cortellini et al. 2018; Miron et al. 2019b). Interestingly, a study that employed a modified L-PRF protocol (2,700 rpm for 12 min) found that the top 4 mL layer was completely devoid of cells, while the majority of cells, amounting to tenfold the cell counts at baseline, were found within the buffy coat layer immediately above the RBC corpuscle layer (Miron 2019b). These cells derived from the buffy coat may secrete up to threefold the amount of growth factors release (PDGF-AA, TGF-B1, and EGF) in comparison to the conventional iPRF protocol (Fujioka-Kobayashi et al. 2020). The PRF obtained from this harvesting technique was named concentrated PRF (C-PRF) and this preparation may exhibit higher growth factor release as well as superior cellular activity.

Data from a recent systematic review of randomized clinical studies demonstrated that the use of PRF in conjunction with open flap debridement resulted in significant improvements in probing depth reduction, attachment level gains, and bone fill (Miron et al. 2021). However, when PRF was used in conjunction with or versus bone grafts/substitutes most of the studies included in the review failed to demonstrate additional benefits of PRF in probing depth reduction or attachment level gain (Miron et al. 2021).

### Enamel Matrix Derivative

Amelogenins are a heterogeneous group of low molecular weight proteins which are the most prevalent (>90%) component of the organic fraction of enamel (Esposito et al. 2004). These proteins promote the adhesion and proliferation of periodontal ligament cells, increased secretion of growth factors (TGF-1, PDGF-AB, IGF-I), production of extracellular matrix (hyalurans, proteoglycans, versican, biglycan and decorin), and mineralization (Gestrelius et al. 1997b; Petinaki et al. 1998). The pool of hydrophobic amelogenins, designated enamel matrix derivative (EMD), are expressed during cementogenesis and have been employed clinically for stimulating periodontal regeneration (Caton

1997). The enamel matrix derivative (EMD), dispersed in propileneglycol-alginate (PGA), is commercially available as Emdogain® (EMD) (Venezia et al. 2004; Zetterstrom et al. 1997) and is a biologic agent for stimulating periodontal regeneration (Sculean et al. 2002b).

The biological effects of EMD appear to replicate the embryonic phases of odontogenesis. After being applied to a previously instrumented root surface, these compounds precipitate and form an unsoluble (Fisher and Termine 1985) layer of proteins which stimulate cementoblasts to deposit new root cementum and promote selective cell repopulation by periodontal ligament cells (Hammaström et al. 1997a; Heijl 1997; Zetterstrom et al. 1997). These events promote the regeneration of the attachment apparatus (Gestrelius et al. 2000; Hammarström et al. 1997b; Hirooka 1998; Minsk 2000) and prevent the apical migration of junctional epithelium (Cochran and Wozney 1999). The clinical use of EMD may result in the formation of new alveolar bone, periodontal ligament, and cementum in bone defects previously contaminated by the bacterial biofilm (Sculean et al. 2015), similarly to true periodontal regeneration (Gestrelius et al 1997a; Heijl 1997; Heden et al. 1999; Rasperin et al. 1999; Silvestri et al. 2003; Fong and Hammastrom 2000).

Results from controlled clinical studies, meta-analyses, and systematic reviews of the treatment of periodontal defects with EMD have demonstrated that this therapy results in additional clinical benefits in relation to significant gains in attachment level, reduction in probing depth and bone gains in comparison with open flap debridement alone (Esposito et al. 2009; Matarasso et al. 2015, 2015; Murphy and Gunsolley 2003; Needleman et al. 2002). These additional clinical outcomes appear to be similar to those reported for guided tissue regeneration with membranes, however, with significant lower frequency of complications (Esposito et al. 2005; Esposito et al. 2009), including less gingival recession, lower frequency of flap dehiscence, and occurrence of abscesses (Crea 2008; Sanz 2004; Silvestri 2003; Zucchelli et al. 2002). Evidence of periodontal regeneration in humans has been reported for the use of EMD alone or combined with autogenous bone, bovine bone mineral (Figures 8.11 to 8.17), bovine bone mineral associated to PRP, bioactive glass, nanocrystalline HA, and biphasic calcium phosphate (Yukna and Mellonig 2000; Windwisch et al 2002; Cochran et al. 2003; Sculean et al. 2003a, 2005b; 2008a, 2008b).

### Platelet-derived Growth Factor—rhPDGF

PDGF (platelet-derived growth factor) is a polypeptide biologic mediator that is intimately related to the processes of bone remodeling with systemic and local actions. This

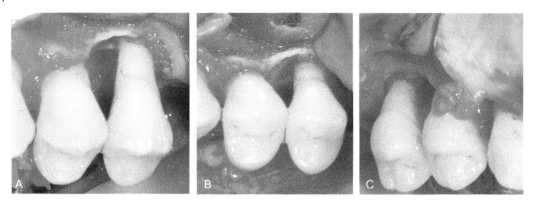

Figure 8.11 Trans surgical view after full-thickness flap reflection and mechanical root treatment (A to C) revealed deep intrabony defect on the mesial and palatal aspects of the maxillary second premolar.

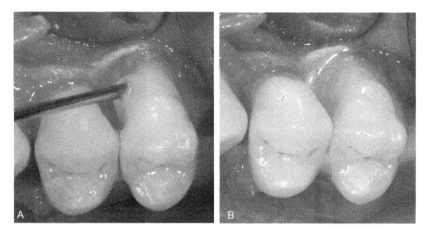

Figure 8.12 Following mechanical instrumentation, the roots were chemically conditioned for 3 min with a 24% EDTA gel (A and B), and then abundantly washed with a saline solution.

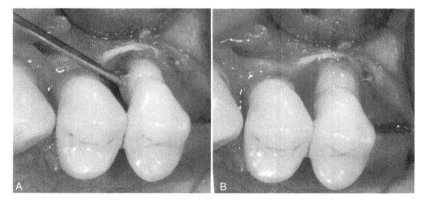

Figure 8.13 An EMD gel (Emdogain®) was applied over the root surfaces (A) and into the bone defect (B).

substance stimulates protein and bone DNA synthesis, and is capable to interact with other hormones and growth factors locally (Canalis et al. 1988). During periodontal regeneration it appears to be related to directed cellular migration of osteoblasts, cementoblasts, periodontal ligament cells, and endothelial cells (Irokawa et al. 2010).

It has been commercially available since 2005 as a synthetic biomaterial (GEM21S®, Lynch Biologics, Franklin, TN), indicated for bone grafting and periodontal regeneration, composed of 0.5 ml of rhPDGF (0.3 mg/ml) and 0.5 cc of β-TCP (β-tricalcium phosphate) (Nevins et al. 2009). The β-TCP is used as a scaffold (Jensen et al. 2006;

Figure 8.14   A particulate bovine xenograft was preconditioned with EMD and carefully packed into the bone defect.

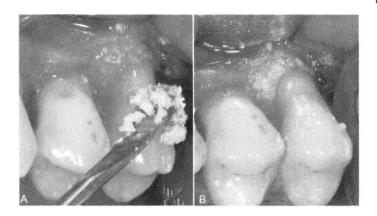

Figure 8.15   A new layer of EMD gel was applied over the grafted area (A) and root surfaces (B).

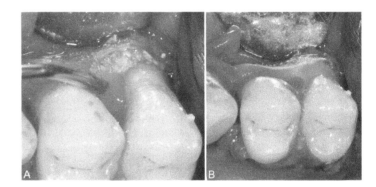

Figure 8.16   The flap was coronally advanced and sutured with interrupted sutures.

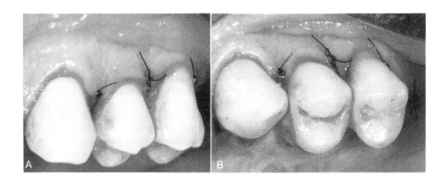

Figure 8.17   Clinical view one year after treatment demonstrated clinically health gingival tissues, absence of bleeding on probing and 2.5 mm probing depth (A). Radiographic evaluation performed five years after treatment revealed significantly increased radiopacity on the mesial aspect of the treated second premolar (B).

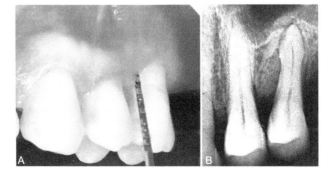

Kondo et al. 2005; Zhang et al. 2010) with well-documented osteoconductive properties in orthotopic sites (Hokugo et al. 2006; Jensen et al. 2006; Ogose et al. 2006; Shirasu et al. 2010). The biological potency and biochemical integrity of rhPDGF-BB is preserved within the β-TCP particles and the release kinetics of rhPDGF-BB from β-TCP is fast and almost complete in the first 72 hours after grafting (Young et al. 2009). GEM 21S® contains more than 1000 times the concentration of PDGF obtained in PRP preparations from the peripheral venous blood from the patient and promote the availability and bioactivity of the PDGF in the periodontal lesions, resulting in significant biological activity, including cell attraction for bone regeneration, proliferation of osteoblasts and cementoblasts, increased angiogenesis, and periodontal ligament formation (Chitguppi 2010; Gamal et al. 2000; Hollinger et al. 2008; Oates et al. 1993). Preclinical studies demonstrated significant regeneration of the periodontal attachment apparatus in dogs with the use of the product (Irokawa et al. 2010).

The efficacy and safety of rhPDGF for the treatment of intrabony defects was established in a randomized controlled multicenter clinical study (Nevins et al. 2003). Additional studies demonstrated that the use of rhPDGF-BB in association with bone grafts/substitutes is effective in enhancing the regeneration of periodontal defects in comparison with the bone grafts used alone (Jayakumar et al. 2011; Nevins et al. 2003, 2009, 2005, 2007, 2013; Ridgway et al. 2008), probably due to the enhanced stimulus of the bone metabolic activity, increased levels of PDGF-AB, VEGF, and ICTP after the local application of the β-TCP scaffold loaded with 0.3 mg/ml or 1.0 mg/ml of rhPDGF at the surgical sites (Cooke et al. 2006; Sarment et al. 2006).

A triple-blind, randomized, controlled clinical trial with 180 patients evaluated two doses of rhPDGF-BB (0.3 and 1.0 mg/ml) combined to β-TCP in the treatment of human intraboby defects, in comparison to β-TCP alone (Nevins et al. 2005). Significant improvement in clinical and radiographic parameters was observed for all the groups; however, both doses of rhPDGF exhibited significantly enhanced linear bone growth and percentage of bone defect fill in comparison to the areas treated with β-TCP alone. The gains in clinical attachment levels were faster in areas treated with 0.3 mg/ml rhPDGFBB+ β-TCP than in areas treated with β-TCP alone. The dose of 0.3 mg/ml rhPDGF-BB was significantly more effective in promoting linear bone growth and bone defect fill than the dose of 1.0 mg/ml rhPDGF-BB (Nevins et al. 2005). Longitudinal follow up of the same patient pool demonstrated additional attachment level gain, linear bone gain, and bone defect fill (Nevins et al. 2013).

In another study, rhPDGF-BB combined with bone allograft as carrier was used to treat interproximal intrabony defects and molar Class II furcation defects in 15 sites with advanced periodontal disease and poor prognosis that required extraction in humans. The defects were grafted with demineralized freeze-dried bone allograft (DFDBA) hydrated with one of three concentrations of rhPDGF-BB (0.5 mg/ml, 1.0 mg/ml, or 5.0 mg/ml), and bloc sections were taken nine months following the surgical procedures. The treated areas exhibited important probing depth reduction, clinical attachment level (CAL) gains, and bone fill of the treated defects. Histologic evaluation of the treated areas after nine months of healing, showed regeneration of a complete periodontal attachment apparatus with new cementum, PDL, and new bone. Similar histologic results were reported in another study (Camelo 2003) demonstrating periodontal regeneration with new bone, cementum, and periodontal ligament formation in humans. Similar results were also reported for human furcation defects treated with DFDBA grafts enhanced with of rhPDGF-BB (Nevins et al. 2003).

### Fibroblast Growth Factor 2 — rhFGF2

Fibroblast growth factors (FGF) are a potent stimulatory of osteoblastic proliferation *in vitro* (Hauschka 1986; Kasperk 1990). FGF2 stimulates human medular cells to form mineralized nodules in vitro, dependent to its mitogenic effects (Noff et al. 1989; Pitaru et al. 1993). Studies in vivo also demonstrated positive effects of FGF in skeletal tissues and systemically administered FGF increased endosteal bone formation in rats (Mayahara et al. 1993; Nakamura et al. 1995). Local injection of FGF-2 increased the volume and mineral content of fracture callus and enhanced the mechanical resistance of the fractured bone (Kawaguchi et al. 1994), increased endosteal bone formation (Nakamura et al. 1997) and local bone mass (Nakamura et al. 1996), as well as stimulated bone healing (Kato et al. 1998). Localized controlled release of FGF-2 in bone defects of diabetic animals demonstrated that it is a potent stimulator of bone healing and appears to be a promising resource to stimulate bone healing in debilitating conditions characterized by compromised healing (Santana and Trackman 2006). Therefore, FGF-2 is a potential candidate as therapeutic molecule due to its anabolic effects on boné tissue that may be an important alternative in regenerative surgeries. Preclinical studies demonstrated that the local application of FGF-2 in periodontal defects result in significative regeneration of the periodontal attachment apparatus (Murakami et al. 1999, 2003; Takayama et al. 2001). Randomized controlled clinical trials demonstrated probing attachment gain and bone regeneration significantly increased for intrabony defects treated with rhFGF-2 in comparison with their respective control areas (Kitamura et al. 2008, 2011; Santana and de Santana 2015). A randomized controlled clinical study (Santana and de Santana 2015) demonstrated that the application of rhFGF-2 in a hyaluronic acid carrier (rhFGF-2/HA), associated with a conservative and minimally invasive periodontal flap approach, demonstrated reduction in probing depth, attachment level gains, and bone gains significantly superior to the control group without the use of biologic mediator. This study demonstrated the important potential of rhFGF-2/HA to optimize the clinical results of minimally invasive surgical techniques in the treatment of periodontal defects.

The systematic review and Consensus Report of the Regeneration Workshop of the American Academy of Periodontology concluded that the use of biologics such as EMD e rhPDGF associated with β-TCP generally enhance bone fill and attachment gain, and also reduce probing depth more effectively than periodontal open flap procedures alone in the treatment of periodontal defects. The clinical effects are similar to those observed for regenerative approaches employing guided tissue regeneration, bovine bone mineral, and DFDBA. It was reported that there is evidence supporting the use of combined application of two or more regenerative therapies, such as bone substitutes, GTR, and biologics and that the results of regenerative therapy are maintained for up to ten years, and that regenerative therapy can improve the prognosis of a treated tooth (Kao et al. 2015; Reynolds et al. 2015).

Contemporary regenerative periodontal therapy can provide meaningful clinical benefits with the use of minimally-invasive flap approaches in conjunction with guided tissue regeneration, bovine xenografts, and decalcified freeze-dried bone allograft (DFDBA). The use of biologics such as enamel matrix derivative, platelet-derived growth factor (rhPDGF), and fibroblast growth factor (rhFGF-2) is an important alternative to enhance periodontal regeneration.

# References

Abd El Raouf, M., Wang, X., Miusi, S. et al. (2017). Injectable-platelet rich fibrin using the low-speed centrifugation concept improves cartilage regeneration when compared to platelet-rich plasma. *Platelets* doi: 10.1080/09537104.2017.1401058.

Anfossi, G., Trovati, M., Mularoni, E. et al. (1989). Influence of propranolol on platelet aggregation and thromboxane B2 production from platelet-rich plasma and whole blood. *Prostaglandins Leukot. Essent. Fat Acids* 36: 1–7.

Babbush, C.A., Kirsch, A., Mentag, P.J., and Hill, B. (1987). Intramobile cylinder (IMZ) two-stage osteointegrated implant system with the intramobile element (IME).Part I. It's rationale and procedure for use. *Int. J. Oral Maxillofac. Surg.* 2: 203–215.

Barnett, J.D., Mellonig, J.T., Gray, J.L., and Towle, H.J. (1989). Comparison of freeze-dried bone allograft and porous hydroxylapatite in human periodontal defects. *J. Periodontol.* 60: 231–237.

Becker, W., Becker, B., and Caffesse, R.G. (1994). A comparison of demineralized freeze-dried bone and autologous bone to induce bone formation in human extraction sockets. *J. Periodontol.* 65: 1128–1133.

Becker, W., Urist, M.R., Tucker, L.M. et al. (1995) Human demineralized freeze-dried bone: inadequate induced bone formation in athymic mice.A preliminary report. *J. Periodontol.* 66: 822–828.

Black, B.S., Gher, M.E., Sandifer, J. et al. (1994). Comparative study of collagen and expanded polytetrafluorethilene membranes in the treatment of human class II furcation defects. *J. Periodontol.* 65: 598–605.

Blumenthal, N.M. (1993). A clinical comparison of collagen membranes with ePTFE membranes in the treatment of human mandibular buccal class II furcation defects. *J. Periodontol.* 64: 925–933.

Bouchard, P., Ouhayoun, J.P., and Nilveus, R.E. (1993). Expanded polytetrafluorethilene membranes and connective tissue grafts support bone regeneration for closing mandibular class II furcations. *J. Periodontol.* 64: 1193–1198.

Bowen, J.A., Mellonig, J.T., Gray, J.L., and Towle, H.T. (1989). Comparison of decalcified freeze-dried bone allograft and porous particulate hydroxyapatite in human periodontal osseous defects. *J. Periodontol.* 60: 647–654.

Bowers, G.M., Chadroff, B., Carnevale, R. et al. (1989a). Histologic evaluation of new attachment apparatus formation in humans. Part III. *J. Periodontol.* 60: 683–693.

Bowers, G.M., Chadroff, B., Carnevale, R. et al. (1989b). Histologic evaluation of new attachment apparatus formation in humans. Part II. *J. Periodontol.* 60: 675–682.

Buchmann, R., Hasilik, A., Heinecke, A., and Lange, D.E. (2001 November). PMN responses following use of 2 biodegradable GTR membranes. *J. Clin. Periodontol.* 28 (11): 1050–1057.

Caffesse, R.G., Domingues, L.E., Nasjletti, C.E. et al. (1990). Furcation defects in dogs treated by guided tissue regeneration (GTR). *J. Periodontol.* 61: 45–50.

Caffesse, R.G., Smith, B.A., Castelli, W.A., and Nasjleti, C.E. (1988). New attachment achieved by guided tissue regeneration in beagle dogs. *J. Periodontol.* 59: 589–594.

Camargo, P.M., Lekovic, V., Weinlaender, M. et al. (2000). A controlled re-entry study on the effectiveness of bovine porous bone mineral used in combination with a collagen membrane of porcine origin in the treatment of intrabony defects in humans. *J. Clin. Periodontol.* 27: 889–896.

Camelo, M., Nevins, M.L., Schenk, R.K. et al. (2003 June). Periodontal regeneration in human Class II furcations using purified recombinant human platelet-derived growth factor-BB (rhPDGF-BB) with bone allograft. *Int. J. Periodontics Restorative Dent.* 23 (3): 213–225.

Canalis, E., McCarthy, T., and Centrella, M. (1988). Growth factors and the regulation of bone remodeling. *J. Clin. Invest.* 81: 277–281.

Castro, A.B., Cortellini, S., Temmerman, A. et al. (2019). Characterization of the leukocyte- and platelet rich fibrin block: release of growth factors, cellular content, and structure. *Int. J. Oral Maxillofac Implants* 34: 855–864. doi: 10.11607/jomi.7275.

Caton, J.G. (1997 March). Overview of clinical trials on periodontal regeneration. *Ann. Periodontol.* 2 (1): 215–222.

Caton, J.G. and Greenstein, G. (1993). Factors related to periodontal regeneration. *Periodontol. 2000* 1: 9–15.

Chitguppi, R. (2010). Enchanced periodontal regeneration through Gem 21S. *KDJ* 33 (1): 29.

Choukroun, J. (2015). Advanced PRF &i-PRF: platelet concentrates or blood concentrates? *J. Periodont. Med. Clin. Pract.* 1: 3.

Choukroun, J., Adda, F., Schoeffler, C., and Vervelle, A. (2001). Une opportunit en paro-implantologie: le PRF. *Implantodontie* 42: e62.

Cochran, D.L., Jones, A., Heijl, L. et al. (2003). Periodontal regeneration with a combination of enamel matrix proteins and autogenous bone grafting. *J. Periodontol.* 74: 1269–1281.

Cochran, D.L. and Wozney, J.M. (1999). Biological mediators for periodontal regeneration. *Periodontol. 2000* 19: 40–58.

Conn, J., Oyasu, R., Welsh, M., and Beal, J.M. (1974). Vicryl(polyglactin 910) synthetic absorbable sutures. *Am. J. Surg.* 128: 19–23.

Conner, H.D. (1996 January). Bone grafting with a calcium sulfate barrier after root amputation. *Compend. Contin. Educ. Dent.* 17 (1): 42, 44, 46.

Cooke, J.W., Sarment, D.P., Whitesman, L.A. et al. (2006). Effect of rhPDGFBB delivery on mediators of periodontal wound repair. *Tissue Eng.* 12: 1441–1450.

Cortellini, P., Pini Prato G., Tonetti M.S. (1995). Periodontal regeneration of human intrabony defects with titanium reinforced membranes. A controlled clinical trial. *J. Periodontol.* 66: 797–803.

Cortellini, P., Nieri, M., Prato, G.P., and Tonetti, M.S. (2008). Single minimally invasive surgical technique with an enamel matrix derivative to treat multiple adjacent intra-bony defects: clinical outcomes and patient morbidity. *J. Clin. Periodontol.* 35: 605–613.

Cortellini, P., Prato, G.P., and Tonetti, M.S. (1995). The modified papilla preservation technique. A new surgical approach for interproximal regenerative procedures. *J. Periodontol.* 66: 261–266.

Cortellini, P., Prato, G.P., and Tonetti, M.S. (1999). The simplified papilla preservation flap. A novel surgical approach for the management of soft tissues in regenerative procedures. *Int. J. Periodontics Restorative Dent.* 19: 589–599.

Cortellini, P. and Tonetti, M.S. (2000). Focus on intrabony defects: guided tissue regeneration (GTR). *Periodontol. 2000* 22: 104–132.

Cortellini, P. and Tonetti, M.S. (2004). Long-term tooth survival following regenerative treatment of intrabony defects. *J. Periodontol.* 75: 672–678.

Cortellini, P. and Tonetti, M.S. (2007a). A minimally invasive surgical technique with an enamel matrix derivative in the regenerative treatment of intra-bony defects: a novel approach to limit morbidity. *J. Clin. Periodontol.* 34: 87–93.

Cortellini, P. and Tonetti, M.S. (2007b). Minimally invasive surgical technique and enamel matrix derivative in intra-bony defects. I: clinical outcomes and morbidity. *J. Clin. Periodontol.* 34: 1082–1088.

Cortellini, S., Castro, A.B., Temmerman, A. et al. (2018). Leucocyte- and platelet-rich fibrin block for bone augmentation procedure: a proof-of-concept study. *J. Clin. Periodontol.* 45: 624–634. doi: 10.1111/jcpe.12877.

Costa-Noble, R., Soustre, E.C., Cardot, S. et al. (1996). Evaluation of bioabsorbable elastin-fibrin matrix as a barrier in surgical periodontal treatment. *J. Periodontol.* 67: 927–934.

Cosyn, J., Cleymaet, R., Hanselaer, L., and De Bruyn, H. (2012). Regenerative periodontal therapy of infrabony defects using minimally invasive surgery and a collagen-enriched bovine-derived xenograft: a 1-year prospective study on clinical and aesthetic outcome. *J. Clin. Periodontol.* 39: 979–986.

Crea, A., Dassatti, L., Hoffmann, O. et al. (2008). Treatment of intrabony defects using guided tissue regeneration or enamel matrix derivative: a 3- year prospective randomized clinical study. *J. Periodontol.* 79: 2281–2289.

Cristgau, M., Bader, N., Schmalz, G. et al. (1998). GTR therapy with bioresorbable membranes. *J. Clin. Periodontol.* 25: 499–509.

Crump, T.B., Rivera Hidalgo, F., Harrison, J.W. et al. (1996). Influence of three membrane types on healing of bone defects. *Oral Surg. Oral Med. Oral Pathol. Oral Radiol. Endod.* 82: 365–374.

De Bruyckere, T., Eghbali, A., Younes, F. et al. (2018). A 5-year prospective study on regenerative periodontal therapy of infrabony defects using minimally invasive surgery and a collagen-enriched bovine-derived xenograft. *Clin. Oral Investig.* 22: 1235–1242.

de Miranda, J.L., Santana, C.M., and Santana, R.B. (2013 January). Influence of endodontic treatment in the postsurgical healing of human Class II furcation defects. *J. Periodontol.* 84 (1): 51–57.

Dragoo, M.R. and Sullivan, H.C. (1973a). A clinical and histological evaluation of autogenous iliac bone grafts in humans. II. External root resorption. *J. Periodontol.* 44: 614–625.

Dragoo, M.R. and Sullivan, H.C. (1973b). A clinical and histological evaluation of autogenous iliac bone grafts in humans. I. Wound healing 2 to 8 months. *J. Periodontol.* 44: 599–613.

Eikholtz, P. and Hausman, E. (1998). Evidence for healing of interproximal intrabony defects after conventional and regenerative therapy: digital radiography and clinical measurements. *J. Periodontal Res.* 33: 156–165.

Esposito, M., Coulthard, P., Thomsen, P., and Worthington, H.V. (2004). Enamel matrix derivative for periodontal tissue regeneration in treatment of intrabony defects: a Cochrane systematic review. *J. Dent. Educ.* 68: 834–844.

Esposito, M., Grusovin, M.G., Coulthard, P., and Worthington, H.V. (2005). Enamel matrix derivative (Emdogain) for periodontal tissue regeneration in intrabony defects. *Cochrane Database Syst. Rev.* 19: CD003875.

Esposito, M., Grusovin, M.G., Papanikolaou, N. et al. (2009 October 7). Enamel matrix derivative (Emdogain(R)) for periodontal tissue regeneration in intrabony defects. *Cochrane Database Syst. Rev.* 4: CD003875. doi: 10.1002/14651858.CD003875.pub3.

Fijnheer, R., Pietersz, R.N., de Korte, D. et al. (1990). Platelet activation during preparation of platelet concentrates: a comparison of the platelet-rich plasma and the buffy coat methods. *Transfusion* 30: 634–638.

Fisher, L. and Termine, J. (1985). Noncollagenous proteins influencing the local mechanisms of calcification. *J. Clin. Orthop.* 200: 362–385.

Fleisher, N., de Waal, H., and Bloom, A. (1988). Regeneration of lost attachment apparatus in the dog using Vicryl absorbable mesh (Polyglactin 910). *Int. J. Periodontics Restorative Dent.* 8(2):44–55.

Flemmig, T.F., Ehmke, B., Bolz, K. et al. (1998). Long-term maintenance of alveolar bone gain after implantation of autolyzed, antigen-extracted, allogenic bone in periodontal intraosseous defects. *J. Periodontol.* 69: 47–53.

Fong, C.D. and Hammarstrom, L. (2000). Expression of amelin and amelogenin in epithelial root sheat remnants of fully formed rat molars. *Oral Surg. Oral Med. Oral Pathol.* 90: 218–223.

Friedlaeder, G.E., Strong, D.M., and Sell, K.W. (1984). Studies on the antigenicity of bone.II. Donor specific anti-HLA antibodies in human recipients of freeze-dried allografts. *J. Bone Jt. Surg.* 66A: 107–111.

Froum, S.J., Ortiz, M., Witkin, R.T. et al. (1976). Osseous autografts. III. Comparison of osseous coagulum-bone blend implants with open curettage. *J. Periodontol.* 47: 287–294.

Fujioka-Kobayashi, M., Miron, R.J., Hernandez, M. et al. (2017). Optimized platelet rich fibrin with the low speed concept: growth factor release, biocompatibility and cellular response. *J. Periodontol.* 88: 112–121.

Fujioka-Kobayashi, M., Katagiri, H., Kono, M. et al. (2020). Improved growth factor delivery and cellular activity using concentrated platelet-rich fibrin (C-PRF) when compared with traditional injectable (i-PRF) protocols. *Clin. Oral. Investig.* 24(12): 4373–4383.

Gamal, A.Y. and Mailhot, J.M. (2000). The effect of local delivery of PDGF-BB on attachment of human periodontal ligament fibroblasts to periodontitis-affected root surfaces–in vitro. *J. Clin. Periodontol.* 27: 347–353.

Garrett, S., Polson, A.M., Stoller, N.H. et al. (1997). Comparison of a bioabsorbable GTR barrier to a non-absorbable barrier in treating human class II furcation defects. A multi-center parallel design randomized single-blind trial. *J. Periodontol.* 68: 667–675.

Gestrelius, S., Andersson, C., Johansson, A.C. et al. (1997). Formulation of enamel matrix derivative for surface coating. Kinetics and cell colonization. *J. Clin. Periodontol.* 24: 678–684.

Gestrelius, S., Andersson, C., Johansson, A.C. et al. (1997a). Formulation of enamel matrix derivative for surface coating. Kinetics and cell colonization. *J. Clin. Periodontol.* 24 (9 Pt 2): 678–684.

Gestrelius, S., Andersson, C., Lidstrom, D. et al. (1997b). In vitro studies on periodontal ligament cells and enamel matrix derivative. *J. Clin. Periodontol.* 24: 685–692.

Gestrelius, S., Lyngstadaas, S.P., and Hammarstrom, L. (2000). Emdogain: periodontal regeneration based on biomimicry. *Clin. Oral Investig.* 4: 120–125.

Gottlow, J. (1993). G.T.R Using bioresorbable and non-resorbable devices: initial healing and long-term results. *J. Periodontol.* 64: 1157–1165.

Gottlow, J., Nyman, S., Lindhe, J., and Karring, T. (1986). New attachment formation in the human periodontium by guided tissue regeneration: case reports. *J. Clin. Periodontol.* 13: 604–616.

Gouldin, A.G., Fayad, S., and Mellonig, J.T. (1996 May). Evaluation of guided tissue regeneration in interproximal defects. (II). Membrane and bone versus membrane alone. *J. Clin. Periodontol.* 23 (5): 485–491.

Graziani, F., Gennai, S., Cei, S. et al. (2012). Clinical performance of access flap surgery in the treatment of the intrabony defect. A systematic review and meta-analysis of randomized clinical trials. *J. Clin. Periodontol.* 39: 145–156.

Hammarstrom, L. (1997a). The role of enamel matrix proteins in the development of cementum and periodontal tissues. *Ciba. F Symp.* 205: 246–260.

Hammarstrom, L. (1997b). Enamel matrix, cementum development and regeneration. *J. Clin. Periodontol.* 24: 658–668.

Hauschka, P.V., Mavrakos, A.E., Iafrati, M.D. et al. (1986). Growth factors in bone matrix. Isolation of multiple types by affinity chromatography on heparin-Sepharose. *J. Biol. Chem.* 261 (27): 12665–12674.

Heden, G., Wennstrom, J., and Lindhe, J. (1999). Periodontal tissue alterations following Emdogain treatment of periodontal sites with angular bone defects: a series of case reports. *J. Clin. Periodont.* 26: 855–860.

Heijl, L. (1997). Periodontal regeneration with enamel matrix derivative in one human experimental defect: a case report. *J. Clin. Periodontol.* 24: 693–696.

Hiatt, W.H., Schallhorn, R.G., and Aaronian, A.J. (1978). The induction of new bone and cementum formation. IV. Microscopic examination of the periodontium following human bone and marrow allograft, autograft and nongraft periodontal regenerative procedures. *J. Periodontol.* 49: 495–512.

Hirooka, H. (1998). The biologic concept for the use of enamel matrix protein: true periodontal regeneration. *Quintessence Int.* 29 (10): 621–630.

Hokugo, A., Sawada, Y., Sugimoto, K. et al. (2006). Preparation of prefabricated vascularized bone graft with neoangiogenesis by combination of autologous tissue and biodegradable materials. *Int. J. Oral Maxillofac Surg.* 35: 1034–1040.

Hollinger, J.O., Hart, C.E., Hirsch, S.N. et al. (2008). Recombinant human platelet-derived growth factor: biology and clinical applications. *J. Bone Joint Surg. Am.* 90 (Suppl 1): 48–54.

Hung, S.L., Lin, Y.W., Wang, Y.H. et al. (2002 August). Permeability of Streptococcus mutants and Actinobacillus actinomycetemcomitans through guided tissue regeneration membranes and their effects on attachment of periodontal ligament cells. *J. Periodontol.* 73 (8): 843–851.

Hurzeler, M.B. and Quinones, C.R. (1993). Autotransplantation of a tooth using guided tissue regeneration. *J. Clin. Periodontol.* 30: 545–548.

Irokawa, D., Ota, M., Yamamoto, S. et al. (2010). Effect of β tricalcium phosphate particle size on recombinant human platelet-derived growth factor-BB-induced regeneration of periodontal tissue in dog. *Dent. Mater. J.* 29: 721–730.

Ivanovic, A., Nikou, G., Miron, R.J. et al. (2014). Which biomaterials may promote periodontal regeneration in intrabony periodontal defects? A systematic review of pre-clinical studies. *Quintessence Int.* 45: 385–395.

Jayakumar, A., Rajababu, P., Rohini, S. et al. (2011). Multi-centre, randomized clinical trial on the efficacy and safety of recombinant human platelet-derived growth factor with beta-tricalcium phosphate in human intra-osseous periodontal defects. *J. Clin. Periodontol.* 38: 163–172.

Jensen, S.S., Broggini, N., Hjorting-Hansen, E. et al. (2006). Bone healing and graft resorption of autograft, an organic bovine bone and beta-tricalcium phosphate. A histologic and histomorphometric study in the mandibles of minipigs. *Clin. Oral Implants. Res.* 17: 237–243.

Kammer, F.M. and Churukian, M.M. (1984). The clinical use of injectable collagen: a three-year retrospective study. *Arch. Otolaryngol.* 110: 93.

Kao, R.T., Nares, S., and Reynolds, M.A. (2015). Periodontal regeneration – intrabony defects: a systematic review from the AAP regeneration workshop. *J. Periodontol.* 86 (2 Suppl): S77–S104.

Kasperk, C.H., Wergedal, J.E., Mohan, S. et al. (1990). Interactions of growth factors present in bone matrix with bone cells: effects on DNA synthesis and alkaline phosphatase. *Growth Factors* 3: 147–158.

Kato, T., Kawaguchi, H., Hanada, K. et al. (1998). Single local injection of recombinant fibroblast growth factor-2 stimulates healing of segmental bone defects in rabbits. *J. Orthop. Res.* 16: 654–659.

Kawaguchi, H., Kurokawa, T., Hanada, K. et al. (1994). Stimulation of fracture repair by recombinant human basic fibroblast growth factor in normal and streptozotocin-diabetic rats. *Endocrinology* 135: 774–781.

Kawahara, H., Hirabayashi, M., and Shikita, T. (1980). Single crystal alumina for dental implants and bone screws. *J. Biomed. Mater. Res.* 14(5): 597–605.

Kim, Y., Nowzari, H., and Rich, S.K. (2013). Risk of prion disease transmission through bovine-derived bone substitutes: a systematic review. *Clin. Implant Dent. Relat. Res.* 15: 645–653.

Kim, Y., Rodriguez, A.E., and Nowzari, H. (2016). The risk of prion infection through bovine grafting materials. *Clin. Implant Dent. Relat. Res.* 18: 1095–1102.

Kitamura, M., Akamatsu, M., Machigashira, M. et al. (2011 January). FGF-2 stimulates periodontal regeneration: results of a multi-center randomized clinical trial. *J. Dent. Res.* 90 (1): 35–40.

Kitamura, M., Nakashima, K., Kowashi, Y. et al. (2008 July 2). Periodontal tissue regeneration using fibroblast growth factor-2: randomized controlled phase II clinical trial. *PLoS One* 3 (7): e2611.

Kobayashi, E., Fluckiger, L., Fujioka-Kobayashi, M. et al. (2016). Comparative release of growth factors from PRP, PRF, and advanced-PRF. *Clin. Oral Investig.* 20: 2353–2360.

Kondo, N., Ogose, A., Tokunaga, K. et al. (2005 October). Bone formation and resorption of highly purified beta-tricalcium phosphate in the rat femoral condyle. *Biomaterials* 26 (28): 5600–5608.

Leknes, K.N., Andersen, K.M., Boe, O.E. et al. (2009). Enamel matrix derivative versus bioactive ceramic filler in the treatment of intrabony defects: 12-month results. *J. Periodontol.* 80: 219–227.

Lekovic, V., Kenney, E.B., Carranza, F.A., and Martignoni, M. (1991 December). The use of autogenous periosteal grafts as barriers for the treatment of Class II furcation involvements in lower molars. *J. Periodontol.* 62 (12): 775–780.

Listgarten, M.A. and Rosenberg, M.M. (1979). Histological study of repair following new attachment procedures in human periodontal lesions. *J. Periodontol.* 50: 333–344.

Lu, H.K., Ko, M.T., and Wu, M.F. (2004 January 15). Comparison of Th1/Th2 cytokine profiles of initial wound healing of rats induced by PDCM and e-PTFE. *J. Biomed. Mater. Res.* 68B (1): 75–80.

Luepke, P.G., Mellonig, J.T., and Brunsvold, M.A. (1997). A clinical evaluation of a bioresorbable barrier with and without decalcified freeze-dried bone allograft in the treatment of molar furcations. *J. Clin. Periodontol.* 24: 440–446.

Lundgren, D., Laurell, L., Gottlow, J. et al. (1995 July). The influence of the design of two different bioresorbable barriers on the results of guided tissue regeneration therapy. An intra-individual comparative study in the monkey. *J. Periodontol.* 66 (7): 605–612.

Magnusson, I., Batich, C., and Collins, B.R. (1988). New attachment formation following controlled tissue regeneration using biodegradable membranes. *J. Periodontol.* 59: 1–7.

Marx, R.E. (2004). Platelet-rich plasma: evidence to support its use. *J. Oral Maxillofac Surg.* 62: 489–496.

Matarasso, M., Iorio-Siciliano, V., Blasi, A. et al. (2015). Enamel matrix derivative and bone grafts for periodontal regeneration of intrabony defects. A systematic review and meta-analysis. *Clin. Oral Investig.* 19: 1581–1593.

Mattson, J.S., McLey, L.L., and Jabro, M.H. (1995). Treatment of intrabony defects with collagen membrane barriers.Case reports. *J. Periodontol.* 66: 635–645.

Maurer, P.K. and McDonald, J.V. (1985 September). Vicryl (polyglactin 910) mesh as a dural substitute. *J. Neurosurg.* 63 (3): 448–452.

Mayahara, H., Ito, T., Nagai, H. et al. (1993). In vivo stimulation of endosteal bone formation by basic fibroblast growth factor in rats. *Growth Factors* 9: 73–80.

Meadows, C.L., Gher, M.E., Quintero, G., and Lafferty, T.A. (1993). A comparison of polylactic acid granules and decalcified freeze-dried bone allograft in human periodontal osseous defects. *J. Periodontol.* 64: 103–109.

Mellado, J.R., Salkin, L.M., Freedman, A.L. et al. (1995). A comparative study of ePTFE periodontal membranes with and without decalcified freeze-dried bone allografts for the regeneration of interproximal intraosseous defects. *J. Periodontol.* 66: 751–755.

Mellonig, J.T. (1984). Decalcified freeze-dried bone allografts as an implant material in human periodontal defects. *Int. J. Periodontics Restorative Dent.* 4: 41–55.

Mellonig, J.T. (1999). Enamel matrix derivative for periodontal reconstructive surgery: technique and clinical and histologic case report. *Int. J. Periodontics Restorative Dent.* 19: 8–19.

Mellonig, J.T., Bowers, G., and Baily, R. (1981a). Comparison of bone graft materials. I. New bone formation with autografts and allografts determined by strontium 85. *J. Periodontol.* 52: 291–296.

Mellonig, J.T., Bowers, G., and Branham, G. (1982). Histologic evaluation of autograft-allograft composites. *J. Dent. Res.* 61 (Spec Issue): 1442.

Mellonig, J.T., Bowers, G., and Cotton, W. (1981b). Comparison of bone graft materials. I. New bone formation

with autografts and allografts: a histological evaluation. *J. Periodontol.* 52: 297–302.

Mellonig, J.T., Bowers, G., Levy, R.A. et al. (1983). Radionucleotide and histological evaluation of marrow-allograft composites. *J. Dent. Res.* 62 (Spec Is): 1208.

Minsk, L. (2000). The role of enamel matrix proteins in periodontal regeneration. *Compend. Contin. Educ. Dent.* 21: 210–214.

Miron, R.J., Chai, J., Zheng, S. et al. (2019a). A novel method for evaluating and quantifying cell types in platelet rich fibrin and an introduction to horizontal centrifugation. *J. Biomed. Mater. Res. A* 107: 2257–2271.

Miron, R.J., Chai, J., Zhang, P. et al. (2019b). A novel method for harvesting concentrated platelet-rich fibrin (C-PRF) with a 10-fold increase in platelet and leukocyte yields. *Clin. Oral Investig.* doi: 10.1007/s00784-019-03147-w.

Miron, R.J., Fujioka-Kobayashi, M., Hernandez, M. et al. (2017). Injectable platelet rich fibrin (i-PRF): opportunities in regenerative dentistry. *Clin. Oral Investig.* 21: 2619–2627.

Miron, R.J., Moraschini, V., Fujioka-Kobayashi, M. et al. (2021 May). Use of platelet-rich fibrin for the treatment of periodontal intrabony defects: a systematic review and meta-analysis. *Clin. Oral Investig.* 25 (5): 2461–2478.

Miron, R.J., Pinto, N.R., Quirynen, M., and Ghanaati, S. (2019b). Standardization of relative centrifugal forces (RCF) in studies related to platelet rich fibrin. *J. Periodontol.* doi: 10.1002/JPER.18-0553. [Epub ahead of print].

Miron, R.J., Zhang, Q., Sculean, A. et al. (2016). Osteoinductive potential of 4 commonly employed bone grafts. *Clin. Oral Investig.* 20: 2259–2265.

Murakami, S., Takayama, S., Ikezawa, K. et al. (1999). Regeneration of periodontal tissues by basic fibroblast growth factor. *J. Periodontal Res.* 34: 425–430.

Murakami, S., Takayama, S., Kitamura, M. et al. (2003). Recombinant human basic fibroblast growth factor (bFGF) stimulates periodontal regeneration in class II furcation defects created in beagle dogs. *J. Periodontal Res.* 38: 97–103.

Murphy, K.G., (1996). Interproximal tissue maintenance in GTR procedures: description of a surgical technique and 1-year reentry results. *Int. J. Periodontics Restorative Dent.* 16 (5): 463–477.

Murphy, K.G. and Gunsolley, J.C. (2003 December). Guided tissue regeneration for the treatment of periodontal intrabony and furcation defects. *A Systematic Review. Ann. Periodontol.* 8 (1): 266–302.

Nakamura, K., Kurokawa, T., Kato, T. et al. (1996). Local application of basic fibroblast growth factor into the bone increases bone mass at the applied site in rabbits. *Arch. Orthop. Trauma. Surg.* 115: 344–346.

Nakamura, K., Kurokawa, T., Kawaguchi, H. et al. (1997). Stimulation of endosteal bone formation by local intraosseous application of basic fibroblast growth factor in rats. *Rev. Rhum. Engl. Ed.* 64: 101–105.

Nakamura, T., Hanada, K., Tamura, M. et al. (1995 March). Stimulation of endosteal bone formation by systemic injections of recombinant basic fibroblast growth factor in rats. *Endocrinology* 136 (3): 1276–1284.

Needleman, I., Tucker, R., Giedrys-Leeper, E., and Worthington, H. (2002). A systematic review of guided tissue regeneration for periodontal infrabony defects. *J. Periodont. Res.* 37: 380–388.

Needleman, I., Tucker, R., Giedrys-Leeper, E., and Worthington, H. (2005). Guided tissue regeneration for periodontal intrabony defects — a Cochrane systematic review. *Periodontol. 2000* 37: 106–123.

Needleman, I., Worthington, H.V., Giedrys-Leeper, E., and Tucker, R. (2006 April 19). Guided tissue regeneration for periodontal infra-bony defects. *Cochrane Database Syst. Rev.* (2): CD001724. doi: 10.1002/14651858.CD001724.pub2.

Nevins, M., Camelo, M., Nevins, M.L. et al. (2003). Periodontal regeneration in humans using recombinant human platelet-derived growth factor-BB (rhPDGF-BB) and allogenic bone. *J. Periodontol.* 74: 1282–1292.

Nevins, M., Giannobile, W.V., McGuire, M.K. et al. (2005). Platelet-derived growth factor stimulates bone fill and rate of attachment level gain: results of a large multicenter randomized controlled trial. *J. Periodontol.* 76: 2205–2215.

Nevins, M., Hanratty, J., and Lynch, S.E. (2007). Clinical results using recombinant human platelet-derived growth factor and mineralized freeze-dried bone allograft in periodontal defects. *Int. J. Periodontics Restorative Dent.* 27: 421–427.

Nevins, M., Kao, R.T., McGuire, M.K. et al. (2013). Platelet-derived growth factor promotes periodontal regeneration in localized osseous defects: 36-month extension results from a randomized, controlled, double-masked clinical trial. *J. Periodontol.* 84: 456–464.

Nevins, M.L., Camelo, M., Schupbach, P. et al. (2009). Human histologic evaluation of mineralized collagen bone substitute and recombinant platelet-derived growth factor-BB to create bone for implant placement in extraction socket defects at 4 and 6 months: a case series. *Int. J. Periodontics Restorative Dent.* 29: 129–139.

Noff, D., Pitaru, S., and Savion, N. (1989 July 3). Basic fibroblast growth factor enhances the capacity of bone marrow cells to form bone-like nodules in vitro. *FEBS Lett.* 250 (2): 619–621.

Novaes, Jr A.B. (1992). Regeneração tecidual guiada: desenvolvimento da membrana nacional. *Periodontia* 1: 20–23.

Novaes, Jr A.B., Moraes, N., and Novaes, A.B. (1990a). "Biofill" membrana biológica nacional para regeneração tecidual guiada. *Revista Brasileira de Odontologia* 47: 25–28.

Novaes, Jr A.B., Moraes, N., and Novaes, A.B. (1990b). Uso do Biofill como membrana biologica no tratamento de lesao de furca com e sem a utilizacao da hidroxiapatita porosa. *Revista Brasileira de Odontologia* 47: 29–32.

Numabe, Y., Hiroshi, I., Hayashi, H. et al. (1993). Epithelial cell kinetics with atecollagen membranes: a study in rats. *J. Periodontol.* 64: 706–712.

Nyman, S., Lindhe, J., Karring, T., and Rylander, H. (1982). New attachment following surgical treatment of periodontal disease. *J. Clin. Periodontol.* 9: 280–286.

Oates, T.W., Rouse, C.A., and Cochran, D.L. (1993). Mitogenic effects of growth factors on human periodontal ligament cells in vitro. *J. Periodontol.* 64: 142–148.

Ogose, A., Kondo, N., Umezu, H. et al. (2006). Histological assessment in grafts of highly purified beta-tricalcium phosphate (OSferion) in human bones. *Biomaterials* 27: 1542–1549.

Oliveira, R.C., Oliveira, F.H.G., Cestari, T.M. et al. (2008). Morfometric evaluation of the repair of critical-size defects using demineralized bovine bone and autogenous bone grafts in rat calvaria. *Clin. Oral Implants Res.* 19: 749–754.

Oreamuno, S., Lekovic, V., Kenney, E.B. et al. (1990). Comparative clinical study of porous hydroxyapatite and decalcified freeze-dried bone in human periodontal defects. *J. Periodontol.* 61: 399–404.

Oxford, G.E., Quintero, G., Stuller, C.B., and Gher, M.E. (1997 July). Treatment of 3rd molar-induced periodontal defects with guided tissue regeneration. *J. Clin. Periodontol.* 24 (7): 464–469.

Pearson, G., Rosens, R., and Deporter, D. (1981). Preliminary observations on the usufulness of a decalcified freeze-dried cancellous bone allograft material in periodontal surgery. *J. Periodontol.* 52: 55–59.

Peltier, L.F. (1959 March). The use of plaster of Paris to fill large defects in bone. *Am. J. Surg.* 97 (3): 311–315.

Petinaki, E., Nikolopoulos, S., and Castanas, E. (1998). Low stimulation of peripheral lymphocytes, following in vitro application of Emdogain. *J. Clin. Periodontol.* 25: 715–720.

Pfeifer, J., Van Swol, R.L., and Ellinger, R. (1989). Epithelial exclusion and tissue regeneration using a collagen membrane barrier in chronic periodontal defects: a histologic study. *Int. J. Periodontics Restorative Dent.* 9: 263–272.

Pietruska, M.D. (2001). A comparative study on the use of Bio-Oss and enamel matrix derivative (Emdogain) in the treatment of periodontal bone defects. *Eur. J. Oral Sci.* 109: 178–181.

Pini Prato, G.P., Clauser, C., and Cortellini, P. (1995). Resorbable membranes in the treatment of human buccal recession. A nine-case report. *Int. J. Periodontics Restorative Dent.* 15: 259–268.

Pitaru, S., Kotev-Emeth, S., Noff, D. et al. (1993). Effect of basic fibroblast growth factor on the growth and differentiation of adult stromal bone marrow cells: enhanced development of mineralized bone-like tissue in culture. *J. Bone Miner. Res.* 8: 919–929.

Pitaru, S., Tal, H., Soldinger, M. et al. (1988). Partial regeneration of periodontal tissues using collagen barriers: initial observations in the canine. *J. Periodontol.* 59: 380–386.

Pitaru, S., Tal, H., Soldinger, M., and Noff, M. (1987). Collagen membranes prevent the apical migration of epithelium during periodontal wound healing. *J. Periodontal Res.* 22: 331–333.

Polson, A.M., Southard, G.L., Dunn, R.L. et al. (1994). Periodontal healing after GTR with Atrisorb barrier in beagle dogs. *J. Dent. Res.* 73: 380.

Polson, A.M., Southard, G.L., Dunn, R.L. et al. (1995). Initial study of guided tissue regeneration in class II furcation defects after use of a biodegradable barrier. *Int. J. Periodontics Restorative Dent.* 15: 43–55.

Posthlewaite, A.E., Seyer, J.M., and Kang, A.H. (1978). Chemotactic attraction of human fibroblasts to type I, II and III collagens and collagen-derived peptides. *Proc. Natl. Acad. Sci. U.S.A.* 75: 871–875.

Pretzl, B., Kim, T.S., Steinbrenner, H. et al. (2009) Guided tissue regeneration with bioabsorbable barriers III 10-year results in infrabony defects. *J. Clin. Periodontol.* 36: 349–356.

Quattlebaum, J., Mellonig, J.T., and Hansel, N. (1988). Antigenicity of freeze-dried cortical bone allograft in human periodontal osseous defects. *J. Periodontol.* 59: 394–397.

Quintero, G., Mellonig, J.T., and Gambill, V. (1982). A six month clinical evaluation of decalcified freeze-dried bone allograft in human periodontal defects. *J. Periodontol.* 53: 726–730.

Rankow, H.R. and Kassner, P.R. (1996). Endodontic applications of guided tissue regeneration in endodontic surgery. *J. Endod.* 22: 34–43.

Rasperin, G., Ricci, G., and Silvestri, M. (1999). Surgical technique for treatment of infrabony defects with enamel matrix derivative (Emdogain): 3 case reports. *Int J. Periodont. Rest. Dent.* 19: 579–587.

Renvert, S., Garrett, S., Shallhorn, R.G., and Egelberg, J. (1985). Healing after treatment of periodontal intraosseous defects. III. Effect of osseous grafting and citric acid conditioning. *J. Clin. Periodontol.* 12: 441–455.

Retzepi, M., Tonetti, M., and Donos, N. (2007 October). Comparison of gingival blood flow during healing of simplified papilla preservation and modified Widman flap surgery: a clinical trial using laser Doppler flowmetry. *J. Clin. Periodontol.* 34 (10): 903–911.

Reynolds, M.A., Aichelmann-Reidy, M.E., Branch-Mays, G.L., and Gunsolley, J.C. (2003). The efficacy of bone replacement grafts in the treatment of periodontal osseous defects. A systematic review. *Ann. Periodontol.* 8: 227–265.

Reynolds, M.A., Kao, R.T., Camargo, P.M. et al. (2015). Periodontal regeneration – intrabony defects: a consensus report from the AAP regeneration workshop. *J. Periodontol.* 86 (2 Suppl): S105–107.

Richardson, C.R., Mellonig, J.T., Brunsvold, M.A. et al. (1999). Clinical evaluation of Bio-Oss: a bovine-derived xenograft for the treatment of periodontal osseous defects in humans. *J. Clin. Periodontol.* 26: 421–428.

Ridgway, H.K., Mellonig, J.T., and Cochran, D.L. (2008). Human histologic and clinical evaluation of recombinant human platelet-derived growth factor and beta-tricalcium phosphate for the treatment of periodontal intraosseous defects. *Int. J. Periodontics Restorative Dent.* 28: 171–179.

Rummelhart, J.M., Mellonig, J.T., Gray, J.L., and Towle, H.J. (1989). A comparison of freeze-dried bone allograft and demineralized freeze-dried bone allograft in human periodontal osseous defects. *J. Periodontol.* 60: 655–663.

Santana, R.B., de Mattos, C.M., Francischone, C.E., and Van Dyke, T. (2010). Superficial topography and porosity of an absorbable barrier membrane impacts soft tissue response in guided bone regeneration. *J. Periodontol.* 81: 926–933.

Santana, R.B., de Mattos, C.M., and Van Dyke, T. (2009). Efficacy of combined regenerative treatments in human mandibular class II furcation defects. *J. Periodontol.* 80: 1756–1764.

Santana, R.B. and de Santana, C.M. (2015). Human intrabony defect regeneration with rhFGF-2 and hyaluronic acid – a randomized controlled clinical trial. *J. Clin. Periodontol.* 42: 658–665.

Santana, R.B. and Santana, C.M.M. (2013). Use of guided tissue regeneration in the treatment of a severe endodontic–periodontic lesion: a 15-year follow-up case report. *Clin. Adv. Periodontics* 3: 10–13.

Santana, R.B. and Trackman, P.C. (2006). Controlled release of fibroblast growth factor 2 stimulates bone healing in an animal model of diabetes mellitus. *Int. J. Oral Maxillofac Implants* 21: 711–718.

Santana, R.B. and Van Dyke, T.E. (1999). The response of human buccal maxillary furcation defects to combined regenerative techniques–two controlled clinical studies. *J. Int. Acad Periodontol.* 1 (3): 69–77.

Sanz, M., Tonetti, M.S., Zabalegui, I. et al. (2004). Treatment of intrabony defects with enamel matrix proteins or barrier membranes: results from a multicenter practice-based clinical trial. *J. Periodontol.* 75: 726–733.

Sarment, D.P., Cooke, J.W., Miller, S.E. et al. (2006). Effect of rhPDGF-BB on bone turnover during periodontal repair. *J. Clin. Periodontol.* 33: 135–140.

Scanttlebury, T.V. (1993). 1982–1992: A decade of technology development for guided tissue regeneration. *J. Periodontol.* 64: 1129–1137.

Scheyer, E.T., Velasquez-Plata, D., Brunsvold, M.A. et al. (2002). A clinical comparison of a bovine-derived xenograft used alone and in combination with enamel matrix derivative for the treatment of periodontal osseous defects in humans. *J. Periodontol.* 73: 423–432.

Schwartz, Z., Mellonig, J.T., Carnes, D.L., Jr et al. (1996 September). Ability of commercial demineralized freeze-dried bone allograft to induce new bone formation. *J. Periodontol.* 67 (9): 918–926.

Schwartz, Z., Somers, A., Mellonig, J.T. et al. (1998). Ability of commercial demineralized freeze-dried bone allograft to induce new bone formation is dependent on donor age but not gender. *J. Periodontol.* 69: 470–478.

Scott, T.A., Towle, H.J., Assad, D.A., and Nicoll, B.K. (1997). Comparison of bioabsorbable laminar bone membrane and non-resorbable ePTFE membrane in mandibular furcations. *J. Periodontol.* 68: 679–686.

Sculean, A., Barbe, G., Chiantella, G.C. et al. (2002a). Clinical evolution of an enamel matrix protein derivative combined with a bioactive glass for the treatment of intrabony periodontal defects in humans. *J. Clin. Periodont.* 73: 401–408.

Sculean, A., Chiantella, G.C., Arweiler, N.B. et al. (2008a). Five-year clinical and histologic results following treatment of human intrabony defects with an enamel matrix derivative combined with a natural bone mineral. *Int. J. Periodontics Restorative Dent.* 28: 153–161.

Sculean, A., Chiantella, G.C., Windisch, P. et al. (2002b). Clinical evaluation of an enamel matrix protein derivative (Emdogain) combined with a bovine-derived xenograft (Bio-Oss) for the treatment of intrabony periodontal defects in humans. *Int. J. Periodontics Restorative Dent.* 22: 259–267.

Sculean, A., Nikolidakis, D., Nikou, G. et al. (2015). Biomaterials for promoting periodontal regeneration in human intrabony defects: a systematic review. *Periodontol. 2000* 68: 182–216.

Sculean, A., Nikolidakis, D., and Schwarz, F. (2008b). Regeneration of periodontal tissues: combinations of barrier membranes and grafting materials—Biological foundation and preclinical evidence: a systematic review. *J. Clin. Periodontol.* 35 (Suppl. 8): 106–116.

Sculean, A., Pietruska, M., Schwarz, F. et al. (2005a). Healing of human intrabony defects following regenerative periodontal therapy with an enamel matrix protein derivative alone or combined with a bioactive glass. A controlled clinical study. *J. Clin. Periodontol.* 32: 111–117.

Sculean, A., Windisch, P., Keglevich, T. et al. (2003a). Clinical and histologic evaluation of human intrabony defects treated with an enamel matrix protein derivative combined with a bovine-derived xenograft. *Int. J. Periodontics Restorative Dent.* 23: 47–55.

Sculean, A., Windisch, P., Keglevich, T., and Gera, I. (2003b). Histologic evaluation of human intrabony defects following non-surgical periodontal therapy with and without application of an enamel matrix protein derivative. *J. Periodontol.* 74: 153–160.

Sculean, A., Windisch, P., Keglevich, T., and Gera, I. (2005b). Clinical and histologic evaluation of an enamel matrix protein derivative combined with a bioactive glass for the treatment of intrabony periodontal defects in humans. *Int. J. Periodontics Restorative Dent.* 25: 139–147.

Sculean, A., Windisch, P., Szendröi-Kiss, D. et al. (2008c). Clinical and histologic evaluation of an enamel matrix derivative combined with a biphasic calcium phosphate for the treatment of human intrabony periodontal defects. *J. Periodontol.* 79: 1991–1999.

Shaffer, C.D. and App, G.R. (1971 November). The use of plaster of paris in treating infrabony periodontal defects in humans. *J. Periodontol.* 42 (11): 685–690.

Shigeyama, Y., D'Errico, J.A., Stone, R., and Sommerman, M.J. (1995). Commercially-prepared allograft material has biological activity in vitro. *J. Periodontol.* 66: 478–487.

Shirasu, N., Ueno, T., Hirata, Y. et al. (2010). Bone formation in a rat calvarial defect model after transplanting autogenous bone marrow with beta-tricalcium phosphate. *Acta Histochem.* 112 (3): 270–277.

Siciliano, V.I., Andreuccetti, G., Siciliano, A.I. et al. (2011). Clinical outcomes after treatment of non-contained intrabony defects with enamel matrix derivative or guided tissue regeneration: a 12-month randomized controlled clinical trial. *J. Periodontol.* 82: 62–71.

Silvestri, M., Sartori, S., Rasperini, G. et al. (2003). Comparison of infrabony defects treated with enamel matrix derivative versus guided tissue regeneration with a nonresorbable membrane. *J. Clin. Periodontol.* 30: 386–393.

Sottosanti, J.S. (1992 March). Calcium sulfate: a biodegradable and biocompatible barrier for guided tissue regeneration. *Compendium* 13 (3): 226–228, 230, 232–234.

Sottosanti, J.S. (1993 June-July). Aesthetic extractions with calcium sulfate and the principles of guided tissue regeneration. *Pract. Periodontics Aesthet. Dent.* 5 (5): 61–69.

Sottosanti, J.S. (1995 Fall). Calcium sulfate-aided bone regeneration: a case report. *Periodontal Clin. Investig.* 17 (2): 10–15.

Spagnuolo, A. and Bissada, N. (1995). The regenerative potential of a resorbable composite barrier in the treatment of periodontitis with severe horizontal bone loss. *J. Dent. Res.* 74 (spec Issue): 98. (abbst 685).

Stahl, S.S., Froum, S.J., and Kushner, L. (1983). Healing responses of human intraosseous lesions following the use of debridement, grafting and citric acid root treatment. II. Clinical and histologic observations: one year postsurgery. *J. Periodontol.* 54: 325–338.

Steiner, S.S., Crigger, M., and Egelberg, J. (1981). Connective tissue regeneration to periodontally diseased teeth. II. Histologic observations of cases following replaced flap surgery. *J. Periodontal Res.* 16: 109–116.

Takayama, S., Murakami, S., Shimabukuro, Y. et al. (2001). Periodontal regeneration by FGF-2 (bFGF) in primate models. *J. Dent. Res.* 80: 2075–2079.

Takei, H., Yamada, H., and Hau, T. (1989). Maxillary anterior esthetics. Preservation of the interdental papilla. *Dent. Clin. North Am.* 33: 263–273.

Thakare, K. and Deo, V. (2012 December). Randomized controlled clinical study of rhPDGF-BB + β-TCP versus HA + β-TCP for the treatment of infrabony periodontal defects: clinical and radiographic results. *Int. J. Periodontics Restorative Dent.* 32: 689–696.

Trombelli, L. and Calura, G. (1993 December). Complete root coverage of denuded root surface using expanded polytetrafluoroethylene membrane in conjunction with tetracycline root conditioning and fibrinfibronectin glue application: case reports. *Quintessence Int.* 24 (12): 847–852.

Trombelli, L., Heitz-Mayfield, L.J., Needleman, I. et al. (2002). A systematic review of graft materials and biological agents for periodontal intraosseous defects. *J. Clin. Periodontol.* 29 (Suppl 3): 117–135.

Trombelli, L., Simonelli, A., Schincaglia, G.P. et al. (2012 January). Single-flap approach for surgical debridement of deep intraosseous defects: a randomized controlled trial. *J. Periodontol.* 83 (1): 27–35.

Turner, D. and Mellonig, J.T. (1981). Antigenicity of freeze-dried bone allograft in periodontal osseous defects. *J. Periodontal Res.* 16: 89–99.

Urist, M.R. (1965). Bone formation by autoinduction. *Science* 150: 893–899.

Urist, M.R. and Dowell, T.A. (1968). Inductive substratum for osteogenesis in pellets of particulate bone matrix. *Clin. Orthop.* 61: 61–78.

Urist, M.R., Dowell, T.A., Hay, P.H. et al. (1967). Inductive substrates for bone formation. *Clin. Orthop.* 53: 243–254.

Varela, H.A., Souza, J.C.M., Nascimento, R.M. et al. (2019). Injectable platelet rich fibrin: cell content, morphological, and protein characterization. *Clin. Oral Investig.* 23: 1309–1318.

Venezia, E., Goldstein, M., Boyan, B.D., and Schwartz, Z. (2004 November 1). The use of enamel matrix derivative in the treatment of periodontal defects: a literature review and meta-analysis. *Crit. Rev. Oral Biol. Med.* 15 (6): 382–402.

Vernino, A.R., Jones, F.L., Holt, R.A. et al. (1995). Evaluation of the potential of a polylactic acid barrier for correction of periodontal defects in baboons: a clinical and histologic study. *Int. J. Periodontics Restorative Dent.* 15: 85–100.

Vernino, A.R., Ringeisen, T.A., Wang, H.L. et al. (1998 December). Use of biodegradable polylactic acid barrier materials in the treatment of grade II periodontal furcation defects in humans—Part I: a multicenter investigative clinical study. *Int. J. Periodontics Restorative Dent.* 18 (6): 572–585.

Vernino, A.R., Wang, H.L., Rapley, J. et al. (1999 February). The use of biodegradable polylactic acid barrier materials in the treatment of grade II periodontal furcation defects in humans—Part II: a multicenter investigative surgical study. *Int. J. Periodontics Restorative Dent.* 19 (1): 56–65.

Vitkus, R. and Meltzer, J.A. (1996). Repair of a defect following the removal of a maxillary adenomatoid tumor using guided tissue regeneration. A case report. *J. Periodontol.* 67: 46–50.

Waerhaug, J. (1978). Healing of the dento-epithelial junction following subgingival plaque control. I. As observed in human biopsy material. *J. Periodontol.* 49: 1–8.

Waldrop, T.C. and Semba, S.E. (1993). Closure of oroantral communication using guided tissue regeneration and an absorbable gelatin membrane. *J. Periodontol.* 64: 1061–1066.

Wallace, S.C., Gellin, R.G., Miller, M.C., and Mishkin, D.J. (1994). Guided tissue regeneration with and without decalcified freeze-dried bone in mandibular class II furcation invasions. *J. Periodontol.* 66: 244–254.

Wang, X., Zhang, Y., Choukroun, J. et al. (2017). Behavior of gingival fibroblasts on titanium implant surfaces in combination with either Injectable-PRF or PRP. *Int. J. Mol. Sci.* 18: 331. doi: 10.3390/ijms18020331.

Wang, X., Zhang, Y., Choukroun, J. et al. (2018). Effects of an injectable plateletrich fibrin on osteoblast behavior and bone tissue formation in comparison to platelet-rich plasma. *Platelets* 29: 48–55. doi: 10.1080/09537104.2017.1293807.

Wend, S., Kubesch, A., Orlowska, A. et al. (2017). Reduction of the relative centrifugal force influences cell number and growth factor release within injectable PRF based matrices. *J. Mater. Sci. Mater. Med.* 28: 188. doi: 10.1007/s10856-017-5992-6.

Wikesjo, U.M., Lim, W.H., Thomson, R.C., and Hardwick, W.R. (2003 July). Periodontal repair in dogs: gingival tissue occlusion, a critical requirement for GTR? *J. Clin. Periodontol.* 30 (7): 655–664.

Windisch, P., Sculean, A., Klein, F. et al. (2002). Comparison of clinical, radiographic, and histometric measurements following treatment with guided tissue regeneration or enamel matrix proteins in human periodontal defects. *J. Periodontol.* 73: 409–417.

Yamagami, A., Kotera, S., Ehara, Y., and Nishio, Y. (1988). Porous alumina for free standing implants. Part I. Implant design and in vivo animal studies. *J. Prosthet. Dent.* 59: 689–695.

Yamaoka, S.B., Mellonig, J.T., Meffert, R.M. et al. (1996). Clinical evaluation of demineralized-unicortical-ilium -strips for guided tissue regeneration. *J. Periodontol.* 67 (8): 803–815.

Young, C.S., Ladd, P.A., Browning, C.F. et al. (2009 December 16). Release, biological potency, and biochemical integrity of recombinant human platelet-derived growth factor-BB (rhPDGF-BB) combined with Augment(TM) Bone graft or GEM 21S beta-tricalcium phosphate (beta-TCP). *J. Control Release* 140 (3): 250–525.

Yukna, R.A., Krauser, J.T., Callan, D.P. et al. (2002). Thirty-six month follow-up of 25 patients treated with combination anorganic bovine-derived hydroxyapatite matrix (ABM)/cell-binding peptide (P-15) bone replacement grafts in human infrabony defects. I. Clinical findings. *J. Periodontol.* 73: 123–128.

Yukna, R.A. and Mellonig, J.T. (2000). Histologic evaluation of periodontal healing in humans following regenerative therapy with enamel matrix derivative: a 10-case series. *J. Periodontol.* 71: 752–759.

Zetterstrom, O., Andersson, C., Eriksson, L. et al. (1997). Clinical safety of enamel matrix derivative (Emdogain) in the treatment of periodontal defects. *J. Clin. Periodont.* 24: 697–704.

Zhang, M., Wang, K., Shi, Z. et al. (2010). Osteogenesis of the construct combined BMSCs with beta-TCP in rat. *J. Plast. Reconstr. Aesthet. Surg.* 63: 227–232.

Zucchelli, G., Bernardi, F., Montebugnoli, L., and De, M. (2002). Enamel matrix proteins and guided tissue regeneration with titanium-reinforced expanded polytetrafluoroethylene membranes in the treatment of infrabony defects: a comparative controlled clinical trial. *J. Periodontol.* 73: 3–12.

# 9

# Surgical Versus Nonsurgical Treatment of Periodontitis

*Annika Kroeger and Thomas Dietrich*

## Introduction

The treatment of periodontal disease is divided in four steps: initial diagnosis and patient motivation, cause-related nonsurgical therapy, optional surgical intervention, followed by supportive periodontal care. Central aspect of all these stages is the aim to remove (or control) pathogenic biofilm to establish a favorable environment (Lisa J. A. Heitz-Mayfield 2005). There are a variety of adjunctive measures (such as antibiotics and other antiseptic modalities) that may be considered during each step. The relevance of these is discussed in other chapters in this book. This chapter therefore focuses on the relative effectiveness and related issues of surgical versus nonsurgical periodontal therapy.

The understanding of the etiopathogenesis of periodontitis and associated diseases has developed significantly in recent years. These changes are most prominently reflected in the 2018 Classification of Periodontal Diseases (Caton et al. 2018). Notwithstanding the development of novel therapeutics, mechanical debridement remains at the core of the treatment of periodontitis (Sanz et al. 2020). However, the relative effectiveness of surgical vs. nonsurgical approaches is continuously discussed and the subject of ongoing research.

## Evidence-based Outcomes

Antczak-Bouckoms et al. was one of the first publications relating to investigation of relative effectiveness of surgical versus nonsurgical methods of treatment of periodontal disease (Antczak-Bouckoms et al. 1993). This meta-analysis included the results of five randomized controlled trials deemed suitable by the authors. All studies compared similar treatments: modified Widman flap versus scaling and root planing under local anesthesia.

Interestingly, the authors highlighted the importance of choice of outcome measures. When considering reduction of probing depths as the goal of therapy, the surgical treatment groups exhibited superior outcomes. Attachment levels, on the other hand, improved more in the nonsurgical treatment group. Overall, all these differences between groups became smaller over follow-up time and were nonsignificant after 5 years. Only the deepest initial pocket probing depths (>6 mm) showed improvement after 5 years in the surgical versus the nonsurgical group. However, this difference was limited to around 0.5 mm.

The findings of two further systematic reviews published in 2002 (L. J. A. Heitz-Mayfield 2002; Hung and Douglass 2002) are consistent with the previously mentioned work. A further review paper attempts to reconcile the minor differences between the results of the three published systematic reviews (Lisa J. A. Heitz-Mayfield 2005).

The most recent systematic review on the topic was conducted by Sanz-Sanchez et al. in preparation for the EFP S3-level guideline (Sanz et al. 2020; Sanz-Sanchez et al. 2020). This review included 36 randomized controlled trials investigating the effectiveness of subgingival instrumentation versus access flaps in reduction of probing depths. Consistent with previous reviews, the results confirmed that the surgical approach is superior in terms of probing depth reduction in deep pockets both in the short and long term. Probing depths of initially moderately deep pockets (4–6 mm) benefit from greater probing depth reduction with a surgical approach in the short term, but this difference becomes negligible in the long-term follow ups (see Figure 9.1).

All of these systematic reviews and their results have to be interpreted with caution. The high variability of included studies—such as sample sizes, patient selection, follow-up times, treatment modalities, chosen outcome measures—pose a limitation on comparability and generalizability. There also have been suggestions that nonsurgical approaches are more promising on single rooted teeth

*Practical Periodontal Diagnosis and Treatment Planning*, Second Edition. Edited By Serge Dibart and Thomas Dietrich.
© 2024 John Wiley & Sons, Inc. Published 2024 by John Wiley & Sons, Inc.

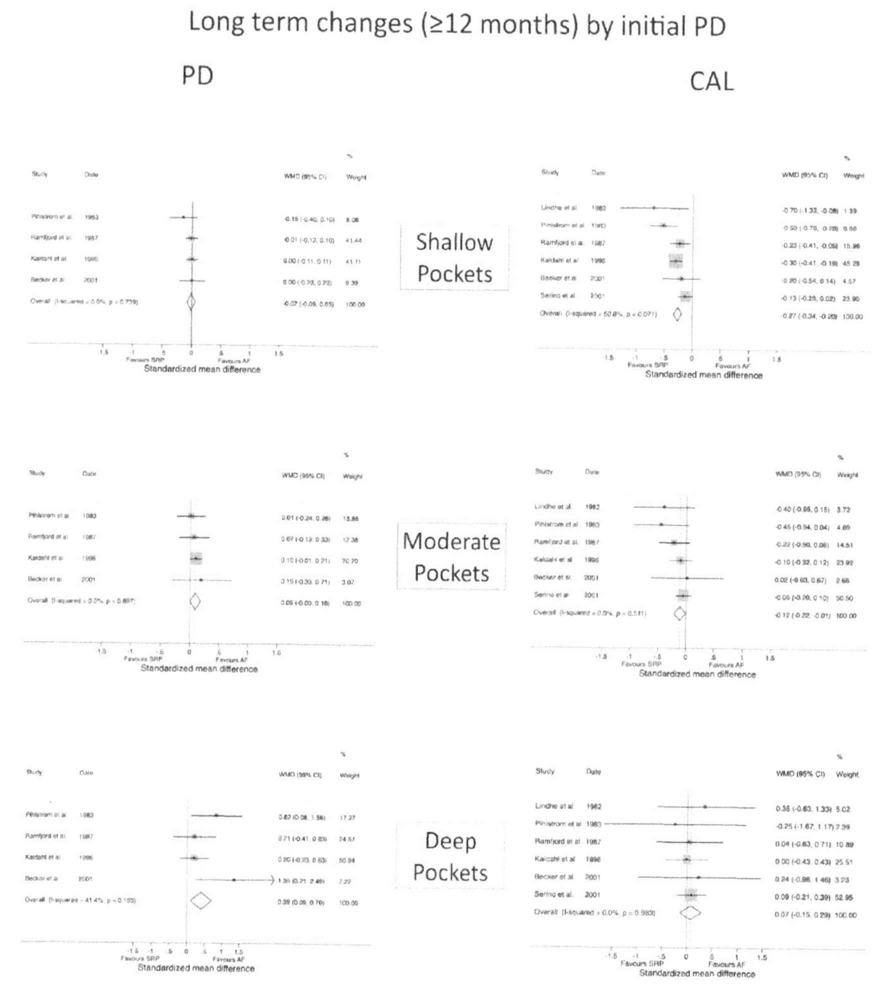

Figure 9.1 Results Overview from the systematic review by Sanz-Sanches et al. (Sanchez et al., 2020 / John Wiley & Sons.): forest plots of studies investigating the long-term (≥12 months) difference in probing depth change (PD) and clinical attachment level (CAL) between access flap procedures (AF) and subgingival instrumentation (SRP). The rectangles represent the individual results for each study, in this case the standardized mean difference in mm between AF and SRP. The size of the rectangle represents the weighting given to the study in the meta-analysis and is directly related to the precision of the study. The horizontal line extending from each square represents the 95% confidence interval (95% CI). The diamond at the bottom is the pooled value from the meta-analysis. The center of the diamond is the summary value and the horizontal points represent the 95% CI. When the diamond is to the left of the zero line the outcome is in favor of SRP, to the right of the zero line the outcome is in favor of AF.

with initially moderately deep or deep pockets (Sanz-Sanchez et al. 2020).

Nonetheless, it can be concluded that in deep pockets, i.e., initial probing depths of 7 mm or more, surgical approaches are superior in terms of probing pocket depths reduction compared to nonsurgical approaches.

## Author's Views/Comments

As stated above, the goal of periodontal therapy may be defined as "to arrest the inflammatory disease process by removal of the subgingival biofilm and establish a local environment and microflora compatible with periodontal health"

(Heitz-Mayfield 2005). While this is a sensible definition in light of our current understanding of the pathogenesis of periodontitis, it does not lend itself to the assessment of success or failure of any periodontal intervention.

In terms of objective clinical periodontal outcomes, we may define the goals of periodontal therapy to be—at least in the short-term—the reduction or elimination of periodontal pockets and the prevention of further attachment loss. Periodontal pocket depth and attachment loss have several characteristics that, for clinicians, make them almost intuitive endpoints to measure success or failure of periodontal therapy. Firstly, periodontal pocket depth and attachment loss are literally defining signs of periodontitis, given that periodontitis is defined as a chronic inflammatory disease characterized by loss of attachment (and the associated pocketing). Secondly, the assessment of periodontal pocket depth and clinical attachment loss is relatively straightforward, both in clinical practice as well as in clinical studies. Thirdly, clinical attachment level and in particular periodontal pocket depth are relatively sensitive to nonsurgical or surgical periodontal interventions in the short-term, i.e., the clinician can almost immediately (i.e., within weeks to a few months) see an effect (benefit) of his or her intervention. It is therefore hardly surprising that the bulk of the available clinical trials on the effects of surgical vs. nonsurgical periodontal therapy used periodontal probing depth and clinical attachment levels as outcome measures.

However, for patients suffering from periodontitis, probing pocket depth and attachment levels in and of themselves may be entirely irrelevant. They only become tangible when they cause symptoms such as recession, malodor, or bad taste, or when they result in tooth loss. A better definition of the goals of periodontal therapy would, therefore, make reference to patient-centered, tangible outcomes such as oral-health-related quality of life, or hard, tangible endpoints such as tooth loss. Therefore, probing pocket depth and clinical attachment level are what is called surrogate outcomes, because they are explicitly or implicitly used as surrogates for hard, tangible outcomes such as tooth loss.

Results from studies using surrogate endpoints generally must be cautiously interpreted, because they may not necessarily be generalized to the hard endpoints of interest (Hujoel 2004). For example, serum cholesterol and blood pressure are surrogate endpoints for interventions to reduce cardiovascular disease risk. Because serum cholesterol and blood pressure are strong risk factors for cardiovascular disease, it would generally be expected that treatments effective in reducing serum cholesterol or blood pressure will also have beneficial effects on cardiovascular disease. While this may be true for many interventions, some interventions that effectively reduce serum cholesterol may actually increase cardiovascular disease risk through a different pathway. Hence, surrogate endpoints need to be carefully validated, and there may always be uncertainty as to whether the effectiveness of a specific intervention as assessed with a surrogate endpoint holds for a true endpoint.

Tooth loss is one tangible endpoint relevant to periodontal therapy, and based on common sense and clinical experience, one may argue that attachment levels and probing depth are valid surrogate endpoints for assessing the effect of periodontal therapy on tooth loss risk. Indeed, it is difficult to think of a scenario in which progressive attachment loss would not ultimately result in tooth loss. Therefore, if

flap surgery is superior to nonsurgical therapy in terms of both probing depth and attachment level in initially deep pockets (7+ mm), does common sense not dictate to go for surgical therapy to reduce tooth loss risk? Unfortunately, it may not be that straightforward. For example, surgical therapy will result in more severe recession, which in turn may be associated with an increased risk for root caries and subsequent tooth loss. Furthermore, nonsurgical therapy may be preferable over surgical therapy with regard to other tangible endpoints, such as esthetics (recession) and hypersensitivity.

So, what then is the evidence for residual probing depth or other surrogate periodontal parameters to be associated with tooth loss or patient-centered outcomes in periodontitis patients? In their excellent recent review, Loos and Needleman found that, "surprisingly, virtually absent are reports that use these commonly applied periodontal probing measures (pockets ≤4 mm, residual probing depth, change in probing depth [...]) after completion of the active periodontal treatment, subsequently to be used as new baseline measures" to evaluate their impact on tooth survival, need for retreatment and oral health-related quality of life (Loos and Needleman 2020). Notably, data from one cohort study in Switzerland demonstrated that, indeed, residual pocket depth ≥6 mm and full-mouth bleeding scores of 30% or more were associated with an increased risk of tooth loss (Matuliene et al. 2008).

To further complicate things, when considering the evidence regarding the effectiveness of nonsurgical vs. surgical periodontal therapy, the clinician faces the formidable dilemma that either form of treatment may be more efficient depending on whether probing pocket depth or clinical attachment level is chosen as the (surrogate) endpoint of interest. The conclusion that (1) surgical therapy provides a greater benefit than nonsurgical therapy if the objective is reduction of probing depth, and (2) nonsurgical therapy provides a greater benefit for shallow and moderate initial pockets (up to 6 mm) but not for deep pockets (7+ mm) in terms of attachment level, is hardly satisfying and not particularly helpful in decision making (Heitz-Mayfield 2005).

The scenario is equivalent to a hypothetical intervention that increases LDL cholesterol levels but lowers blood pressure. In this case a physician would have to choose whether he considers blood pressure or LDL cholesterol to be more important. While there may be a specific patient for whom a physician could make such a decision, the surrogate endpoints are clearly not useful in assessing the benefit of this hypothetical intervention with respect to cardiovascular disease. Such evidence could only come from a clinical trial using true disease endpoints. In any case, it is unlikely that an intervention that lowers blood pressure and increases LDL cholesterol would be a popular, first line treatment to prevent cardiovascular disease in patients with high blood pressure. Therefore, in the absence of robust evidence from clinical trials regarding the effects of surgical vs. nonsurgical therapy on tooth mortality and/or other patient-centered outcomes, it may not be justifiable to prescribe surgical therapy universally, even for deep sites.

It is often argued that probing depth reduction (and therefore surgical therapy) has priority because shallow sites are easier to maintain by the patient, hygienist, and dentist in the long term. As Loos and Needleman put it: "Deep residual pockets form a favourable niche for biofilms dominated by asaccharolytic, proteolytic and anaerobic pathobionts. [...] These subgingival dysbiotic microcosms in deep residual pockets after therapy re-challenge the periodontitis patients who have already demonstrated to have an aberant immune response." Thus, while acknowledging the extremely thin evidence base, they conclude that "the achievement of shallow periodontal pockets (≤4 mm) that do not bleed on probing in patients with full-mouth bleeding scores <30% confers the highest chance of stability of periodontal health and lowest risk of tooth loss." It should be noted, however, that this conclusion does not immediately translate in the—seemingly equivalent—conclusion that surgical treatment is preferred over nonsurgical treatment. Again, robust trial evidence is needed to assess the validity of this assertion. Another important limitation of the available evidence is that studies have been exclusively conducted in university settings, i.e., under ideal conditions with few time constraints and often very frequent, intensive follow-up care with a highly motivated, selected patient population. Hence, it is uncertain whether these conclusions can be generalized to general or periodontal practice settings.

Nonsurgical therapy and flap surgery are, strictly speaking and in current periodontal practice, not true treatment alternatives, because nonsurgical therapy is almost invariably performed initially, i.e., practically all patients diagnosed with periodontitis initially receive nonsurgical periodontal therapy (Sanz et al. 2020). Accordingly, only some of the studies included in the systematic reviews compared nonsurgical vs. surgical therapy without any pretreatment scaling, while the majority of studies conducted nonsurgical treatment in all groups and then either compared surgery to no treatment or surgery to a second nonsurgical treatment (Sanz et al. 2020; Sanz-Sanchez et al. 2020).

In a given clinical situation, the relevant clinical question to be discussed with the patient would be whether or not the likely benefits of flap surgery outweigh the likely adverse effects when compared to continued maintenance

therapy after nonsurgical therapy, including, when necessary, repeated subgingival instrumentation. If the expected benefits of surgery outweigh the expected adverse effects, the next question to be discussed with the patient is whether the net benefit of surgery over maintenance justifies its additional cost.

This is not merely an academic discussion. Importantly, there is no need to make a decision for or against surgical therapy before initial therapy from a periodontal perspective. Rather, whether or not surgical therapy is necessary and if so, on what teeth, should be decided only after the results of nonsurgical therapy have been evaluated. In this context it is important to remember that the conclusions drawn from clinical trials refer to population averages, i.e., periodontal surgery results in greater pocket depth reduction and better clinical attachment levels in deep pockets on average. For most treatment outcomes, considerable interindividual variability exists, i.e., many patients respond unexpectedly well to nonsurgical therapy, and additional surgery would not be expected to yield significant benefits (Figure 9.2.). In fact, it was shown almost 40 years ago that "there is no certain magnitude of initial probing pocket depth where nonsurgical periodontal therapy is no longer effective" (Badersten et al. 1984). Others may respond unexpectedly poorly to nonsurgical therapy and surgical therapy may have to be considered, even in shallow or moderately deep pockets.

The evidence for an association between periodontitis and systemic disease may also have implications on the choice of treatment in some periodontitis patients. For example, a recent study included surgical treatment to facilitate rapid pocket elimination in a randomized trial on the effects of periodontal treatment on metabolic control of diabetes in diabetic patients with periodontitis (D'Aiuto et al. 2018).

In summary, the relative effectiveness of surgical vs. nonsurgical periodontal therapy depends on the initial disease level (initial pocket depth). There is robust evidence from clinical trials that in the short term, surgical periodontal therapy results in better outcomes in terms of probing depth reduction and, in deep sites with initial probing depths greater than 6 mm, better outcomes in terms of clinical attachment levels, compared to nonsurgical therapy. However, the relevance of these benefits in the long term with regard to tooth loss and other outcomes relevant to the patient, including any adverse effects of surgical vs. nonsurgical therapy, is uncertain. In the absence of such evidence, it may be prudent to offer nonsurgical therapy as a first line treatment to every patient with periodontitis, irrespective of initial disease levels, and to consider surgical therapy in cases in which the response to nonsurgical therapy was unsatisfactory.

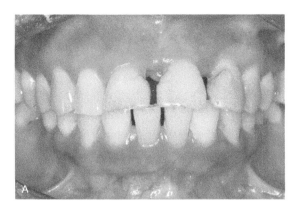
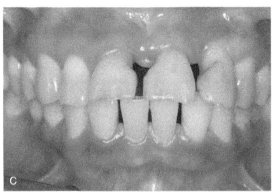
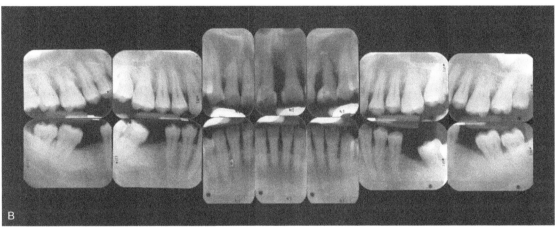
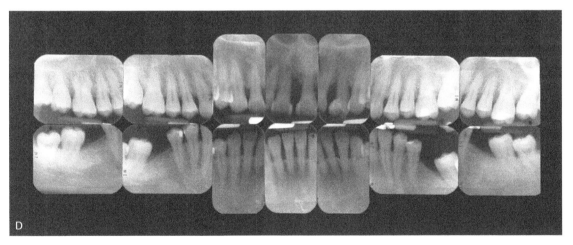

Figure 9.2   37-year-old female patient, nonsmoker, medically fit. A, Clinical and B, radiographic status at the time of presentation to the university clinic. Note the massive bone and attachment loss of maxillary incisors. The maxillary right central incisor has a 9-mm pocket mesially; pocket depths are up to 6 mm at the other incisors. The patient received nonsurgical periodontal therapy with hand and sonic instruments combined with systemic antibiotics (375 mg amoxicillin and 250 mg metronidazole tds for seven days). The patient was recalled every three months for supportive periodontal therapy, at which time the sites with probing depths of 4 mm and bleeding on probing and all sites with probing depths of 5+ mm were instrumented with ultrasonic instruments. C, After 17 months of therapy no probing depths greater than 3 mm remain and D, there is radiographic evidence of bony repair. Case courtesy of Drs. Walter and Krastl. Full case report: Walter C and Krastl G. 2007. Quintessence, 58, 1085–1096.

## References

Antczak-Bouckoms, A., Joshipura, K., Burdick, E., and Tulloch, J.F. (1993). Meta-analysis of surgical versus non-surgical methods of treatment for periodontal disease. *J. Clin. Periodontol.* 20 (4): 259–268.

Badersten, A., Nilveus, R., and Egelberg, J. (1984). Effect of nonsurgical periodontal therapy. II. Severely advanced periodontitis. *J. Clin. Periodontol.* 11 (1): 63–76.

Caton, J.G., Armitage, G., Berglundh, T. et al. (2018). A new classification scheme for periodontal and peri-implant diseases and conditions – Introduction and key changes from the 1999 classification. *J. Clin. Periodontol.* 45 (Suppl 20): S1–S8.

D'Aiuto, F., Gkranias, N., Bhowruth, D. et al. TASTE Group. (2018 December). Systemic effects of periodontitis treatment in patients with type 2 diabetes: a 12 month, single-centre, investigator-masked, randomised trial. *Lancet Diabetes Endocrinol.* 6 (12): 954–965.

Heitz-Mayfield, L.J.A. (2005). How effective is surgical therapy compared with nonsurgical debridement? *Periodontol. 2000* 37: 72–87.

Heitz-Mayfield, L.J.A., Trombelli, L., Heitz, F. et al. (2002). A systematic review of the effect of surgical debridement vs non-surgical debridement for the treatment of chronic periodontitis. *J. Clin. Periodontol.* 29 (Suppl 3): 92–102. discussion 160–62.

Hujoel, P.P. (2004). Endpoints in periodontal trials: the need for an evidence-based research approach. *Periodontol. 2000* 36: 196–204.

Hung, H.-C. and Douglass, C.W. (2002). Meta-analysis of the effect of scaling and root planing, surgical treatment and antibiotic therapies on periodontal probing depth and attachment loss. *J. Clin. Periodontol.* 29 (11): 975–986.

Loos, B.G. and Needleman, I. (2020). Endpoints of active periodontal therapy. *J. Clin. Periodontol.* 47: 61–71.

Matuliene, G., Pjetursson, B.E., Salvi, G.E., et al. (2008). Influence of residual pockets on progression of periodontitis and tooth loss: Results after 11 years of maintenance. *J. Clin. Periodontol.* 35: 685–695. https://doi.org/10.1111/j.1600-051X.2008.01245.x.

Sanz, M., Herrera, D., Kebschull, M. et al. (2020). Treatment of stage I-III periodontitis – The EFP S3 level clinical practice guideline. *J. Clin. Periodontol.* n/a (n/a): 4–60.

Sanz-Sanchez, I., Montero, E., Citterio, F. et al. (2020). Efficacy of access flap procedures compared to subgingival debridement in the treatment of periodontitis. A systematic review and meta-analysis. *J. Clin. Periodontol.* doi: 10.1111/jcpe.13259.

# 10

# Supportive Periodontal Therapy
*Praveen Sharma*

## Introduction

The 2017 World Workshop classification recognizes periodontitis as a condition, for which patients retain a lifelong susceptibility. With this in mind, clinicians should think of "management" of periodontitis, as opposed to "treatment" of periodontitis. This is similar to other, chronic, noncommunicable diseases, such as diabetes. Most patients with diabetes "manage" their condition, often via a mixture of pharmacological and non-pharmacological means. In a similar fashion, patients with periodontitis also manage their condition, this time using almost exclusively non-pharmacological means (mechanical disruption of plaque biofilm). Having this conversation with patients at the outset of treatment is recommended to obtain informed consent and to empower patients to manage their disease. As part of this process, the lifelong nature of management of periodontitis should be stressed. In practice, the lifelong management of periodontitis takes different forms and needs to be personalized to the individual patient.

After the phase of active periodontal therapy (APT), patients are entered into the maintenance phase of treatment called supportive periodontal therapy (SPT) or supportive periodontal care (SPC). With this support in place, most patients can expect to retain most teeth (Carvalho et al. 2021). The evidence supporting SPT and the steps involved in delivering SPT are detailed below.

## Technique

1) **Duration of recall**

Just as periodontal disease and therapy is highly individualized between patients, so is the recall therapy. The recall interval should be titrated for individual patients based on analyses of factors such as probing pocket depth (PPD), plaque levels, and risk factor control over time (Sanz et al. 2020). These are discussed in more detail below. Initially, a short (3–6 month) recall interval may be prudent (Ramseier et al. 2019). If the patient maintains stability in their periodontal condition, this can be relaxed to a longer (6–12 month) interval. If, however, the longer interval leads to a recurrence of unstable periodontal disease, the interval can be shortened again. In addition, patients with rapidly progressing disease (Grade C) may warrant a shorter recall interval compared with patients with slower progressing disease (Grade A) (Carvalho et al. 2021). This dynamic assessment of recall interval would be very familiar to practitioners. Finally, as outlined below, not all steps need to be followed at all intervals. For example, a patient with less-than-ideal plaque control may be seen at 3-month intervals for a plaque score and reinforcement of oral hygiene instructions as well as a generalized supragingival professional mechanical plaque removal (PMPR) and then seen every 6–12 months for a 6-point pocket chart measuring PPD (± recession) and bleeding on probing. Similarly, the division of these appointments can be shared between the specialist, dentist, and hygienist.

2) **Anamnesis**

Thorough anamnesis should comprise a summary of the patient's experience of any "side effects" of treatment. As part of the informed consent process, prior to commencing APT, patients would be warned about the short-term side effects including soreness and the longer-term side effects, mainly recession and the sequelae of recession including sensitivity, aesthetic compromise, and increased risk of root caries. It is important to ask non-leading, open-ended questions at this point. If patients encounter these side effects after being informed of them, they are much more likely to respond positively and see these as signs of improving periodontal health. During SPT, this information will be updated and important points reiterated, to continuously engage with the patient to ensure compliance

*Practical Periodontal Diagnosis and Treatment Planning,* Second Edition. Edited by Serge Dibart and Thomas Dietrich.
© 2024 John Wiley & Sons, Inc. Published 2024 by John Wiley & Sons, Inc.

and to modify the approach to SPT as necessary. As for any recall appointment, updating the medical and social histories can provide an update on some risk factors and their control. This is very important and is discussed in detail below. Finally, the dental care practitioner should then elicit the patient's oral hygiene routine, in their own words. Well-motivated and experienced patients can usually tell the practitioner exactly which interdental brush (brand and color/size) they use in each interdental space.

3) **Risk factor management**
Risk factors in periodontitis can be classified as modifiable/non-modifiable. The effect of the non-modifiable risk factors can be mitigated to some extent by improving oral hygiene on the part of the patient. Among the modifiable risk factors, the level of plaque control is paramount and all other risk factors operate via affecting either plaque and/or host-response. Plaque control can be gleaned from the anamnesis as well as using disclosing dye to visualize plaque and use a score/index to quantify this. A plaque score is relatively straightforward to use but lacks the detail that might be captured in various plaque indices. The plaque score is also readily summarized as a percentage and is easy for patients to understand and see longitudinal changes in. These changes in plaque score over time can be used as an important motivator for the patient. Following from plaque control, update on other modifiable risk factors and their control (such as tobacco use, diabetes control, diet and stress) is usually elicited in updating the medical/social history of the patient. While the assessment/management of individual risk factors is beyond the scope of this chapter, it is important for the patient and practitioner to recognize the importance of risk factors and their control as, without this dimension, periodontal therapy may not sufficiently manage the patient's disease (Ramseier et al. 2020).

4) **Reassessment of periodontal health measures**
Opportunity should be taken at some, if not all, SPT visits to reassess the periodontal health measures collected at baseline. This usually involves a 6-point pocket charting recording, at 6 sites per tooth, usually mesio-, mid-, and distobuccal and palatal/lingual per tooth, the PPD (± recession) and bleeding on probing. This allows for the classification of periodontal disease as stable/in remission/unstable (Chapple et al. 2018) and allows for further management as necessary. Once the 6-point chart is completed, mobility of individual teeth can be reassessed. This is usually followed by a full mouth plaque score/index as mentioned in the risk factor sec-

tion above. The disclosed mouth can then be used as a tool to reinforce oral hygiene instruction as detailed below.

5) **Reinforcement of oral hygiene instructions (OHI)**
Reinforcement of detailed, tailored OHI both in the use of electric/manual toothbrushes and interdental cleaning is a key component of the SPT visits (Sanz et al. 2020). OHI can be tailored to the individual patient using the patients' disclosed mouth to highlight areas of good plaque control and areas where the plaque control may be less than ideal. This can be correlated with the patient's 6-point pocket charting as areas of poor plaque control will often show a worse response to treatment. The reinforcement of OHI is important as it is the twice daily disruption of the biofilm on the tooth surfaces which will limit the negative effect on the periodontium. This has been demonstrated by several experimental gingivitis studies where volunteers are advised not to clean a section of the mouth and the deterioration in gingival health (up to development of gingivitis which is reversed with the resumption of OH) is noted. One way of reinforcing OHI is, using the disclosed mouth, demonstrating OH techniques to the patient using their own OH aids (toothbrush, interdental brush as well as any other aids) and asking the patient to demonstrate the technique back to the healthcare practitioner.

6) **Generalized supragingival PMPR**
PMPR performed on a regular basis by dental care practitioners should form a part of each SPT visit (Sanz et al. 2020). This can be performed following the OHI demonstrated on the patient's disclosed mouth. Removal of any plaque retentive factors, commonly calculus, reduces the rate of plaque buildup and can help with prevention of relapse of disease (Axelsson and Lindhe 1981).

## Evidence-based Outcomes

In 2014, Costa et al. reported the findings from a five-year prospective cohort study (Costa et al. 2014). In this, the authors reported following a cohort of 256 patients who had completed APT and were enrolled for SPT. The cohort was divided into "regular compliers" (RC), which included patients who attended all scheduled SPT appointments, and "irregular compliers" (IC), which included patients who missed any SPT visits but continued to attend sporadically with a maximum of 18 months between visits. At the end of the study, ICs had a more than threefold increase in odds of tooth loss, compared with RCs (OR:3.13; 95% CI:1.45 to 4.98). Other factors associated with an increased odds of tooth loss included male gender (OR: 1.86; 95% CI: 1.18 to 6.34), smoking (OR: 4.42; 95% CI: 2.01 to 12.78), diabetes (OR: 2.73; 95% CI: 1.09 to 6.69), and probing depth between 4 and 6 mm up to 10% of sites (OR: 3.47; 95% CI: 2.02 to 11.64).

An updated systematic review published in 2021 (Carvalho et al. 2021) supports the notion of low rate of tooth loss in patients enrolled in SPT. The authors demonstrated that, with SPT, the average rate of tooth loss can be very low (0.12 teeth per year, 95% CI: 0.10 to 0.14).

## Conclusion

In conclusion, the importance of regular SPT is key in the maintenance of periodontal health and tooth retention. SPT needs to be tailored, both in its interval as well as the contents, and therefore duration, of the visit. Patients should be informed of the need for lifelong SPT from the outset of treatment and should be on board with this. With an SPT plan in place, most patients should expect to keep most teeth in the long term.

## References

Axelsson, P. and Lindhe, J. (1981). The significance of maintenance care in the treatment of periodontal-disease. *J. Clin. Periodontol.* 8 (4): 281–294.

Carvalho, R., Botelho, J., Machado, V. et al. (2021). Predictors of tooth loss during long-term periodontal maintenance: an updated systematic review. *J. Clin. Periodontol.* 48 (8): 1019–1036.

Chapple, I.L.C., Mealey, B.L., Van Dyke, T.E. et al. (2018). Periodontal health and gingival diseases and conditions on an intact and a reduced periodontium: consensus report of workgroup 1 of the 2017 World Workshop on the Classification of Periodontal and Peri-Implant Diseases and Conditions. *J. Clin. Periodontol.* 45: S68–S77.

Costa, F.O., Lages, E.J.P., Cota, L.O.M. et al. (2014). Tooth loss in individuals under periodontal maintenance therapy: 5-year prospective study. *J. Periodont. Res.* 49 (1): 121–128.

Ramseier, C.A., Nydegger, M., Walter, C. et al. (2019). Time between recall visits and residual probing depths predict long-term stability in patients enrolled in supportive periodontal therapy. *J. Clin. Periodontol.* 46 (2): 218–230.

Ramseier, C.A., Woelber, J.P., Kitzmann, J. et al. (2020). Impact of risk factor control interventions for smoking cessation and promotion of healthy lifestyles in patients with periodontitis: a systematic review. *J. Clin. Periodontol.* 47: 90–106.

Sanz, M., Herrera, D., Kebschull, M. et al. (2020). Treatment of stage I–III periodontitis – The EFP S3 level clinical practice guideline. *J. Clin. Periodontol.* 47: 4–60.

## 11

# Dental Implants Therapy
*Serge Dibart and Lorenzo Montesani*

## Introduction

The history of implants and their surgical placement, indications, healing process, etc. have been discussed in great detail in a previous book (Dibart 2007). The purpose of this chapter is a little bit more challenging. What evidence do we have that the treatments we are rendering are really necessary or effective? And if so, how effective? We looked at systematic reviews in our attempt to answer these questions in light of the most recent evidence-based research literature available. Such reviews of the existing literature can be found in various databases (MEDLINE, Cochrane, EMBASE). Several authors have described the value of systematic reviews in dental research, and as a result they have been recognized as powerful research tools in evidence-based dentistry. Systematic reviews are inherently less biased, more reliable, and more valid than narrative reviews (Bader 2004; Carr 2002). The treatment decisions we make need to be based on the scientific study of clinical outcomes taken from properly documented and executed clinical research.

## Indications

Implant therapy is aimed at replacing natural teeth that have been lost in the past or had to be recently extracted, leaving an area edentulous. So let us look at a few reasons why we would need to extract natural teeth. The decision to extract is made when the restorability of the tooth is in doubt. The usual scenario involves incipient or recurrent caries, trauma, endodontic failure, root fracture, and periodontal disease.

## Evidence-based Outcomes

### The Tooth Extraction Dilemma: Root Canal Therapy, Fixed Partial Denture, or Implant-supported Crown?

There are enormous benefits in retaining a natural tooth; we have to remember that we, as periodontists, have the duty to preserve the natural dentition as long as possible and that dental implants, as wonderful as they are, may never replace fully natural teeth. The advantages of retaining a natural tooth include:

- Preservation of the alveolar bone
- Preservation of the papilla
- Preservation of pressure perception
- Preservation of natural structures (crown, root)
- Lack of movement of the surrounding teeth

Torabinejad et al., in 2007, after a thorough systematic review of the literature, tried to compare the long-term success rate of endodontic treatment vs. fixed partial denture (FPD) or implant-supported crown (ISC). This proved to be an arduous task, because the evidence identified by the authors did not permit them to definitively answer all of the questions posed. The evidence available for answering the questions came from mainly indirect comparisons, hence the warning that these conclusions are tentative and that there is a need for additional studies.

The concept of success is also reported differently in the literature when we compare the outcomes of RCT, FPD, or implant-supported crowns (ISC). An implant that has had some marginal bone loss and is still functional is not generally considered a failure, whereas FPD's failure can be reported as presence of recurrent decay, root fracture, porcelain fracture, loss of retention, etc. The endodontic literature is far more precise in documenting/defining success and failure. Because RCT is aimed at treating an existing disease, the evaluation of a successful outcome via radiographic monitoring or patient's lack of symptoms is much easier.

In Torabinejad's analysis, looking at 6+ years follow-up, the weighted survival data indicated that in patients with periodontally sound teeth having pulpal and/or periradicular pathosis, root canal therapy resulted in a survival rate of 97% (Table 11.1). The same rate (97%) was also found for extraction and replacement of a missing tooth with an implant. On the other hand, an extraction and replacement with FPD had a survival rate of 82%, well below that of RCT and ISC at six years. The authors also reported that FPD success rates continued to drop steadily over time beyond 60 months. This was confirmed by another review of the literature, by Salinas et al. (2004), which stated that at 15 years the rate of survival of the FPD had dropped to 69%, whereas at 11 years the cumulative success rate for implants was 93% (Naert et al. 2000). This indicates that an implant-supported crown would be the better choice when deciding on how to restore a missing tooth in a dentition.

In 2007, Stavropoulou and Koidis conducted a systematic review of the literature to test the hypothesis that the placement of a prosthetic crown on an endodontically treated tooth was associated with improved survival rates. They found that the cumulative survival rates after 10 years for RCT with crowns and RCT without crowns were 81 ± 12% and 63 ± 15%, respectively. Hence, the necessity to crown the teeth that have been endodontically treated.

**Author's Views/Comments:** The longevity of the classical treatment—RCT, possible crown lengthening when needed, and prosthetic crown—depends on the quality of each of the steps performed by the general dentist or the specialists involved. Not all dentists are created equal, hence the variability of long-term success/survival. It is much easier and less technique-sensitive to remove a questionable tooth and place an implant followed by a crown. That being said, we have to emphasize the better soft tissue esthetics when a natural tooth is kept as well as the overall shorter treatment time.

## Dental Implant Placement: Immediate, Immediate Delayed, or Conventional Delayed Placement?

Dental implants can be placed in fresh extraction sockets, just after tooth extraction. These are called immediate implants. They have the advantage of shortening the treatment time for the patient as well as reducing the number of surgical procedures. They also can be placed without raising a flap in most cases. The disadvantages are enhanced risk of infection and failure, the presence of a gap between the implant and alveolus, and the necessity sometimes of bone grafting (Rosenquist 1997; Takeshita et al. 1997). An alternative is the immediate-delayed option. These implants are placed in the healing socket after four to eight weeks to allow for the soft tissue healing that will permit primary closure of the coronal gingiva when using a two-stage system. Finally, conventional or delayed implants are those placed several months after extraction in a partially or completely healed socket.

Esposito et al. (2008), after a very thorough review of the existing literature, found only two randomized control trials (Lindeboom et al. 2006; Schropp et al. 2003) that could be used to shed some light on which therapeutic conduct to adopt (Table 11.2). They concluded that based on

Table 11.1 Comparative long-term survival rates of root canal treatment plus crown, root canal treatment without crown, implant-supported crown, and fixed partial denture.

| Treatment option | 6 years | 10 years | 11 years | 15 years |
|---|---|---|---|---|
| Root canal treatment with crown | 97% | 81 ± 12% | | |
| Root canal treatment without crown | | 63 ± 15% | | |
| Implant-supported crown | 97% | | 93% | |
| Fixed partial denture | 82% | | | 69% |

Table 11.2 Failure rate comparison between immediate, immediate delayed, and delayed implants.

| Study | Immediate | Immediate delayed | Delayed |
|---|---|---|---|
| Lindeboom, 2006 N = 50 | 2/25 (8%) | | 0/25 (0%) |
| Schropp, 2003 N = 44 | | 2/22 (9%) | 1/22 (4.5%) |

the outcome from these two well-designed and -conducted studies, immediate and immediate delayed implants were viable treatment options. Looking at the raw numbers, these groups both had more implant failures and complications than the delayed implant group. Esposito et al. mentioned that patients prefer immediate delayed implants, which may provide a better esthetic outcome, even though they might be associated with increased failures and complication rates. They also mentioned that there is not enough reliable evidence supporting or refuting the need for augmentation procedures at immediate implant placements in fresh extraction sockets and that there is no reliable evidence supporting the efficacy of platelet-rich plasma (PRP) in conjunction with implant placement. Finally, they emphasized the fact that these are only preliminary results and that more randomized, controlled trials are necessary to confirm these findings.

**Author's Views/Comments:** All of these options are viable, but immediate implants are quite technique/operator-sensitive. They seem to be more prone to complication/failure when compared to the delayed implants. If one does not have much experience with implant placement, one should do many delayed placements before attempting the immediate implant placement.

## Is Antibiotherapy Justified to Prevent Implant Failures?

We routinely give patients antibiotics to avoid complications, but with the alarming increase in antibiotic-resistant bacteria, is this reasonable? Are we really helping the patient or are we helping ourselves to a better night's sleep? Once again, let us look at the pertinent literature. Esposito et al. (2009), in the Cochrane database of systematic reviews of 2008, tried to identify suitable randomized, controlled trials to assess the effects of prophylactic antibiotics for implant placement vs. no antibiotics or placebo administration. They found no randomized, controlled trial that could pass rigorous scrutiny (some had flaws in the methodology, others had flaws in data extraction, etc.). They concluded that there is no appropriate scientific evidence to recommend or discourage the use of prophylactic systemic antibiotics to prevent complications and failures of dental implants. They stated, "It seems sensible to recommend the use of prophylactic antibiotics for patients at high and moderate risk for endocarditis, patients with immunodeficiencies, metabolic diseases, irradiated in the head and neck area and when an extensive or prolonged surgery is anticipated." This implies that every single healthy patient who receives an implant may not necessarily need to be premedicated and that antibiotherapy should be reserved for medically compromised patients

and those undergoing long or traumatic procedures (multiple implant placement, external sinus lifts, guided bone regeneration, bloc grafts, surgery performed in infected sites, etc.).

In a 2009 update, Esposito et al. concluded that there was some evidence suggesting that 2 g of amoxicillin given orally on hour preoperatively significantly reduced failures of dental implants placed in ordinary conditions. Various prophylactic systemic antibiotic regimens are available, and the current recommendation is to keep the prophylaxis short (i.e., a single dose of amoxicillin—2 g—given one hour prior to surgery) with the understanding that with each administration, adverse events may occur, ranging from diarrhea to life-threatening allergic reactions.

**Author's Views/Comments:** I personally believe that we are too quick in prescribing antibiotics. But this is also a reflection on the type of litigious society we are living in—40% of the world's lawyers practice in the USA! In my opinion, a good presurgical intraoral rinse with chlorhexidine, followed by thorough cleansing of the skin (lips, nose, cheeks, etc.), and the use of surgical drapes and aseptic surgical technique should cut down on the use of antibiotics tremendously, especially when the patient is healthy and the procedure is short and atraumatic (i.e., single implant placement).

## When Should Implants Be Loaded?

Primary implant stability and lack of micro-movements are considered to be two of the main factors necessary for achieving predictable high success of osseointegrated oral implants (Albrektsson et al. 1981). The presence of micro-movements during the healing period may impair successful osseointegration of the implant by allowing a soft tissue interface to develop between the bone and the implant (Brunski et al. 1979), hence the original recommendation to keep the implants load-free during the healing period (three to four months for the mandible and six to eight months for the maxilla) (Branemark et al. 1977). With the current desire to reduce the length of treatment, achieve better esthetics, and reduce the annoyance of removable temporaries, we are restoring and loading the implants at a different pace. The immediately placed implant can be restored immediately (within 72 hours) and can be occlusally loaded or not (immediate provisionalization). The early loading of an implant takes place six to eight weeks after surgical placement; finally, the conventional loading takes place according to Branemark's recommendations.

Whether implants can be loaded immediately after their placement or months later has important clinical repercussions. Patients like to leave the office with teeth, and do not enjoy wearing a transitional partial denture while waiting for the process of osseointegration to take place. Furthermore, in this fast-paced society, short treatment times are appealing to the patient and dentist alike—so is this a viable option? Esposito et al. (2007) conducted a systematic review of the subject and retained 11 articles out of the 20 originally selected. They found no statistically significant difference at six months to one year follow-up between the various loading regimens.

An interesting finding that is directly correlated to the success of immediate loading is the initial insertion torque of the implant. In fact, Ottoni et al. (2005) demonstrated a strong correlation between implant failures and the initial insertion torque of the implant. Nine of the 10 immediate nonocclusal load implants inserted with a 20 Ncm torque failed, vs. only one failure out of 10 placed with an insertion torque of 32 Ncm torque (90% failure vs. 10%!) (Table 11.3). This demonstrates the imperative need to have a high degree of primary stability at implant insertion for a successful immediate or early loading procedure.

Another question that comes to mind is: Is immediate nonocclusion loading safer than immediate occlusal loading, where there is full occlusal contact with the opposing dentition? Lindeboom et al. attempted to answer this question in a randomized, controlled trial in 2006. They concluded that there is no statistically significant difference nor clinical increased failure when comparing immediate occlusal loading and nonocclusal loading.

**Author's Views/Comments:** It is important to use caution when reading the abovementioned findings, because the number of patients and trials is relatively small and the follow-up period short (six months to one year). There is a need for more randomized, controlled studies to gain the definitive answers. This being said, and reviewing the relevant current literature, one notices that in the very successful trials only the "ideal" patients were recruited, using stringent selection criteria and being treated by very skilled operators. Therefore, the chances of failure were minimized. When less experienced operators were involved, failure rates could be as high as 42% (Tawse-Smith et al. 2002). One constant seems to be the necessity of a high degree of primary stability (torque value of at least 32 Ncm) for the immediate loading to be successful. This could be achieved during the surgical phase by "under preparing"

Table 11.3 Correlation of insertion torque values and failure rates of immediate nonocclusal load implants. Adapted from Ottoni et al., 2005.

| Torque value | Failure rate |
| --- | --- |
| 20 Ncm | 90% |
| 32 Ncm | 10% |

the osteotomy site and inserting the implant slowly, avoiding unnecessary heating of the bone. Another critical component, in my opinion, is the control of the occlusion and the necessity of avoiding lateral forces and excessive load after provisionalization.

**What about Peri-Implant Diseases?**

A recent systematic review based on a European consensus conference revealed that the prevalence of peri-implant mucositis and peri-implantitis ranges from 19 to 65%! (Derks and Tomsai 2015). This rather high percentage makes peri-implantitis and peri-implant mucositis a common complication of dental implant therapy. Treatment of peri-implantitis may not be as predictable or as long lasting as the surgical treatment of compromised teeth (Carcuac et al. 2020; Jepsen et al. 2016). We have to keep that in mind and not be quick to condemn teeth with modest amounts of caries, need for endodontic or periodontal therapy. Our practice pattern needs to change to retain more natural teeth given the excellent long-term track record of successful therapy for tooth preservation (Giannobile and Lang 2016).

## References

Albrektsson, T., Branemark, P.I., Hansson, H.A., and Lindstrom, J. (1981). Osseointegrated titanium implants. Requirements for ensuring a long lasting, direct bone to implant anchorage in man. *Acta. Orthopedica. Scandinavica.* 52 (2): 155–170.

Bader, J.D. (2004). Systematic reviews and their implications for dental practice. *Tex. Dent. J.* 121: 380–387.

Branemark, P.I., Hansson, B.O., Adell, R. et al. (1977). *Osseointegrated Implants in the Treatment of the Edentulous Jaw. Experience from a 10 Year Period.* Stockholm: Almqvist and Wiskell International.

Brunski, J.B., Moccia, A.F., Pollack, S.R. et al. (1979). The influence of functional use of endosseous dental implant on the tissue-implant interface. 1. Histological aspects. *J. Dent. Res.* 58 (10): 1953–1969.

Carcuac, O., Derks, J., Abrahamsson, I. et al. (2020 November). Risk for recurrence of disease following surgical therapy of peri-implantitis – A prospective longitudinal study. *Clin. Oral Implants Res.* 31 (11): 1072–1077. doi: 10.1111/clr.13653. Epub 2020 Sep 14).

Carr, A.B. (2002). Systematic review of the literature: the overview and meta analysis. *Dent. Clin. North Am.* 46: 79–86.

Derks, J. and Tomsai, C. (2015). Peri-implant health and disease: a systematic review of current epidemiology. *J. Clin. Periodontol.* 42 (Suppl. 16): S158–S171.

Dibart, S. (2007). *Practical Advanced Periodontal Surgery*. Blackwell Publishing.

Esposito, M., Grusovin, M.G., Talati, M. et al. (2008). Interventions for replacing missing teeth: antibiotics at dental implant placement to prevent complications. Cochrane Database of Systematic Reviews.

Esposito, M., Grusovin, M.G., Talati, M. et al. (2009). Interventions for replacing missing teeth: antibiotics at dental Implant placement to prevent complications. Cochrane Database of Systematic Reviews. Issue 2.

Esposito, M., Grusovin, M.G., Willings, M. et al. (2007). Interventions for replacing missing teeth: different times for loading dental implants. Cochrane Database of Systematic Reviews, Issue 2.

Giannobile, W.V. and Lang, N.P. (2016 January). Are dental implants a panacea or should we better strive to save teeth? *J. Dent. Res.* 95 (1): 5–6. doi: 10.1177/0022034515618942.

Jepsen, K., Jepsen, S., Laine, M.L. et al. (2016 January). Reconstruction of peri-implant osseous defects: a multicenter randomized trial. *J. Dent. Res.* 95 (1): 58–66. doi: 10.1177/0022034515610056. Epub 2015 Oct 8.).

Lindeboom, J.A., Tjiook, Y., and Kroon, F.H. (2006). Immediate placement of implants in periapical infected sites: a prospective randomized study in 50 patients. *Oral Surg. Oral Med. Oral Pathol.* 101 (6): 705–710.

Naert, I., Koutsikakis, G., Duyk, J. et al. (2000). Biologic outcome of single-implant restorations as tooth replacements: a long-term follow-up study. *Clin. Impl. Dent. Relat. Res.* 2: 209.

Ottoni, J.M., Oliveira, Z.F., Mansini, R., and Cubral, A.M. (2005). Correlation between placement torque and survival of single tooth implants. *IJOMI* 20 (5): 769–776.

Rosenquist, B. (1997). A comparison of several methods of soft tissue management following the immediate placement of implants into extraction sockets. *IJOMI* 12 (1): 43–51.

Salinas, T.J., Block, M.S., and Sadan, A. (2004). Fixed partial denture or single tooth implant restoration? Statistical considerations for sequencing and treatment. *J. Oral Maxillofac. Surg.* 62 (9): 2–16.

Schropp, L., Kostopoulos, L., and Wenzel, A. (2003). Bone healing following immediate versus delayed placement of titanium implants into extraction sockets: a prospective clinical study. *IJOMI* 18 (2): 189–199.

Takeshita, F., Tyama, S., Ayukawa, Y. et al. (1997). Abscess formation around a hydroxyapatite coated implant placed into the extraction socket with autogenous bone graft. A histological study using light microscopy, image processing and confocal laser scanning microscopy. *J. Perio.* 68 (3): 299–305.

Tawse-Smith, A., Payne, A.G., Kumara, R., and Thomson, W.M. (2002). Early loading of unsplinted implants supporting mandibular overdentures using a one-stage operative procedure with two different implant systems: a 2-year report. *Clin. Implant Dent. Relat. Res.* 4 (1): 33–42.

# 12

## Digital Integration of Implant Surgery Workflow

*Jeremy Kernitsky and Massimo Di Battista*

## Basic Concepts in Digital Dentistry

The origins of digital dentistry can be traced to almost 40 years ago, when the first dental restoration was milled using computer aided-design (CAD) and computer aided-manufacturing (CAM) by the first commercial CAD/CAM system: CEREC (Dentsply, Sirona) (Mörmann 2006). Since then, many advancements have been made in digital dentistry, but most of the basic principles stand the test of time. Most workflows in digital dentistry start from a process known as digitization, which consists of transporting diagnostic information into the digital world through various modalities. For instance, bone structures can be digitized by obtaining a cone-beam computed tomography (CBCT) providing a Digital Imaging and Communications in Medicine (DICOM) file, while teeth and soft tissue can be digitized by a variety of optical scanners to create a jaw replica in the form of a stereolithography (STL) file.

The digitized files have different functions and properties during the CAD-CAM process. For example, a DICOM file is a tridimensional volume rendering of an area of interest and its resolution is determined by the voxel size (Bankman 2000). This tridimensional visualization is nothing but a hologram and does not contain digital information on the surface geometry of the bone. In other words, this means that the boundaries of the imaged anatomical structures are not registered in the digital world. This type of imaging study (DICOM) is useful for diagnostic purposes, such as bone volume measurement and screening for pathology. However, due to the lack of surfaces in this type of file, it cannot be modified or integrated into a digital workflow without first identifying and extracting surfaces through segmentation.

An STL file, which is another type of 3D file, represents a surface and can be modified. Due to their versatility and the fact that they can be modified, STL files are used extensively in digital dentistry.

Segmentation is a process that allows obtaining an STL file from the original DICOM file. It is generally defined as the identification of all the voxels (or pixels) that belong to the object of interest or its boundary. Among the many existing segmentation methods, the preferred one is called "threshold segmentation." As implied by the name, threshold segmentation involves separating the object of interest (bone and teeth) from the rest of the volume (soft tissues and background) utilizing a cutoff radio-opacity value: the threshold (Bankman 2000). Some digital implant software will not let users set a specific threshold value, instead providing them with predetermined settings corresponding to different thresholds (e.g., bone, soft tissue, endo, etc.), while other software will let the user decide of the threshold themselves. Figure 12.1 represents different thresholds of the same CBCT.

Another important concept is superposition, which is defined as the process of placing an object over another. In the context of implant dentistry this is mostly done to superimpose an intraoral scan (or a scan of an impression) to the CBCT. This process is also referred to as "merging." This is beneficial because intraoral scans have a better resolution and fewer artifacts than CBCT images, especially for dental structure. The image of the dentition provided by a CBCT is not accurate enough to fabricate a surgical template that will precisely fit on teeth. By superimposing both files, the clinician gets the best of both worlds, high accuracy and anatomy visualization. Merging the scans also adds diagnostic value because it allows for more accurate visualization of the soft-tissue thickness. Unless the CBCT was acquired with cheek retractors in place (Januário et al. 2008), the facial soft tissue of the patient will most likely be contacting the cheeks at time of acquisition and will therefore be indistinguishable from them

*Practical Periodontal Diagnosis and Treatment Planning*, Second Edition. Edited by Serge Dibart and Thomas Dietrich.
© 2024 John Wiley & Sons, Inc. Published 2024 by John Wiley & Sons, Inc.

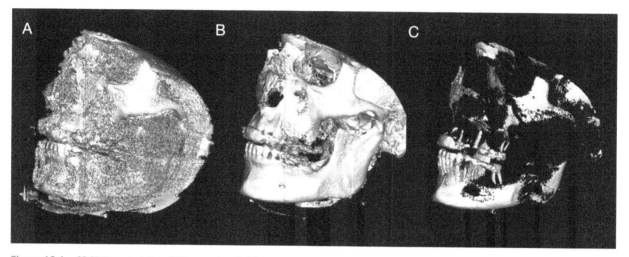

**Figure 12.1** CBCT Thresholding. Different thresholds are applied to the same CBCT dataset. (A) represents a too low thresholds; therefore, soft tissue and artifacts are visible. (B) represents an adequate threshold; the surface created represents mostly hard tissue. (C) represents a too high threshold; major parts of the hard tissue are missing.

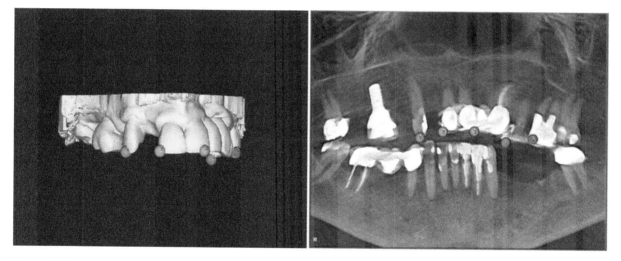

**Figure 12.2** The merging procedure. Reference points are highlighted on the STL surface of the intraoral scan (right) and a reconstructed panoramic image (left). The software then uses an algorithm to match both and gives the user the option to verify the merge. While the concept remains the same, other software systems have different ways of doing this, for example matching points to a 3D reconstruction of the CBCT instead of a panoramic image. To ensure a successful merge, it is recommended to have points on both sides of the arch.

on the resulting imaging study. When the intraoral scan is overlayed atop the CBCT, the thickness of the soft tissue becomes evident (Figure 12.3).

The STL files cannot be directly superimposed to the DICOM files; a surface must be extracted from the DICOM first. Most modern implant planning software will do this automatically for the clinician. Once the STL of the intraoral scan has been superimposed to the surface extracted from the DICOM file, the intraoral scan will be backwardly superimposed to the DICOM. In order to minimize the introduction of error in the treatment plan, it is primordial to ensure that the merging of the two surfaces is done accurately. The most

common way of doing this for dentate patients is by selecting and matching multiple reference points on the DICOM and the intraoral scan as shown in Figure 12.2. The relation of both scans can then be compared by evaluating the adaptation of the outline of the intraoral scan to the anatomical structure of the CBCT as shown in Figure 12.3.

Once the CBCT dataset is merged with the STL of the intraoral structures, the clinician can start planning for the implant treatment plan. Having the CBCT and the intraoral scan allows all the steps of implant planning, such as the digital wax-up, the surgical planning, and the design and manufacture of a surgical guide.

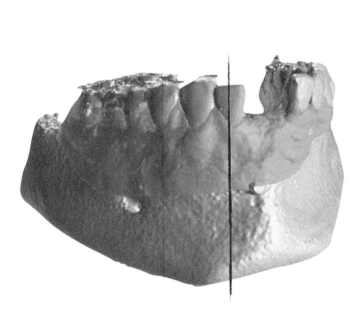
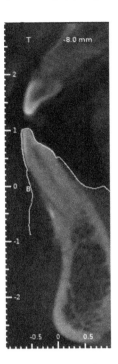

**Figure 12.3** Superimposition of intraoral scan and CBCT. (A)The STL surface of the intraoral scan (green) superimposed over the surface extracted from the CBCT (gray). (B) The outline of the intraoral scan (green) backwardly superimposed to the CBCT (grayscale). The tight adaptation of the outline around the tooth indicates a successful merge. Note that the soft tissue thickness is perceivable (distance between green line and bone).

## Surgical Planning: From Analog Static to Computer Generated Guides, Dynamic Surgery (Navigation and Robotic Placement)

### Digital Diagnostic Wax-up

One of the most notable paradigm shifts in modern implant dentistry is the "restoratively driven" concept. This is a treatment philosophy based around the fact that the only purpose of dental implants is to support a restoration, therefore the implant position should be mainly driven by the restorative plan and not the anatomy of the patient (Orentlicher et al. 2012). The surgical-restorative team must start with the end result in mind, i.e., the planned restoration, and the fixture(s) should be placed in the ideal position according to this plan.

From that perspective, the first step of implant planning, after patient assessment and interview, should be the diagnostic wax-up. Early protocols involved mounting casts, carving a physical wax-up, and subsequently scan it to merge with the CBCT (Kourtis et al. 2012). Later, fully digital protocols where a tooth is selected from a premade tooth bank and added onto the STL file of the intraoral scans were described (Lee et al. 2012). Although this method had the advantage of being fully digital, the fact

that teeth were from predetermined shapes meant that occlusion was not accounted for in the planning.

With modern advances in computer-assisted design and manufacturing (CAD/CAM), the planning, design, and manufacture of dental restoration are now routinely in most dental offices and educational institutions (Mörmann 2006). The technology used for these can be applied for the planification of ideal restorations for implant therapy. Dano et al. (2018) describes a fully digital workflow for restorative design and implant planning, as shown in Figure 12.4. This technique has the advantage of both being fully digital and taking occlusion in consideration.

For edentulous patients, since soft tissue is not a reliable indicator for the merging process (as it is not captured accurately in the CBCT) the ideal restoration can be merged to the 3D radiographic images through a process known as a dual scan. This process consists of obtaining a CBCT of the patient wearing an ideal denture that is embedded with radiopaque markers. Subsequently, another CBCT of the denture alone is captured. Two different DICOM files (one of the patient with the denture and one of the denture alone) are exported. The radiographic markers are then used to superimpose both images. This allows for visualization of the ideal denture teeth position in relation to the bone. A surface (STL file) can then be extracted from the denture scan and used as a framework for a surgical guide.

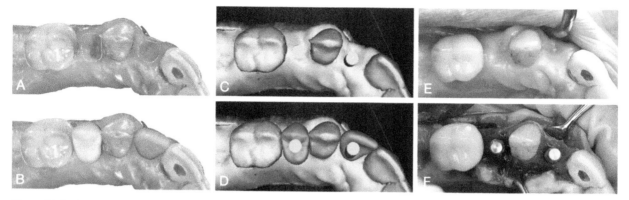

**Figure 12.4** From diagnostic wax-up to implant placement. (A) The intraoral scan with the approximate position of the CEJ traced. The digital wax-up is then computed and shown in (B). The implant planning based on these restorations is depicted in (C) and (D). This is done in the implant planning software and the CBCT is examined to confirm that the anatomy allows this placement. (E) and (F) represent the surgical procedure.

Currently, a multitude of guidance systems in dental implantology are available. They can be divided in two major categories: static and dynamic guidance. Static guides are characterized by the use of a physical template based on the digital plan, which is usually made of an acrylic material. This plan cannot be modified, and its accuracy is affected by multiple factors including but not limited to: planning software, distortion of the initial intraoral scan (STL) or DICOM, process of manufacturing of the guide, and most importantly the supporting or stabilization method of the guide intraorally (Ozan et al. 2009; Tahmaseb et al. 2018). Literature shows that tooth-supported guides usually offer superior precision over bone supported or mucosa supported (Ozan 2009). Surgical guides can be designed to be used for every step of the surgical procedure (fully guided) or to be used for one or some of the drills only (partially guided). As a rule of thumb, given the guide is fitting properly, fully guided surgery will be more accurate than partially guided surgery. It is also important to keep in mind that partially guided surgery is still significantly more accurate than free-hand surgery (Younes 2018). Static guides are the most common guidance method used but are subject to inaccuracy of on average 0.9 mm (up to 2 mm) and 2 degrees if a fully guided protocol is followed (Younes et al. 2018).

Static guides usually present as perforated arch-shaped templates. The perforations allow osteotomy drills and implants to pass in a restricted fashion, therefore limiting the range of motion of the operator to the desired position of the implant. These perforations are sometimes fitted with metallic sleeves to increase rigidity and further limit the range of motion. Usually, the sleeve will be of the diameter of the largest drill or of the implant attachment. Adaptors with the same external diameter as the sleeve, but with a smaller internal diameter also known as "drill keys" or "drill spoons" will be fitted inside the sleeves during osteotomy preparation to accommodate smaller drills and guide the entirety of the surgery.

Dynamic guidance consists of installing a fixture through either a navigation system or robotic guidance. These both allow for intraoperative modification of the surgical plan, hence the name "dynamic." In general, both methods will allow for a full digital workflow without the need for a physical guide. This eliminates the main drawback of physical guides, which is the inability to perform the surgical procedure immediately after planning (because of the time needed to manufacture the guide). Furthermore, not having a physical guide also allows for better access to the surgical site, facilitating visualization and irrigation.

Based on available evidence, both methods can achieve levels of accuracy similar to fully guided static guides, if not more. However, as these technologies are fairly new and are still being developed, more evidence is required (Bolding et al. 2021; Rawal et al. 2022; Stefanelli et al. 2019). That said, to this date there is no system that is 100% accurate. Consequently, the surgeon must still verify the accuracy of the guidance system throughout the implant surgery.

## Static Implant Guidance

### Tooth-borne Guide

Tooth-supported templates are the most accurate type of static guides (Dawson et al. 2009). They are therefore preferred when the conditions allow for their use. The surgical template must be stable and not present any deformation while under pressure in order to provide adequate precision for the implant placement. Caution must be exerted while treating a large edentulous area or a distal end. It has been shown that the quality and the location of teeth supporting the surgical guide influence the accuracy. However, for single implant sites, there is no benefit in covering more than four teeth adjacent to the surgical site or more than three posterior teeth. Including more teeth might increase the chances of misfit. Span of the guide for longer edentulous areas need to be evaluated in a case-by-case fashion (El Kholy et al. 2019).

Most digital implant software suites have an extension for the design of surgical templates. After the implant planning, the clinician will need to select a sleeve diameter and position based on the case and implant type. Then, the perimeter of the guide has to be selected. Care must be taken not to include too much soft tissue, as this can interfere with the stability of the guide. Retention must also be adequately assessed, as a too retentive guide might not sit, and a poorly retentive guide might move during the surgical procedure. Once the template is designed, it can then be manufactured in-house via either milling, 3D printing, or outsourced to a third party.

Figure 12.5 shows an immediate implant installed with a tooth-supported template. In immediate maxillary implant cases, the use of a guide is preferred because it reduces facial drift of the implant during placement compared to freehand surgery (Chen et al. 2018). A facially positioned implant might be detrimental to the overall success of the case because it can prevent the use of a screw-retained restoration or can result in the screw hole being in an unaesthetic position. The use of guided surgery also allows the preoperative preparation of a provisional restoration to be "picked up" after the placement, such as in Figure 12.5.

This workflow can also be modified for the template to be supported by prepared crown or bridge abutment teeth. In some cases of full-arch rehabilitation, the edentulous spaces can be temporarily restored by provisional bridges. To do so, the abutment teeth must be reduced before implant placement. If the provisional restorations are made with a radiolucent material, e.g., polymethylmethacrylate (PMMA), they will not be captured by the CBCT, therefore merging with an intraoral scan of the provisional teeth will be impossible. To address this, it is possible to merge the CBCT with an intraoral scan of the prepared abutment teeth, leading to the fabrication of an abutment teeth-supported guide. This also has the advantage of allowing the making and modifying of a new digital wax-up based on the abutment teeth and therefore gives more flexibility to the clinician. Figure 12.6 shows a scan that has been obtained with a PMMA provisional restoration, and Figures 12.7 and 12.8 show the workflow of a prepared teeth-borne surgical guide.

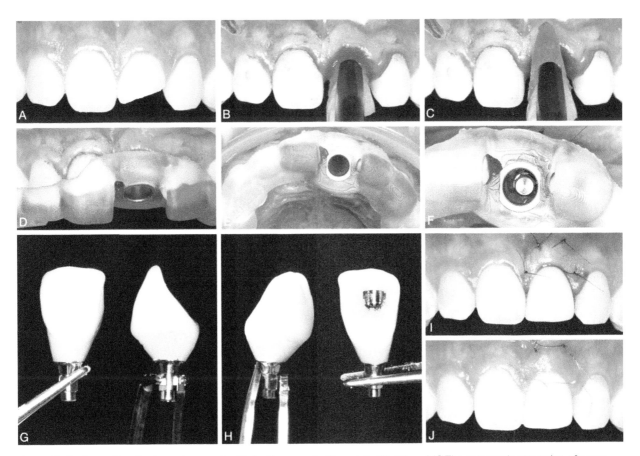

**Figure 12.5** Immediate implant placement with tooth-supported template. (A), (B), and (C)The atraumatic extraction of a non-restorable vertically fractured central incisor. (D) and (E) The surgical guide in situ. (F) The implant in final position. (G) and (H) The provisional restoration. (I) Immediate outcome. (J) 2 weeks post-surgery. Courtesy of Dr. Elias Exarchos.

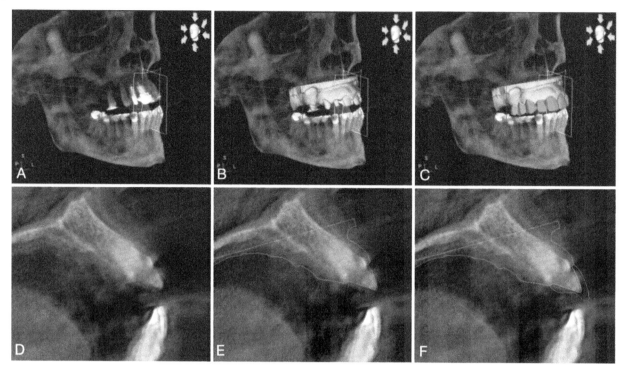

**Figure 12.6** Merging CBCT with scan of prepared teeth. This CBCT was captured with a PMMA provisional restoration. Note that the provisional is not visible on any of the images due to its radiolucency. (A)3D reconstruction of the CBCT. (B) 3D reconstruction of the CBCT with the merged scan of abutment teeth. (C) 3D reconstruction of the CBCT with the merged scan of abutment teeth and a digital wax-up. (D), (E), and (F) Cross-sectional views of A, B, and C.

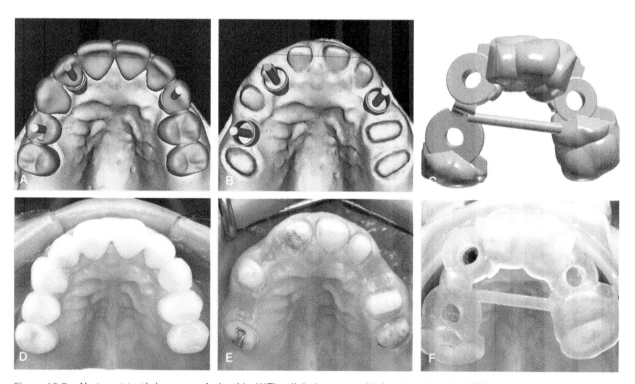

**Figure 12.7** Abutment teeth-borne surgical guide. (A)The digital wax-up with implant planning. (B) The implant planning on the digital cast of the abutment teeth. (C) The designed surgical guide. (D) The provisional restoration made with the digital wax-up. (E) Prepared teeth and edentulous areas. (F) The surgical guide in situ.

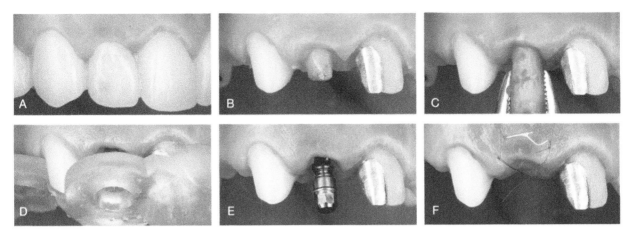

**Figure 12.8** Immediate implant placement with abutment teeth-borne surgical guide. (A) Provisional restoration in place preoperatively. (B) Tooth preparations exposed and cleaned after removal of provisional restoration. (C) Atraumatic extraction of the maxillary lateral incisor. (D) Surgical guide in situ. (E) Final implant position. (F) Site closed with collagen matrix after bone grafting.

## Mucosa-supported Guide

Mucosa-supported surgical templates are useful in cases where tooth-borne options are not suitable, such as fully edentulous patients. Utilization of this type of guide has been shown to deliver more accurate implant positions than freehand surgery (Vercruyssen et al. 2014). They rely on the mucosa for support, but fixation pins extending into the bone can be added to increase retention. The use of fixation pins may help in reducing facio-lingual deviation of the implants (Verhamme et al. 2015) but might result in a shallower implant placement apico-coronally than planned. This is believed to be a result of most templates not seating all the way, leading to an implant placed about 0.5 mm too coronal on average. If pins aren't used to stabilize a template, the template is subject to movement due to the mucosa being compressed by the pressure occurring during osteotomy presentation. This allows the implant to go deeper and therefore closer to the planned depth, but it also causes the neck of the implant to be placed more facially (Pessoa et al. 2022). To help seating the template while utilizing fixation pins, the template should be made to resemble a denture (with functional occlusal surfaces), allowing the patient to bite down on the template and the template to be anchored while in occlusion (Figure 12.10). One of the main advantages of fixation pins is that once they are placed, they can serve as a landmark for the guide position. This way, the guide can be used after the reflection of a flap without the need for the support of the crestal tissues, such as shown in Figure 12.11.

Since these templates are usually designed following the "dual scan" described earlier in this chapter, they are based off a denture. This allows for the template to be positioned in the mouth not only based on the relation of the soft tissues and the intaglio of the guide, but also the patient's occlusion (Figure 12.9). The patient can be asked to bite down on the guide while the fixation pins are being

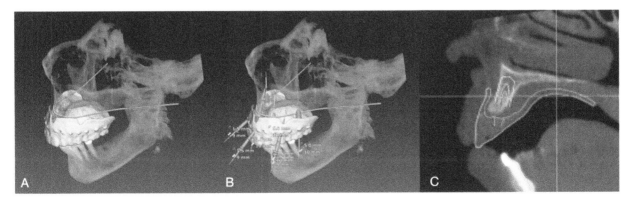

**Figure 12.9** Restoratively driven surgical treatment planning of maxillary full arch implant-supported overdenture. (A) Merging of both the scans of the "dual scan" procedure. The denture is positioned in its ideal position relative to the bony structure of the patient using radiographic markers. (B) Implant planning based on the merged restoration. Note the use of fixation pins. (C) Cross-sectional view of the implant planning. External surface of the denture is traced in cyan, intaglio in pink, implant position in blue, and implant safety zone in yellow.

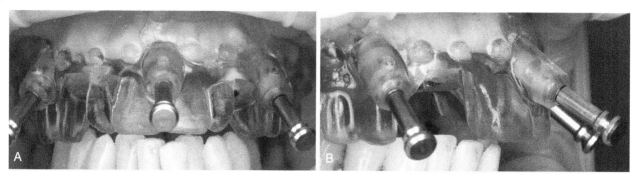

**Figure 12.10** Surgical template in situ. (A) and (B) depict the template in situ with anchor pins. Note the dental anatomy reproduced in the template, allowing the patient to bite on the template to ensure proper position.

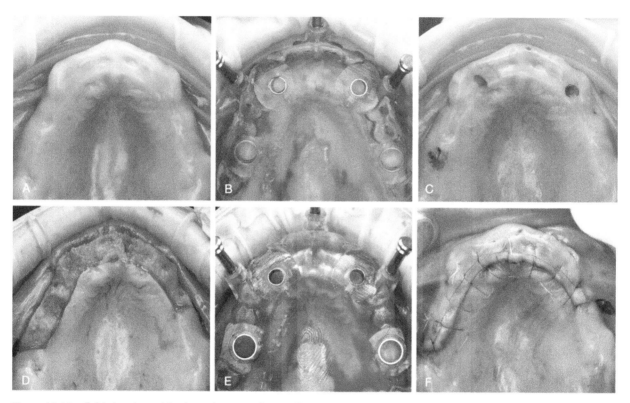

**Figure 12.11** Guided endosteal implant placement for maxillary full arch implant-supported overdenture. (A) Preoperative situation. (B) The guide is secured in position with three guide pins. (C) A Thompson stick can be used through the perforations in the guide to note the desired implant placement and guide flap reflection. (D) Flap reflected. (E) The surgical template is repositioned over the reflected flap and the anchor pins are set in their previous position. (F) Immediate postoperative situation.

installed, leading to compression of the mucosa and theoretical reduction of error in placement.

**Bone-supported Guide**

Bone-supported surgical templates are made from a process that is somewhat different to other templates described earlier in this chapter. The part that adapts to the patient, in this case on the bone, is made from the segmentation of a CBCT alone, rather than merging with an intraoral scan or

dual scan. As mentioned previously, the merging process of the CBCT+STL helps to create a more accurate jaw replica, which leads to superior adaptation of the guide. The segmentation process for these needs to be as good as possible, making the process more arduous and steepening the learning curve. These factors affect the overall outcome, as literature shows that these guides are less precise than tooth-supported or mucosa-supported options (Tahmaseb et al. 2018). These templates can still be planned based on the future restoration. To do so, a wax-up of the planned dentition of the patient is merged with the current dentition and super-imposed to the CBCT data. The implants are then planned accordingly, such as shown in Figure 12.13.

The reason that these guides are still used today is because tooth-borne guides or muco-supported guides are not applicable to every situation, for example, for a case of a patient in an unstable terminal dentition for which immediate implants with bone reduction are planned. The teeth in this case are going to be extracted during the procedure and the bone will be reduced, making them impossible to use as template abutments. The mucosa is also not ideal, because this situation complicates the dual scan protocol and, since teeth are present at the time of planning, there is not going to be mucosal support from the alveolar ridge.

In some situations, bone-supported templates can also offer more versatility than other options, such as when there is a need for combined procedures. Anchoring the framework of a surgical guide on bone allows for multiple attachments to be fitted in order to do multiple procedures at once. The guide can be fitted with a bone reduction template to be used immediately after extraction of remaining dentition, then to a bone reduction template, then to an implant placement template and subsequently serve as a guide for the pickup of an immediate implant-supported full arch restoration (Yang et al. 2021). Figures 12.12 to 12.18 depict this workflow.

### Manufacturing

There are several methods available to the clinician to manufacture surgical templates after computer-assisted design (CAD). These manufacturing techniques (CAM) can be divided in two main categories: subtractive manufacturing (milling) and additive manufacturing (3D printing). Subtractive methods involve starting from a block of material and shaving it down until it reaches the desired shape. Additive manufacturing involves, in this case, hardening a polymerizable material layer-by-layer in order to create the template (Galante and Rubio 2021). Additive and subtractive manufacturing methods have

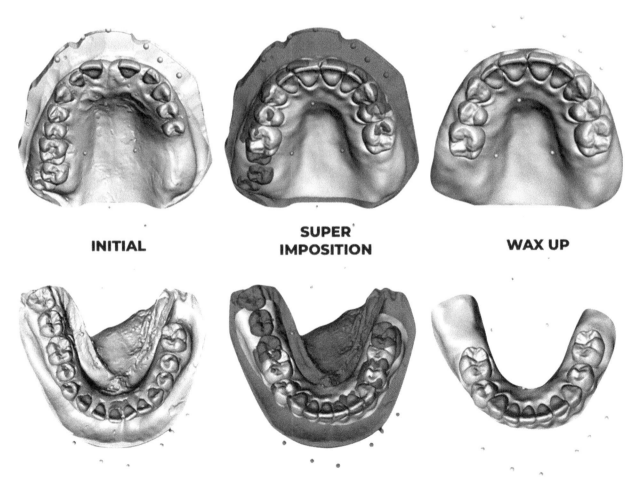

**INITIAL**  **SUPER IMPOSITION**  **WAX UP**

**Figure 12.12**  Merged wax-up/terminal dentition. This figure shows superimposition of the current dentition of the patient and the planned implant-supported restoration.

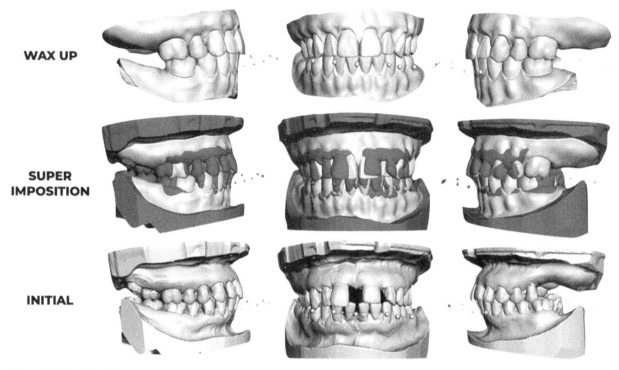

Figure 12.12   **(Cont'd)**

been shown to produce guides of similar accuracy (Henprasert et al. 2020). For surgical templates, milling is usually done with a dental CAD-CAM mill, while 3D printing is usually done with a 3D printer (Figures 12.19, 12.20).

### Milling

Milling surgical templates (subtractive manufacturing) is generally made utilizing PMMA. As mentioned previously, the accuracy has been shown to be similar clinically to 3D printing. However, in vitro studies showed that this process can be made to a very high level of precision, potentially more than 3D-printed templates (Liu et al. 2022).

The template can be milled either from a dental laboratory and returned to the clinician, or by a chairside CAM mill fitted with acrylic burs. The latter is advantageous to a clinician if they already own the necessary hardware; however, such mills are much more expensive than 3D printers. Milling a guide in-office usually takes about 20–30 minutes, as opposed to more than 2 hours for 3D-printed guides. Compared to their 3D-printed counterparts, milled guides do not require post-processing. The process of milling a guide is generally simpler than 3D printing, as the mill does not require to be adjusted as much as a 3D printer. The resulting surgical templates are also more stable dimensionally, as 3D-printed templates can morph with time if they are stored improperly. The milling process,

however, is also limited by the allowed bur axis of the machine used, which makes certain angles or undercuts impossible to be accurately reproduced.

### 3D Printing

3D printing, or additive manufacturing, is the most popular option for manufacturing surgical templates. 3D printing is advantageous because it has a smaller up-front cost and is more space effective for in-office production. The cost can be even further reduced by utilizing a consumer grade 3D printer, which has been shown to produce templates of a similar accuracy to that of a high-end device (Wegmüller et al. 2021). While a lot of different technologies are available to accomplish this, most of in-office printed surgical templates were made with either laser-based stereolithography (SLA) or Digital Light Processing (DLP) (Galante and Rubio 2021). Both methods involve photo-curing a layer-by-layer to end up making a 3D object. SLA uses a laser beam that is directed to the resin to create the desired shape, whereas DLP projects the whole image of each layer on the build area utilizing a projector screen.

Although purpose-made dental surgical guide resin is biocompatible when post-processing is carefully made according to the manufacturer's instruction, the material can be toxic and detrimental to cell viability if the instructions aren't followed carefully (Kurzmann et al. 2017).

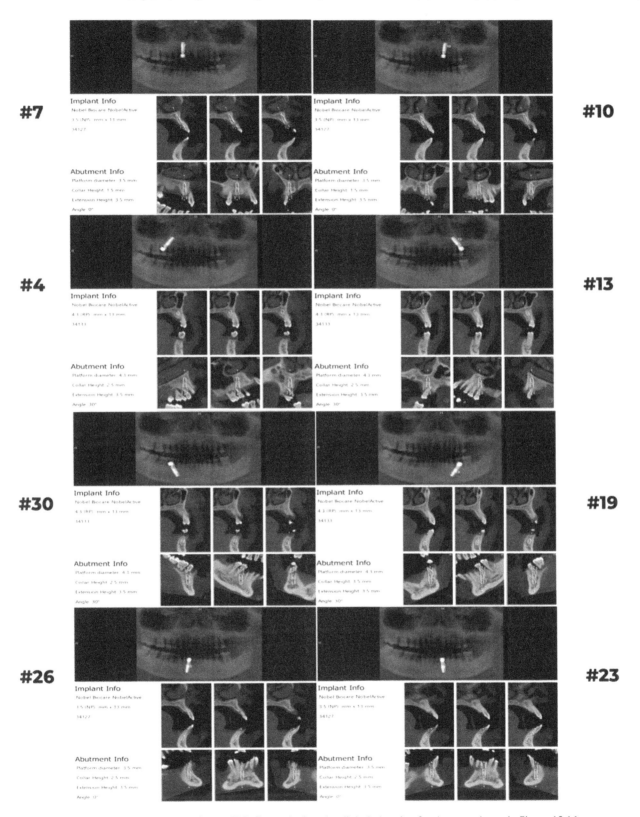

**Figure 12.13** Implant planning in software. This figure depicts the digital planning for the case shown in Figure 12.16.

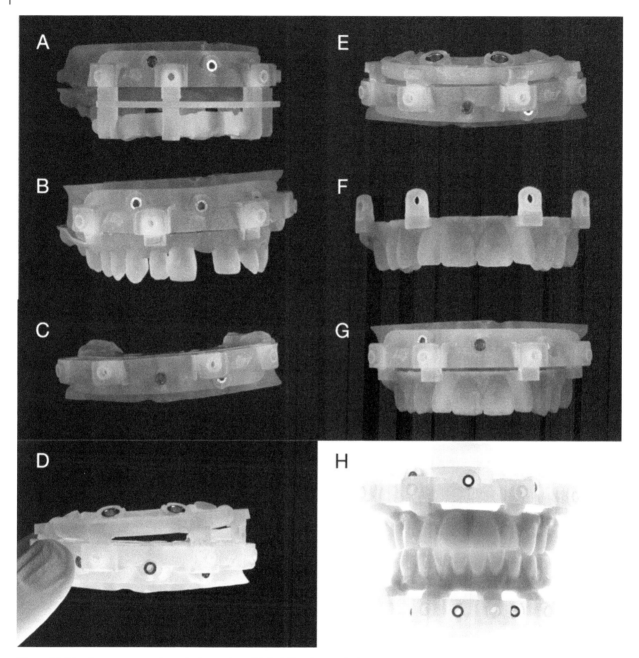

Figure 12.14 Bone-supported surgical template. (A) Stabilization of the bone-supported guide via a tooth-supported attachment prior to dental extractions. (B) Bone-supported guide attached apical to the patient's current dentition. (C) Bone-supported guide attached to the maxilla model after the suggested bone reduction. (D) and (E) Attachment of the bone-supported guide to the implant fully guided attachment. (F) and (G) With an attachment of the planned dentition, to be used as an intermediary splint. (H) Interim restorations for both arches attached to the bone-supported guide to be picked up.

## Dynamic Implant Guidance

### Navigation Systems

The navigation method, or optical navigation system, consists of a device tracking the clinician's handpiece utilizing optical systems. Optical markers are placed on the patient and on the handpiece. The navigation system utilizes camera to locate and relate both markers in 3D space. The system then transposes the movements of the handpiece onto the CBCT data and displays in real time the position of the drill relative to the bone. As with the conventional guide protocol, the CBCT data can also be superimposed by the merged STL file of the intraoral scan with the wax-up of the ideal tooth position, as well as the planned implant position.

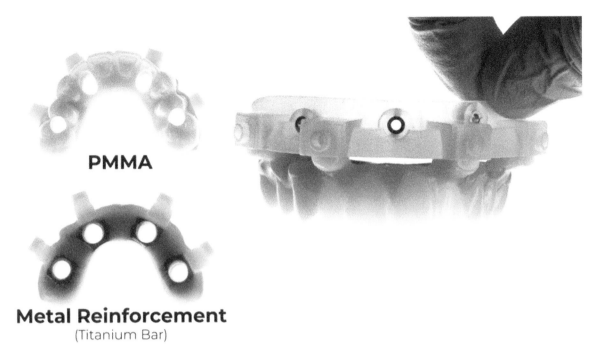

**Figure 12.15** Interim prosthesis. This figure depicts the interim prosthesis. Note the metal reinforcements and the attachments to the surgical template, for guided pickup.

Prior to implantology, similar systems were used in other surgical disciplines, such as otorhinolaryngology and spine surgery, as well as interventional radiology. At the time of writing this chapter, seven different systems for surgical navigation are commercially available (Galante and Rubio 2021).

The main advantage of surgical navigation is that it allows placement of an implant without any physical template. Since the implant is placed without the constraints of a physical template, the tactile feedback, as well as the irrigation, is maintained during the osteotomy and implant placement. This elimination of the physical template from the workflow also means that the surgical plan can be changed at any time during the procedure, and that there is no need to take the time to design and manufacture the template (Figure 12.21). Some limited evidence shows that when operated by an experienced user, this technique could be more even more precise than tooth-supported guides (Stefanelli et al. 2019). Another advantage is that these systems can be useful for other surgical procedures than implant placement, such as extraction of root tips or removal of hardware. Different handpieces can be used with the system; it is therefore also possible to use a piezoelectric knife in a guided fashion, such as for performing Piezocision (Dibart 2020). The main limitations of these systems are the steep learning curve, the technique sensitivity, and the lack of constraint preventing to go off-track (Block 2017; Gargallo-Albiol 2019).

**Robotic Systems**

The robotic system, which is another type of dynamic guidance, has additional advantages over the navigation system, such as the use of haptic guidance and a significant reduction in the surgical time. Limited evidence shows that robotically assisted implant placement has an accuracy comparable to the best implementation of static guides (Bolding 2021). The absence of a physical guide also allows for more irrigation during osteotomy and leads to less clutter in the surgical field (Figure 12.22). Robotics also present some drawbacks such as the cost of equipment, additional training, and potential errors as the scans are superimposed to each other, and lastly has a loss of tactile sensitivity as the guidance system is rigid.

To this date, there is only one FDA-approved system: the YOMI robot (Wu et al. 2019). This robot uses a "tracking arm" connected to an intraoral splint (Figure 12.22) in order to use as a reference for the 3D location of the patient's anatomical structures. The intraoral splint can be toothborne for dentate patients, and temporarily screwed in bone for edentulous patients. A CBCT is taken preoperatively the day of surgery with the intraoral splint installed and attached to a radiographic reference, called the "fiducial

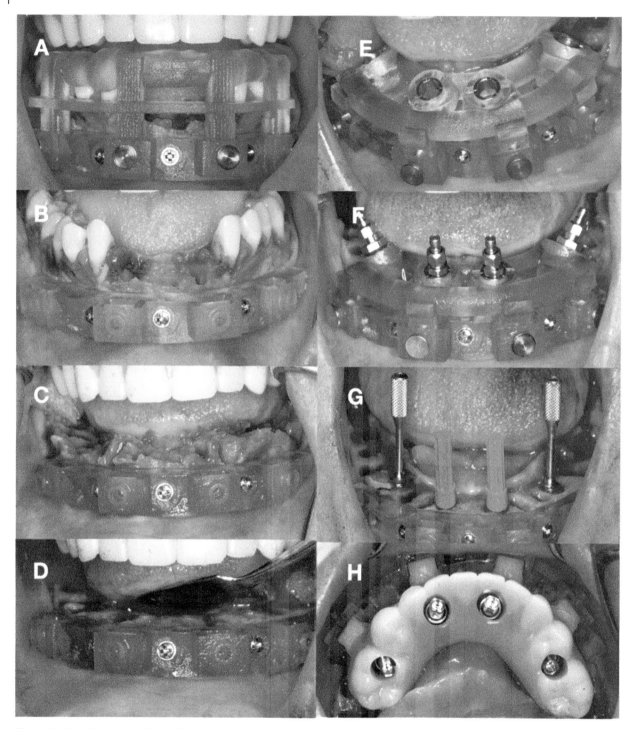

Figure 12.16    Clinical workflow with bone-supported template. (A) Stabilization of the bone-supported guide via use of a tooth-supported attachment to the existing dentition. (B) Stabilized bone-supported guide prior to extractions and flap reflection. (C) Full mandibular arch extractions, prior to bone reduction. (D) Bone reduction following the bone-supported guide. (E) Implant guidance attachment stabilized by the bone-supported guide. (F) Mandibular implants placed with a fully guided protocol. (G) Placement of multi-unit abutments as established in the surgical plan. (H) Mandibular interim prosthesis attached to the bone-supported guide ready for pickup. Notice the centered emergence of the temporary abutments through the predesigned access holes in the interim prosthesis.

Figure 12.17 One week follow-up post-surgery. Notice the interim maxillary and mandibular prosthesis adequately occluding against each other, and the uneventful healing of the patient.

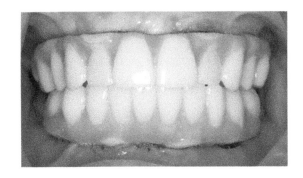

Figure 12.18 Orthopantomographs of the case in Figures 12.12 through 12.17. (A) Preoperative. (B) Immediate postoperative, placement of eight implants with the immediate load of both maxillary and mandibular interim prosthesis.

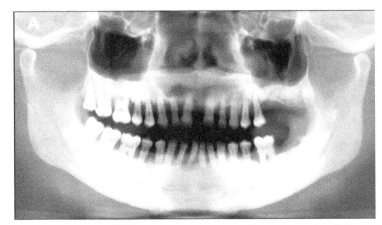

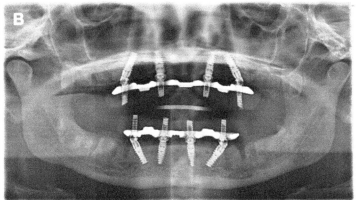

Figure 12.19 Manufacturing devices for surgical templates. (A) A desktop 3D printer, for additive manufacturing. (B) Chairside CAD-CAM mill, for subtractive manufacturing.

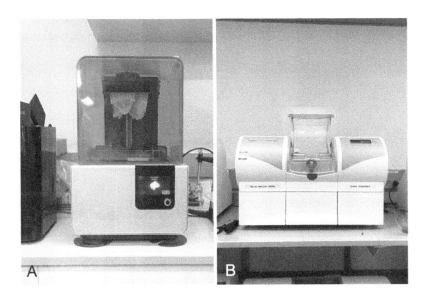

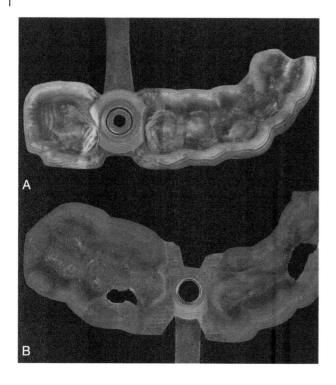

Figure 12.20 Milled and 3D-printed surgical templates. (A) Milled surgical template (subtractive manufacturing). (B) 3D-printed surgical template (additive manufacturing). Both guides are shown with drill keys inserted.

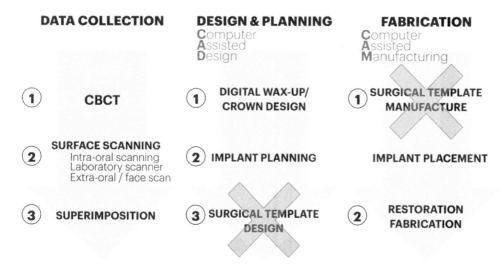

Figure 12.21 Implant surgery workflow for dynamic guidance. This figure depicts the conventional workflow for creating a physical guide, with some "X's" placed over the elements that can be skipped by utilizing a dynamic guidance system.

array." This CBCT can then be merged with a previously taken CBCT to import a surgical plan made prior. Figure 12.22 shows the workflow and operator position while utilizing the robot for surgery. The operator can then confirm that the robot is correctly locating the patient's structures by touching a preselected landmark. This process is known as

"passing landmark" (Talib et al. 2022). The software will also give the user the accuracy at which landmark is passed, giving insight on the accuracy of the whole process and the amount of intraoperative precautions to be taken. After this process, the operator advances the handpiece close to the surgical site and enters "guided mode." In "guided mode"

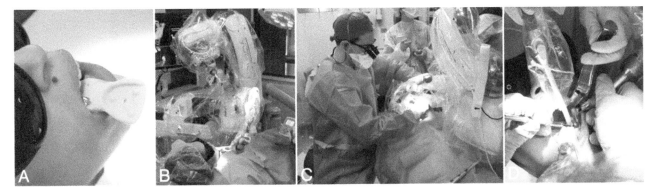

Figure 12.22 Robotically guided implant placement procedure. (A) The splint in situ. (B) The robot set up for surgery. Note the connection between the guidance arm and the splint. (C) The operator in position. (D) The relatively small size of the handpiece and the lack of physical surgical template allows for proper retraction, visualization, and irrigation.

the handpiece will lock in the desired implant placement axis and will only permit movement in that direction. The user then uses a standard implant motor foot control to control the drill and create the osteotomy. It is important to note that the operator remains in control of the advancement of the drill in the osteotomy axis during the whole procedure. A closer view of the software and clinical view can be appreciated in Figure 12.23

Although there is currently not yet enough evidence to establish a precise accuracy range for robotic surgery, early results are promising (Bolding and Reebye 2021). Figure 12.24 shows a case where two implants were placed in the esthetic zone, and then scanned with an intraoral scanner and compared with the planned position utilizing quality control software. One implant was placed with less than 2 degrees or 2 mm of variation from the plan in any given direction while the other one had less than 1 degree or 1 mm of variation from the plan in any direction.

The accuracy of robotic surgery appears to be unaltered by the number and disposition of remaining teeth, which offer significant advantage. This not only allows for implant placement with more accuracy for edentulous patients, it can also avoid some of the shortcomings of tooth-supported templates for dentate patients. Surgical templates with free ends, for placement of a distal tooth, have been shown to be less accurate than templates where the edentulous space is surrounded by a tooth on both sides, especially when the guide doesn't incorporate mucosa support (to allow for flap surgery), with angular deviations from the plan varying on average from $4.06 \pm 1.06°$ to $6.56 \pm 0.44°$ depending on the impression technique used (Nagata et al. 2021). These findings were for implants only 1 position distal to the terminal tooth, therefore one can assume that templates for implants 2 to 3 positions distal to the terminal tooth would be even less accurate. This makes a tooth-borne guide a nonreliable

option for placement of implants for a posterior fixed partial denture when no teeth distal to the planned restoration are present. This situation can be addressed by using robotic surgery, as illustrated by the case shown in Figure 12.25. In this case, guided bone regeneration (GBR) at time of implant placement was planned, therefore flapless implant was not advisable because the mucosal punch would be detrimental to primary closure. Reflection of a flap was therefore necessary, making a hybrid tooth-mucosa-supported template not possible for this case. Options are then freehand surgery, which could lead to a suboptimal outcome, as freehand surgery is even less accurate when more than one implant is planned (Choi et al. 2017), or to perform the GBR and the implant placement during separate procedures, which not only adds the burden of another surgery to the patient, but also significantly lengthens the process. Robotic surgery allowed for both procedures to be done simultaneously and in a guided fashion.

## Other Digitally-planned Surgical Procedures in Implantology

### Guided Sinus-Lift

The concepts discussed in this chapters can be extrapolated and used for different procedures. The merging process of a CBCT with and an intraoral scan leaves the clinician with the powerful combination of the view of the patient's anatomy (CBCT) and a very precise and reproducible intraoral reference (intraoral scan). From that, templates can be created for other procedures than implant placement, and implant placement templates can be combined with references for anatomical landmark. A notable application of this is for sinus floor elevation

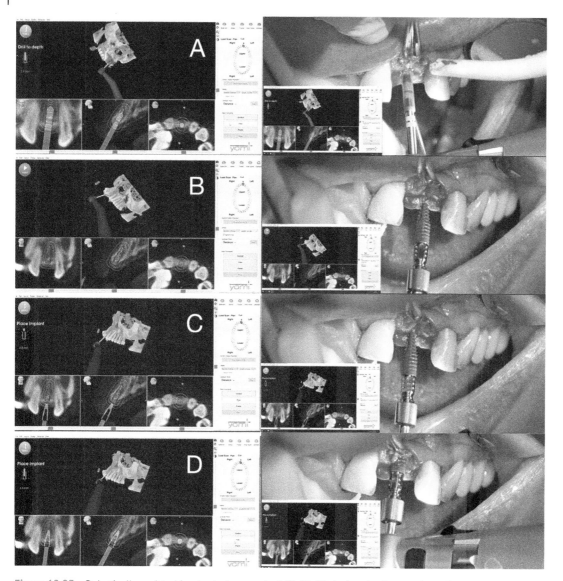

**Figure 12.23** Robotically assisted implant placement of #9. (A) Clinical and software view of a guided osteotomy preparation. (B) Free mode during the approach of the implant to the osteotomy site; notice the green circle. (C) Guided mode has been engaged in the software, giving precise indications of the necessary adjustments for guided placement of the implant. (D) Implant #9 almost place to depth while engaged in guided mode.

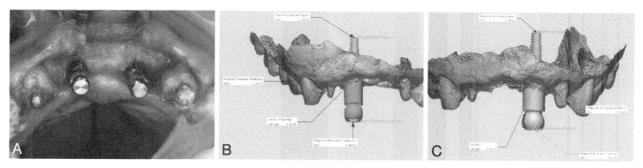

**Figure 12.24** Robotically guided implant placement case. (A) The implants immediately after placement. (B) and (C) Comparison of intraoral scans of the planned implant position (green) and the final implant position (blue). Note the quasi-total superimposition of both samples. Courtesy of Dr. Dmitriy Klass.

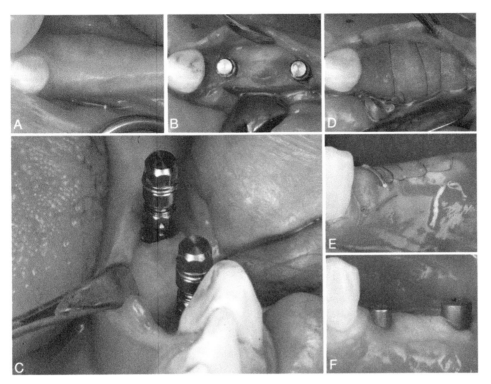

Figure 12.25  Robotically guided implant placement case for a distal end. (A) Preoperative situation. (B) and (C) Implants in situ. (D) Guided bone regeneration was carried out with cortico-cancellous freeze-dried bone allograft and a resorbable cross-linked collagen membrane. (E) After 2 weeks of healing. (F) After second stage surgery and free gingival graft.

templates (Mandelaris and Rosenfield 2008) and sinus floor elevation templates combined to implant placement templates. These can be either bone supported (Osman et al. 2018) or tooth supported (Strbac et al. 2020).

The lateral, or so-called Caldwell-Luc, technique for sinus elevation involves an antrostomy on the posterolateral wall of the maxillary antrum. The location and size of this antrostomy is dictated by anatomical factors and access. Care must be taken not to rupture the maxillary artery (Elian et al. 2005) and avoiding maxillary septa, as they can interfere with the creation and inversion of lateral windows (Pommer et al. 2012). Since both these structures can be appreciated on a CBCT scan, it is recommended to do a radiographic examination before performing a sinus elevation procedure. After thorough radiographic examination, the ideal window design can be transferred clinically by adding it to the surgical template. It is also possible to 3D print the maxilla of the patient to better visualize the structures. This process is depicted in Figure 12.26.

### 3D-Printed Ti-Mesh

As it is a very technique sensitive technique, authors have been constantly refining the guided bone regeneration (GBR) surgical protocol. One of the biggest challenges in GBR is vertical regeneration, because it commands for very

rigid space maintenance. Titanium meshes, or Ti-Meshes, have been used as rigid barriers to maintain space around bone grafts. One main drawback of using them is the need to bend and adapt them to the defect intraoperatively. Nowadays, utilizing digital dentistry concepts, it is possible to utilize CAD/CAM to design a custom Ti-Mesh and have it 3D-printed. This protocol is named CBR (custom bone regeneration). This technique was first used to regenerate alveolar ridge defects (Ciocca et al. 2011; Otawa et al. 2015) and then was used for full jaw reconstruction (Yamada et al. 2014). In addition to reducing chair time by not having to bend the mesh to adapt it directly to the patient's anatomy, the CBR technique has been shown to result in less mesh exposure than the regular GBR technique with Ti-Mesh (Zhou et al. 2021).

Recently, some commercial services became available to simplify this workflow. The clinician can upload the CBCT online through a service and the supplier will design the lattice shaped Ti-Mesh and submit a proposal to the clinician. The clinician can ask for modifications, such as the location of the stabilizing screws or even adding an opening that allows for implant placement. Once the design is finalized, the clinician can order the 3D-printed Ti-Mesh and proceed with the CBR procedure. Figure 12.27 shows the planning and the delivered product, while Figure 12.28 shows the clinical workflow for CBR.

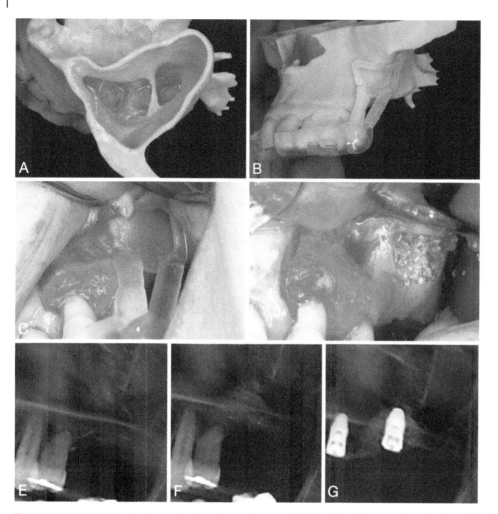

Figure 12.26 Guided antrostomy for sinus floor elevation. (a) 3D print of the maxilla with the guide. Axial view. Note the septum in the sinus. (b) Sagittal view of the 3D-printed guide with the maxilla. (c) Clinical view of the seated guide. (d) The antrostomy has been performed and the sinus is packed with grafting material. (e) Reconstructed orthopantomography showing the pre-op situation, after sinus grafting in (f) and after implant placement in (g). Courtesy of Dr. Sean Lee.

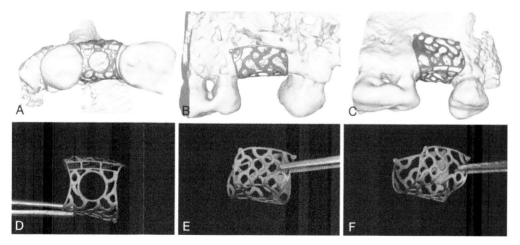

Figure 12.27 Custom Ti-Mesh for custom bone regeneration (CBR). (A), (B), and (C) Different views of the planned mesh in software. (D), (E), and (F) The finalized product, as received from the manufacturer.

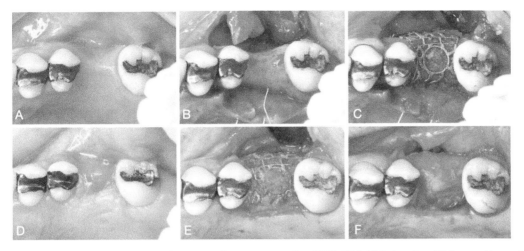

**Figure 12.28** Clinical workflow for custom bone regeneration (CBR). (A) Initial situation. (B) Exposed bone. (C) The Ti-Mesh in situ. (D) The surgical site, after 6 weeks of healing. (E) The regenerated bone with the mesh, after 11 months of healing. (F) The regenerated bone after removal of the mesh. Courtesy of Dr. Sean Lee.

## References

Bankman, I.N. (ed.) (2000). *Handbook of Medical Imaging*. San Diego: Academic Press.

Block, M.S., Emery, R.W., Lank, K., and Ryan, J. (2017). Implant placement accuracy using dynamic navigation. *Int. J. Oral Maxillofac Implants* 32: 92–99.

Bolding, S.L. and Reebye, U.N. (2021 March 5). Accuracy of haptic robotic guidance of dental implant surgery for completely edentulous arches. Epub.

Chen, Z., Li, J., Sinjab, K. et al. (2018). Accuracy of flapless immediate implant placement in anterior maxilla using computer-assisted versus freehand surgery: a cadaver study. *Clin. Oral Implants Res.* 29: 1186–1194.

Choi, W., Nguyen, B.-C., Doan, A. et al. (2017). Freehand versus guided surgery: factors influencing accuracy of dental implant placement. *Implant Dent.* 26: 500–509.

Ciocca, L., Fantini, M., De Crescenzio, F. et al. (2011). Direct metal laser sintering (DMLS) of a customized titanium mesh for prosthetically guided bone regeneration of atrophic maxillary arches. *Med. Biol. Eng. Comput.* 49: 1347–1352.

Dano, D., Stiteler, M., and Giordano, R. (2018). Prosthetically driven computer-guided implant placement and restoration using CEREC: a case report. *Compend. Contin. Educ. Dent.* 39: 311–317.

Dawson, A., Chen, S., Buser, D. et al. (2009). *The SAC Classification in Implant Dentistry*, 1e. Quintessence Publishing Co, Ltd.

Dibart, S. (2020). *Practical Advanced Periodontal Surgery*, 2e. Hoboken: John Wiley & Sons, Inc.

El Kholy, K., Janner, S., Buser, R., and Buser, D. (2019 October 24). Variables affecting the accuracy of static computer-assisted implant surgery: bridging the gap between clinical success and broad application. Epub.

Elian, N., Wallace, S., Cho, S.-C. et al. (2005). Distribution of the maxillary artery as it relates to sinus floor augmentation. *Int. J. Oral Maxillofac Implants* 20: 784–787.

Galante, J.M. and Rubio, N.A. (eds.) (2021). *Digital Dental Implantology: From Treatment Planning to Guided Surgery*, 1e. Springer. 2021.

Gargallo-Albiol, J., Barootchi, S., Salomó-Coll, O., and Wang, H.-L. (2019 September). Advantages and disadvantages of implant navigation surgery. A systematic review. Epub.

Henprasert, P., Dawson, D.V., El-Kerdani, T. et al. (2020). Comparison of the accuracy of implant position using surgical guides fabricated by additive and subtractive techniques. *J. Prosthodont.* 29: 534–541.

Januário, A.L., Barriviera, M., and Duarte, W.R. (2008). Soft tissue cone-beam computed tomography: a novel method for the measurement of gingival tissue and the dimensions of the dentogingival unit. *J. Esthet. Restor. Dent.* 20: 366–373. discussion 374.

Kourtis, S., Skondra, E., Roussou, I., and Skondras, E.V. (2012). Presurgical planning in implant restorations: correct interpretation of cone-beam computed tomography for improved imaging. *J. Esthet. Restor. Dent.* 24: 321–332.

Kurzmann, C., Janjić, K., Shokoohi-Tabrizi, H. et al. (2017). Evaluation of resins for stereolithographic 3D-printed surgical guides: the response of L929 cells and human gingival fibroblasts. Epub.

Lee, C.Y.S., Ganz, S.D., Wong, N., and Suzuki, J.B. (2012). Use of cone beam computed tomography and a laser intraoral scanner in virtual dental implant surgery: part 1. *Implant Dent.* 21: 265–271.

Liu, X., Liu, J., Feng, H., and Pan, S. (2022). Accuracy of a milled digital implant surgical guide: an in vitro study. *J. Prosthet. Dent.* 127: 453–461.

Mandelaris, G.A. and Rosenfeld, A.L. (2008). A novel approach to the antral sinus bone graft technique: the use of a prototype cutting guide for precise outlining of the lateral wall. A case report. *Int. J. Periodontics Restorative Dent.* 28: 569–575.

Mörmann, W.H. (2006 September). The evolution of the CEREC system. Epub.

Nagata, K., Fuchigami, K., Hoshi, N. et al. (2021). Accuracy of guided surgery using the silicon impression and digital impression method for the mandibular free end: a comparative study. *Int. J. Implant Dent.* 7: 2.

Orentlicher, G., Goldsmith, D., and Abboud, M. (2012). Computer-guided planning and placement of dental implants. *Atlas Oral Maxillofac. Surg. Clin. N.* 20: 53–79.

Osman, A.H., Mansour, H., Atef, M., and Hakam, M. (2018). Computer guided sinus floor elevation through lateral window approach with simultaneous implant placement. *Clin. Implant Dent. Relat. Res.* 20: 137–143.

Otawa, N., Sumida, T., Kitagaki, H. et al. (2015). Custom-made titanium devices as membranes for bone augmentation in implant treatment: modeling accuracy of titanium products constructed with selective laser melting. *J. Cranio-Maxillofac Surg.* 43: 1289–1295.

Ozan, O., Turkyilmaz, I., Ersoy, A.E. et al. (2009). Clinical accuracy of 3 different types of computed tomography-derived stereolithographic surgical guides in implant placement. *J. Oral Maxillofacial Surg.* 67: 394–401.

Pessoa, R., Siqueira, R., Li, J. et al. (2022). The impact of surgical guide fixation and implant location on accuracy of static computer-assisted implant surgery. *J. Prosthodont.* 31: 155–164.

Pommer, B., Ulm, C., Lorenzoni, M. et al. (2012). Prevalence, location and morphology of maxillary sinus septa: systematic review and meta-analysis. *J. Clin. Periodontol.* 39: 769–773.

Rawal, S. (2022). Guided innovations: robot-assisted dental implant surgery. *J. Prosthet. Dent.* 127: 673–674.

Stefanelli, L.V., DeGroot, B.S., Lipton, D.I., and Mandelaris, G.A. (2019). Accuracy of a dynamic dental implant navigation system in a private practice. *Int. J. Oral Maxillofac Implants* 34: 205–213.

Strbac, G.D., Giannis, K., Schnappauf, A. et al. (2020). Guided lateral sinus lift procedure using 3-dimensionally printed templates for a safe surgical approach: a proof-of-concept case report. *J. Oral Maxillofacial Surg.* 78: 1529–1537.

Tahmaseb, A., Wu, V., Wismeijer, D. et al. (2018 October). The accuracy of static computer-aided implant surgery: a systematic review and meta-analysis. *Clin. Oral Impl. Res.* 29: 416–435. https://doi.org/10.1111/clr.13346.

Talib, H.S., Wilkins, G.N., and Turkyilmaz, I. (2022 May 31). Flapless dental implant placement using a recently developed haptic robotic system. Epub.

Vercruyssen, M., Cox, C., Coucke, W. et al. (2014). A randomized clinical trial comparing guided implant surgery (bone- or mucosa-supported) with mental navigation or the use of a pilot-drill template. *J. Clin. Periodontol.* 41: 717–723.

Verhamme, L.M., Meijer, G.J., Bergé, S.J. et al. (2015). An accuracy study of computer-planned implant placement in the augmented Maxilla Using Mucosa-supported surgical templates: accuracy of implant placement in the augmented Maxilla. *Clin. Implant Dent. Relat. Res.* 17: 1154–1163.

Wegmüller, L., Halbeisen, F., Sharma, N. et al. (2021). Consumer vs. High-end 3D printers for guided implant surgery – an in vitro accuracy assessment study of different 3D printing technologies. *J. Clin. Med.* 10: 4894.

Wu, Y., Wang, F., Fan, S., and Chow, J.K.-F. (2019). Robotics in dental implantology. *Oral Maxillofac Surg. Clin. North Am.* 31: 513–518.

Yamada, H., Nakaoka, K., Horiuchi, T. et al. (2014). Mandibular reconstruction using custom-made titanium mesh tray and particulate cancellous bone and marrow harvested from bilateral posterior ilia. *J. Plast. Surg. Hand Surg.* 48: 183–190.

Yang, J.-W., Liu, Q., Yue, Z.-G. et al. (2021). Digital workflow for full-arch immediate implant placement using a stackable surgical guide fabricated using SLM technology. *J. Prosthodont.* 30: 645–650.

Younes, F., Cosyn, J., De Bruyckere, T. et al. (2018). A randomized controlled study on the accuracy of free-handed, pilot-drill guided and fully guided implant surgery in partially edentulous patients. *J. Clin. Periodontol.* 45: 721–732.

Zhou, L., Su, Y., Wang, J. et al. (2021). Effect of exposure rates with customized versus conventional titanium mesh on guided bone regeneration: systematic review and meta-analysis. *J. Oral Implantol.* 48: 339–346.

# 13

# Introduction to Minimally Invasive Facial Aesthetic Procedures

*Bradford Towne*

## Overview

Today, neurotoxins and temporary facial fillers are the top cosmetic procedures purchased by the public, replacing more invasive procedures such as face lifts and facial peels. According to a 12-year retrospective analysis conducted by the American Society of Plastic Surgeons, major facial cosmetic procedures declined by 27% in one 3-year period (2006–2009) (Remington 2008), while minimally invasive procedures (MIP) increased during the 12-year study period. Neurotoxin use increased by 680% and soft tissue fillers increased by 205% during the same period (Sandoval et al. 2014). Facial fillers have been available for decades but only in the last dozen years has there been the development of fillers that are technically easy to use, non-allergenic, give predictable results, are easily manipulated and sculpted by the injector, and have minimal risk of complications. Neurotoxins have also been available for years. They were first isolated and potential medical uses described in 1822. The source of the toxin, however, was not isolated until 80 years later (Foster 2014). Neurotoxins for cosmetic use were first approved by the US Food and Drink Administration (FDA) in 2002. Since then they have become the most commonly used cosmetic procedure by far, with soft tissue facial fillers the second most common cosmetic procedure performed.

The clinician that provides his or her patients with cosmetic neurotoxins and soft tissue fillers must have a detailed understanding of facial anatomy and the mechanics of the muscles of facial expression. A thorough appreciation of the aging process, including the physiologic changes that occur to skin, subcutaneous tissues, and muscles of the face, is critical to successfully treating cosmetic patients. This knowledge must be combined with an in-depth understanding of the pharmacology and working properties of the products to be used to restore facial volume. The clinician must also have an appreciation for the artistic qualities of the human facial form to be successful in creating an aesthetically pleasing result for the patient.

## Patient Selection and Assessment

Patient motivation for seeking MIPs varies tremendously but can be divided into three primary sectors. Young patients, generally 18–35, are usually motivated by the desire to augment an area of their face they feel is deficient or not normal. Those in the 35–55 age group are usually seeking rejuvenation and the 55+ are usually looking for restoration. All are looking for MIPs with minimal downtime, providing minimal risks and rapid results.

MIPs are generally procedures with minimal risks and complications when performed correctly and on the right patients. Fortunately, there are few medical contraindications for the use of neurotoxins or facial fillers today. Success in providing MIPs is the result of a careful evaluation of the patient's motivation in seeking treatment as well as a complete facial assessment. Cosmetic patients may have unrealistic expectations of what can be accomplished with MIPs and the clinician must be able to educate the patient about realistic outcomes.

The evaluation begins with the patient describing what they are unhappy with about their face. This provides a starting point for the examination. It provides the clinician with an initial focal point to understand a patient's motivation. For example, a patient may tell the clinician that family and friends tell them they always look angry or tired. A patient may say that their cheeks look flat or hollow. Some patients describe the loss of lip exposure. Each of these complaints provides a starting point for the clinical evaluation. Once the patient's primary concern/complaint and treatment goal is ascertained the clinician can perform a comprehensive facial evaluation and develop treatment recommendations to achieve the patient's goal.

No evaluation is complete without a review of the patient's past medical history, medications, and social history, including sun exposure, smoking, and history of any prior facial cosmetic procedures. The examination should include an assessment of the skin condition using the Glogau Classification of photo aging and wrinkles (Table 13.1).

*Practical Periodontal Diagnosis and Treatment Planning*, Second Edition. Edited by Serge Dibart and Thomas Dietrich.
© 2024 John Wiley & Sons, Inc. Published 2024 by John Wiley & Sons, Inc.

Table 13.1  Glogau Classification of photo aging and wrinkles.

| Group | Classification | Age | Description | Skin characteristics |
|---|---|---|---|---|
| I | Mild | 28 to 35 | No wrinkles | Early photo aging: mild pigment changes, no keratosis, minimal wrinkles, minimal or no make-up |
| II | Moderate | 35 to 50 | Wrinkles in motion (dynamic rhytids) | Early to moderate photo aging: early brown spots visible, keratosis palpable but not visible, parallel smile lines begin to appear, wears some foundation |
| III | Advanced | 50 to 65 | Wrinkles at rest (static rhytids) | Advanced photo aging: obvious discolorations, visible capillaries (telangiectasia), visible keratosis, wears heavier foundation always |
| IV | Severe | 60 to 75 | Only wrinkles | Severe photo aging: yellow–gray skin color, prior skin malignancies, wrinkles throughout, no normal skin, cannot wear make-up because it cakes and cracks |

The physical evaluation should follow the three facial esthetic zones as first described by Leonardo da Vinci. These three zones divide the face horizontally into thirds. The top extends from the top of the forehead to the inferior orbital rim. The midface extends from the inferior orbital rim to the base of the nose. The lower third extends from the nasal base to the chin.

It is useful in this evaluation to have a frontal facial diagram on which the clinician can indicate the location of static and dynamic wrinkles, areas of volume loss, redundant or sagging skin, and deep folds. Consent should be obtained and pretreatment photos and or videos obtained to demonstrate the areas of concern. Videos are particularly useful in demonstrating dynamic vs. static rhytids. Preexisting facial asymmetries should also be noted. This is very important to document so that the patient is made aware of their existence prior to any treatment administration. Once the evaluation is complete, the clinical findings should be reviewed with the patient and treatment recommendations discussed in detail, including the rationale, expected result, and potential risks and complications. If different products are available to treat the same problem, the benefits and risks of each should be reviewed.

## Neurotoxins

Currently there are three neurotoxin products available for cosmetic uses: Botox Cosmetic®, Dysport®, Xeomin®, and Jeuveau®. All of these are derivatives of BoNT A. Use of botulinum toxin type A (BoNT A) derivatives is FDA approved to treat glabellar frown lines. Botox Cosmetic® has been approved for crow's feet treatment. Each derivative has its own specific unit concentration but the results are similar (Rubin 2013).

Common adverse effects at the injection site include pain, bruising, erythema, and edema. The most common general adverse effects are headaches, upper respiratory tract infections, nausea, pain, and flu-like symptoms.

## Temporary and Semipermanent Fillers

The first cosmetic filler used was paraffin in 1899 (Kontis and Rivkin 2009). Its popularity was short lived as the complications associated with its use quickly exceeded the benefits. Today, there are many types of temporary and semipermanent facial fillers available on the market. The most commonly utilized are the hyaluronic acid (HA) fillers. These fillers (Restylane® family, Juvaderm® family, and Belotero®) are composed of micro particles of hyaluronic acid, a naturally occurring substance in our body with the highest concentrations found in the connective tissue and fluid around our eyes and also in some cartilage and joint fluid. HA fillers are synthetically derived and are more concentrated than those naturally found in our bodies. The injected gel provides a volume greater than the volume injected because it is hydrophilic (draws water into the area of injection). It is important not to over-inject because of this delayed phenomenon. The material is slowly degraded over time. The microspheres vary in size by product and the indications for the use of each are based on the desired effect. The small particle sizes are used for wrinkle ablation and the larger sizes for volume replacement.

Another commonly utilized product is hydroxyapatite filler (Radiesse®). This product is composed of microspheres of hydroxyapatite crystal (a component of bone) suspended in a gel matrix. The mechanism of action is immediate volume enhancement (what you see is what you get). Over time the degradation of the hydroxyapatite stimulates collagenesis. Although this new collagen is not permanent it does prolong the benefit of the treatment.

Neither hyaluronic acid nor hydroxyapatite produces an allergic response or requires allergy testing. Most HA products provide 12–18 months of benefit. Hydroxyapatite gel will usually provide 18–24 months of volume enhancement. Both product types are relatively risk free with minimal complications such as bruising (Table 13.2). An important distinction between the two is the reversibility of HA by injecting the treated area with hyaluronidase.

**Table 13.2** Properties of hyaluronic acid fillers and hydroxyapatite filler.

*Hyaluronic acid fillers (Restylane®/Perlane®, Juvaderm®, and Belotero®)*

Lasts 6–12 months (Juvaderm Voluma 18–24 months)

Maximum volume effect takes several days due to hydrophilic volume

Identical in all species and tissues

Isovolemic degradation

No skin test required

Reversible

*Hydroxyapatite filler (Radiesse®)*

Lasts 12–18 months

Provides an immediate volumizing effect

Stimulates the patient's own collagen to produce a satisfying and longer lasting result

Less volume required per equivalent treatment compared to HA fillers to achieve the same result

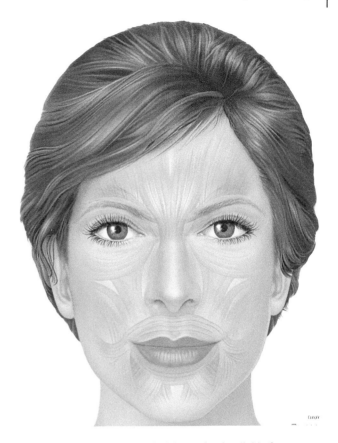

**Figure 13.1** Subcutaneous facial muscles (available from Allergan for providers enrolled in their website). Adapted from botoxcosmetic.com.

## Treatment Sequencing

Treatment sequencing is based on the products to be used and the areas to be treated. Generally, treatment should begin with neurotoxins followed by facial fillers. If both are to be injected into the same area it is best to wait a week after administration of the neurotoxin prior to injecting the fillers. Injecting filler into the area of a hyperkinetic muscle will likely result in the displacement of the filler away from the intended site. Facial fillers placed in the midface to increase volume will elevate the nasolabial folds and lower face. This effect will result in less volume replacement being required when treating the lower face.

Figure 13.1 (which is available from Allergan for providers enrolled in their website) is a useful teaching and treatment planning tool. The clinician can show the patient the areas to be treated and draw out the treatment solution being recommended. The individual muscles to be treated with neurotoxin can be identified along with the injection sites. For fillers, the area to be treated can be highlighted along with the planned injection patterns.

## Neurotoxin Injection Technique

The neurotoxin of choice should be reconstituted following the package insert guidelines. Typically injections are done with a TB or insulin syringe with a 30- or 32-gauge needle. The neurotoxin is measured in units. Vials come in either 50-unit or 100-unit doses. Individual injections sites usually have between 2 and 10 units depending on the product being used. Insertion of the needle is just into the body of the muscle

being treated except when treating crow's feet, when the injection should be subcutaneous due to the orbicularis oculi muscle being very thin and superficial laterally. The most common area of treatment is the vertical glabellae rhytids. These furrows form as the result of the activity of the procerus and corrugator muscles, which pull the lower middle forehead down and toward the center, creating single, double, or triple furrows (also known as the 1s, 11s, and 111s). The crow's feet formed as the result of the contraction of the lateral aspect of the orbicularis oculi is the second most common area of neurotoxin treatment, followed by the forehead.

The glabellar (11s) lines arise from the action of the procerus and corrugator supercilii muscles (Figures 13.2 and 13.3). These muscles tend to be hyperdynamic and when coupled with loss of subcutaneous fat and repetitive creasing result in the development of static wrinkles and potential textural changes. The lines usually appear between the muscle bodies as the subcutaneous fat volume shrinks.

Crow's feet or smile lines (Figure 13.4) are the result of the activity of the lateral aspect of the orbicularis oculi. The muscle's hyperdynamic activity combined with subcutaneous fat loss and repetitive creasing produce textural and static wrinkles lateral to the eye.

**Glabellar complex**

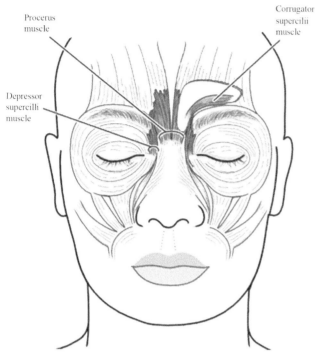

Figure 13.2  The glabellar muscle complex that creates the frown lines.

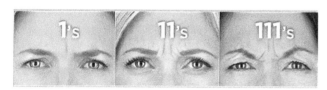

Figure 13.3  Vertical glabellae rhytids: single, double, and triple furrows (also known as the 1s, 11s, and 111s). Adapted from botoxcosmetic.com.

Forehead wrinkles (Figure 13.5) are the result of the action of frontalis muscle. They produce horizontal wrinkles. The wrinkles become deeper and more exaggerated as the result of the loss of subcutaneous fat, photoaging, and loss of dermal elasticity. Repetitive creasing also produces textural changes to the epidermis.

Neurotoxins are measured in units, for example Botox Cosmetic® and Xeomin® come in either 100-unit or 50-unit vials. The recommended reconstitution of a 100-unit vial of Botox Cosmetic® requires the addition of 2.5 cc of nonpreserved sterile saline for injection. This volume yields a concentration of 40 units per 1 cc or 4 units per 0.1 cc. A typical number of units of Botox Cosmetic® recommended for a glabellar injection site is 4 units or 0.1 cc. Use of 1-cc TB syringes or 1-cc insulin syringes is necessary to deliver accurate volume and concentration of the neurotoxin to the sites (Figure 13.6). This volume will produce a small wheal, minimize discomfort, and limit the diffusion radius to about 1 cm. The dose for each site is individualized based on the examination, including

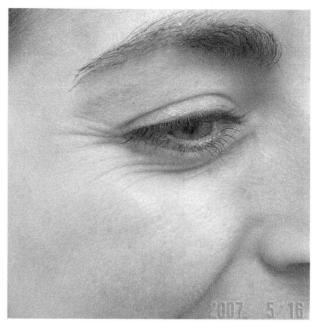

Figure 13.4  Hyperdynamic orbicularis oculi resulting in crow's feet rhytids.

(A)

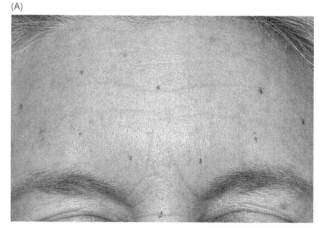

(B)

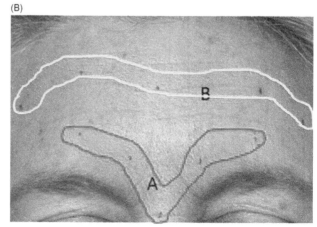

Figure 13.5  Glabellar frown rhytids (A) and horizontal forehead rhytids (B) (the result of frontalis action) with marks indicating planned injection sites of neurotoxin.

Figure 13.6 Specialized TB syringe with plunger tip extending into hub to reduce waste with each syringe, coupled with a 32-gauge needle to minimize the discomfort of injections.

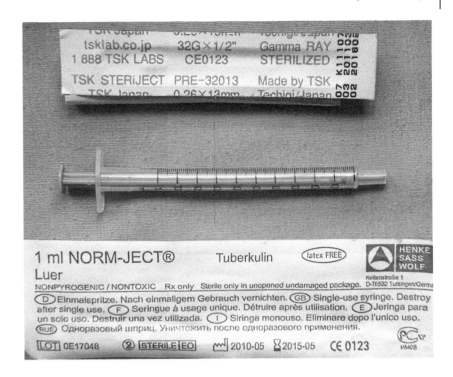

Figure 13.7 Typical injection sites for treatment of the glabellar lines. Adapted from xeominaesthetic.com.

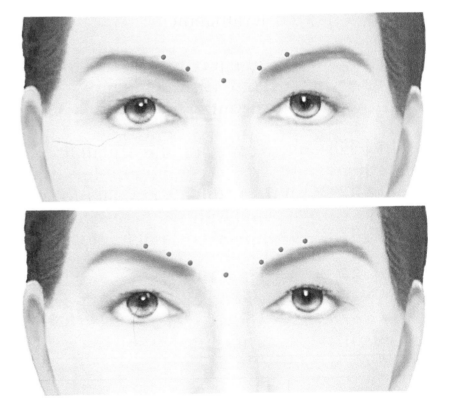

the muscle thickness, degree of hyperkinetic activity, and past patient results. Each product has different suggested dilutent instructions and the clinician should refer to the package insert of each product for those instructions.

When injecting the frown lines (glabellar) there are typically five injection sites that correspond to the bodies of the procerus and corrugator muscles. Figure 13.7 demonstrates the usual locations of these injection sites. It is important to stay 1 cm above the superior orbital rim to avoid diffusion of the product into the upper eyelid. The eyebrow position is a poor landmark to use due to its variable location. The boney orbital rim should always be palpated and the injection given 1 cm above this landmark. The action of the corrugator muscle should be observed as its location may be more vertical in some individuals. Figure 13.8 shows the typical lateral injection site at mid-pupil, with the patient looking straight ahead. Each injection is typically 2–4 units of Botox Cosmetic® or Xeomin® or 5–10 units of Dysport®.

The forehead horizontal lines (Figure 13.9) can also be treated but caution should be observed if injecting at the same time as the glabellar frown lines. If complete frontalis paralysis occurs the patient may present with eyebrow

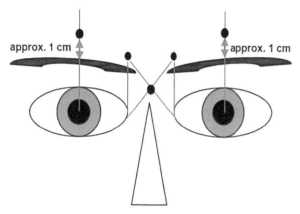

**Figure 13.8** The location of each injection site relative to the eyes. Adapted from xeominaesthetic.com.

ptosis. A couple of centimeters of frontalis should be kept inferiorly untreated to insure that this does not happen.

Crow's feet or smile lines (Figure 13.10) are easily treated at the same time as the glabellar lines. By reducing hyperdynamic activity before static creases develop the occurrence of static wrinkles can be postponed. Care should be taken not to extend the injections into the inferior orbital rim area as this increases the risk of producing a result that looks like a mask, with no animation at all when smiling. Crow's feet are usually treated with a dose of 2 units of Botox Cosmetic® or Xeomin® or 5 units of Dysport® per injection site. The injection of the crow's feet is just subcutaneous due to the superficial position of the orbicularis oculi laterally. Caution should be exercised as there are superficial veins in this area that must be avoided. These veins are often visible when the skin is stretched during the injections. The superior injection is usually at the lateral aspect of the eyebrow, the next is level with the canthus, and the lower is inferiolateral. Each should be 1 cm from the bony orbital rim (Figure 13.11).

Today, there are many off label injection sites in addition to those described above. One of the more dramatic results can be seen in the injection to reduce a "gummy smile." The initial evaluation of the gummy smile is important. Neurotoxin use to treat a gummy smile is only effective when there is hyperactivity of the levator labii superioris alaeque nasi and levator labii superioris and zygomaticus

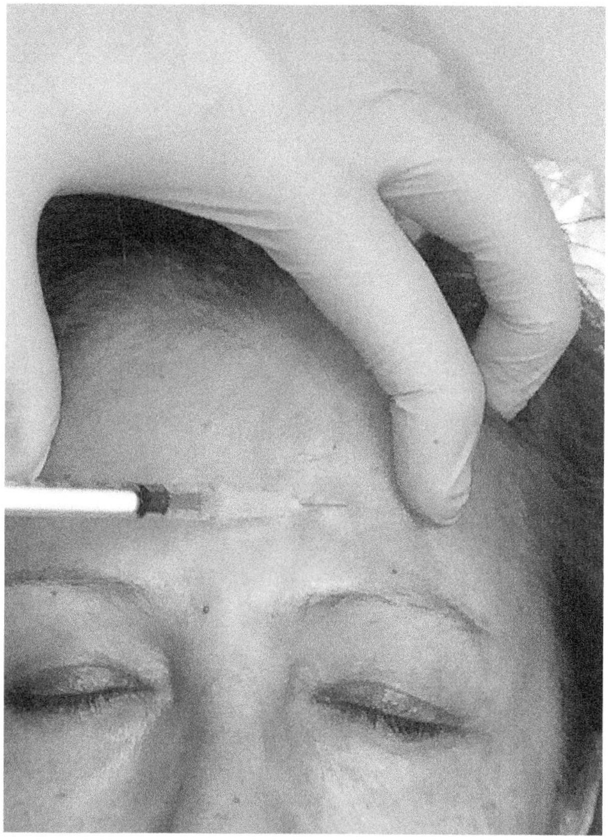

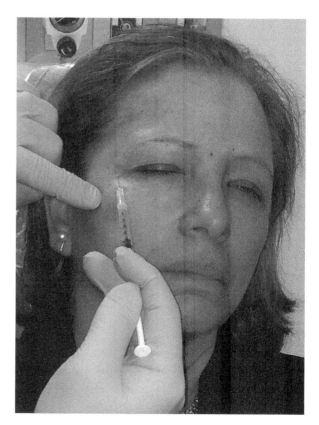

**Figure 13.10** Injection of the orbicularis oculi 1 cm lateral to the orbital rim at the mid-canthus level. It is important to remain quite superficial in this area.

**Figure 13.9** Injection of the left lateral site (corrugator muscle).

**Figure 13.11** Top: 1 week post injection results of neurotoxin ablation of crow's feet showing the left (A) and right (B) preinjections. Bottom: 1 week post injection, left (C) and right (D).

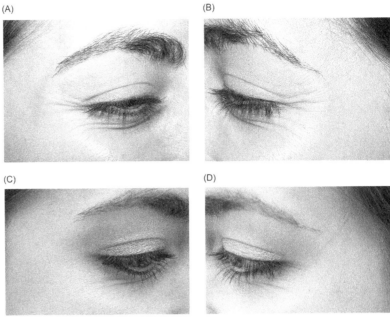

**Figure 13.12** (A) Injection spot is at the coalition of the levator labii superioris alaeque nasi and levator labii superioris and zygomaticus minor (Yonsei point) 1 cm lateral to the lateral ala and 3 cm above oral commissure . (B, C) Before and after photos courtesy of Dr. Lauren E. Fitzgerald.

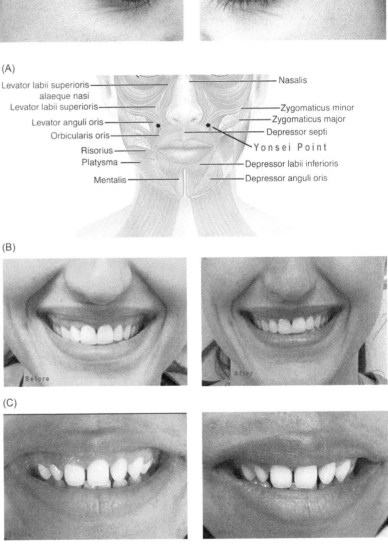

minor. In this condition the patient will have a normal upper lip rest position but excessive elevation upon smiling. If the rest position of the lip is high then treatment with neurotoxin is generally not effective.

Injection is performed bilaterally, typically 1 cm lateral the nasal ala and 3 cm above the oral commissure. This point has been named the "Yonsei Point." Two to three units at this point are generally sufficient (Figure 13.12).

## Treatment of the Midface and Lower Face with Fillers

Volume loss plays a much more important role in aging in the mid and lower face than hyperdynamic muscle activity. When evaluating the midface the fullness of the cheeks should be assessed even though this is not usually an area the patient is aware of. Cheek volume can profoundly affect the appearance of the nasolabial folds, marionette lines, and prejowl sulcus. Deep folds such as the nasolabial and marionette lines are the result of loss of subcutaneous fat from the height of the cheek bones to the inferior border of the mandible. This loss of fat results in skin sags and laxity, creating a tired and older looking face. The combination of this with the loss of the structural framework to support the skin (collagen and elastin) and surface wrinkles further complicates the aging process. Lip volume is an important visual component of the face. Lips, particularly in women, play a major role in defining beauty and youthfulness in most cultures. An upper lip that is a flat, poorly defined white roll with narrowing of the Cupid's bow and lack of fullness of the vermillion border is generally considered deficient and lacking in beauty. Add to this the vertical rhytids associated with aging, volume loss, smoking, and photoaging and you have a very old looking first impression of the face. Neurotoxins cannot address these deficiencies. Augmentations with some form of filler or implants are the only viable solution for treating these volume deficiencies. Even full or modified facelifts ultimately only remove redundant skin and tighten the skin over a volume-deficient face.

The temporary and semipermanent fillers available offer a patient treatment options with reduced risks and complications compared to the fillers available previously, but they yield similar longevity and offer patients minimal downtime for "recovery." For the clinician, the fillers are easy to use and offer predictable results when properly administered, and one class of fillers (HA) are reversible.

Injection techniques are varied and are dependent on both the location of injection and clinician preference. Typical techniques (Figure 13.13) include linear threading, fanning, cross-hatching, and serial puncture.

When using HA for fine wrinkle ablation a linear threading technique usually works best. Injection on withdrawal in usually easier and more comfortable for the patient but there is slightly higher risk of bruising as the needle is pushed forward intradermally. Injection on advancement offers the benefit of a reduced risk of bruising because filler is injected ahead of the needle, opening up a space.

For volume enhancement, several techniques are available. Cross-hatching works particularly well for marionette lines and the mouth corners as well as in the area below the zygoma and zygomatic arch. For the nasolabial folds, midface/cheekbones, and pre-jowl sulcus deep linear

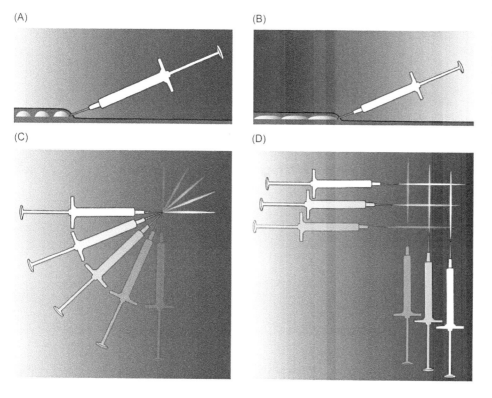

(A)

(B)

(C)

(D)

**Figure 13.13** (A) Serial puncture, (B) linear threading, (C) fanning, and (D) cross-hatching. Rohrich et al., 2007 / The American Society of Plastic Surgeons.

threading or fanning tends to work best. Alternatively, there are clinicians who prefer to inject small intermittent aliquots of filler then massage and shape the product into the area they desire to enhance. Most fillers need to be gently massaged and shaped after placement. This is where an understanding of what constitutes beauty and ideal facial form is critical.

Many patients arrive with a primary complaint of deep nasolabial folds and a flat thin upper lip. Often, in spite of other areas of volume deficits, these are the key areas of concern. The next areas of concern are the marionette lines and pre-jowl sulcus. These areas are usually easy to evaluate for the clinician and injection techniques are straight-forward (Figure 13.14).

In evaluating the nasolabial folds, look at how deep they are. Are the folds narrow or wide? Do they sag over the upper lip? Is there any hyperdynamic activity resulting in the upper lip folding under the midface? Is there any asymmetry? Is the lip flat with vertical rhytids? Is there a white roll? Is the columella well defined or flat? Are there any vertical folds at the corners of the mouth extending toward the inferior border of the mandible? Does the inferior border of the mandible in front of the masseter muscle insertion show a depression?

Once the injection sites have been identified, the product to be used must be selected. HA fillers come in various particle sizes and are available from multiple companies. For fine wrinkles and shallow (intradermal) injections, HA products are always the best choice. Deep volume enhancement can be accomplished with either HA products or the hydroxyapatite product, Radiesse® (Figure 13.15).

The volume of product injected will vary by site and the degree of deficit to be filled. In most cases to treat a patient with moderate nasolabial folds will take at least two 1 cc syringes of HA product or 1.8 cc of Radiesse® (Figure 13.16). There is always a delicate balance of overtreatment vs. undertreatment. It is always better to undertreat and tell the patient that a reassessment will be done in 7–10 days and touch up carried out as needed as opposed to a patient returning complaining of excessive fill. Although HA products are reversible with hyaluronidase, the result is usually the loss of the entire product. Radiesse®, on the other hand, is not reversible. It can be manipulated up to 7 days post injection by warming with moist heat packs

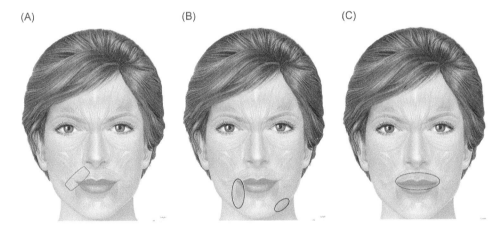

**Figure 13.14** (A) Nasolabial folds injection site, (B) marionette lines and pre jowl sulcus, and (C) upper lip.

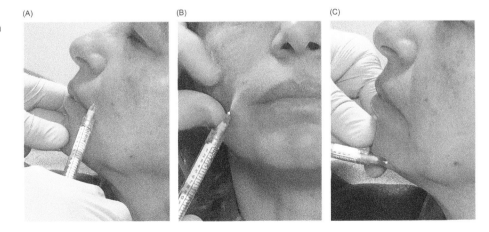

**Figure 13.15** Linear injection on withdrawal technique used in the placement of Radiesse® at the subdermal/dermal junction to provide fill and ablation of (A) nasolabial fold, (B) junction nasolabial fold and marionette line, and (C) prejowl sulcus.

(A)    (B)

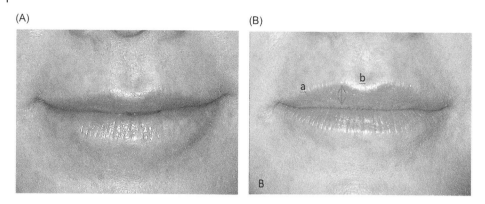

Figure 13.16   A 1.8-ml syringe Radiesse® filler was used to fill the nasolabial folds: (A) pre injection, (B) 1 week post injection. Linear threading and fanning on withdrawal were used to achieve the final result.

(A)    (B)

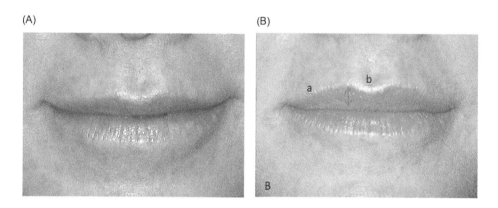

Figure 13.17   (A) Pre injection with topical anesthetic cream on lips (note the reversed ratio of upper lip to lower lip here) and (B) 2 months post injection. Notice the improved definition of the white roll (the junction between the mucosa and the skin). The increased height of the upper lip creates a more balanced relationship with the lower lip. The Cupid's bow has better projection and fullness.

and then massaging, which can disperse some overfill but not eliminate it.

Lip augmentation consists of two components. Definition of the vermillion border by reestablishing the white roll plays a major role in revitalizing the lips. This interrupts fine vertical rhytids from continuing from the skin onto the mucosa and creates a distinct light reflection at the junction of the mucosa and the skin of each lip. In some lips where volume has significantly diminished or in the edentulous patient with a combination of alveolar atrophy and lip sagging, volume enhancement may be appropriate. In the upper lip this is accomplished with the placement of pillows of filler in the body of the lip where the arch of the upper lip is highest bilaterally. The lower lip is augmented with a pillow placed in the body at the mid third of the lip (Figure 13.17).

MIPs such as neurotoxins, and temporary and semipermanent facial fillers, offer patients the opportunity to enhance and restore not only their oral cavity but also the extra-oral facial appearance, allowing a complete facial makeover without undergoing more invasive procedures requiring extensive recovery time. The key motivators for patients seeking aesthetic procedures fall into roughly three categories: augmentation, rejuvenation, and restoration. These vary in the population primarily based on the age range of the individual. Youth seeks augmentation, looking for improvement over what they have, middle age (post children) generally are looking to rejuvenate and bring back what has declined over time, and seniors are looking for the restoration of what has been lost. Awareness of these generational motivators helps clinicians identify what the treatment goals are for their patient. This then helps to customize the treatment plan to reach the patient's objectives. The difficulty is making sure that a patient's desired outcome is achievable and not unrealistic. Treatment should be directed to match the generational timeline. You cannot esthetically take a senior and enhance them in the same way as you would a youthful patient.

# References

Foster, K.A., editor. (2014). Molecular aspects of botulinum neurotoxin. In: *Overview and History of Botulinum Toxin Research, Current Topics in Neurotoxicity*, 1–7. Springer.

Kontis, T. and Rivkin, A. (2009). The history of injectable facial fillers. *Facial Plast. Surg.* 25 (2): 67–71.

Remington, B.K. (2008) Facial contouring and volumization. *Medscape Dermatology*. Remington Laser Centre, Calgary.

Rohrich, R.J., Ghavami, A., and Crosby, M.A. (2007). The role of hyaluronic acid fillers (restylane) in facial cosmetic surgery: review and technical considerations. *Plast. Reconst. Surg.* 120 (6 Suppl): 41S–54S.

Rubin, M. (2013) Neurotoxins: clinical perspective on subtle differences. *Practical Dermatology* January, 29–32.

Sandoval, L., Huang, K., Davis, S. et al. (2014). Trends in the use of neurotoxins and dermal fillers by US physicians. *J. Clin. Aesthet. Dermatol.* 7 (9): 14–19.

14

# Inflammation and Bone Healing around Dental Implants

*Thomas Van Dyke and Sheilesh Dave*

The integration of dental implant materials with bone takes advantage of the fact that bone is able to heal with new bone following injury. Furthermore, it can do so in very close apposition with certain metals and ceramics—for example, titanium or hydroxyapatite—without an intervening layer of less differentiated connective tissue. The implantation of titanium into bone initiates a wound healing process very similar to that which occurs when bone forms via the membranous pathway and later when bone remodels and repairs itself. This chapter reviews the basic processes in bone biology as they relate to bone formation, homeostasis, remodeling, and repair, and finally the events that occur at the bone-implant interface.

## Bone Function and Structure

Among the numerous functions now attributed to bone, structural integrity and protection remain central. Mature bone is made up of two distinct calcified compartments, an outer cortical or compact shell and an inner trabecular or cancellous core. Cortical bone is tightly organized in a series of concentric calcified rings or lamellae organized around a central canal containing blood vessels, lymphatics, nerves, and connective tissue. Embedded in islands or lacunae within these lamellae are osteocytes. Whereas cancellous bone is highly mineralized and poorly vascularized, trabecular bone is much less mineralized but highly vascularized. Trabecular bone is composed of an interconnected latticework of mineralized trabeculae with the trabeculae organized parallel to lines of stress. Again, osteocytes are embedded in lacunae within the trabeculae. The outer layer of cortical bone is sheathed in a specialized connective tissue, periosteum.

Periosteum is composed of an outer fibrous layer and an inner cellular layer. While the outer layer has no osteogenic potential, the inner layer that is in contact with the bone is home to osteoblasts and their precursors as well as

osteoclasts and their precursors. Similarly, the inner endosteal surfaces of trabeculae and cortical bone are also surrounded by a connective tissue layer, endosteum, that again contains osteoblasts and osteoclasts and their progenitor cells.

## Bone Homeostasis

Appearances aside, bone is a dynamic organ undergoing constant remodeling and adaptation in response to mechanical, systemic, and local factors. This process involves the closely coupled destruction of existing bone by osteoclasts followed by deposition of new bone by osteoblasts. If either of these processes—destruction or formation—is interrupted, pathology is observed. Bone multicellular units (BMUs) composed of osteoblasts, osteoclasts, and osteocytes are responsible for maintaining bone homeostasis and for repair and regeneration following injury.

## Osteoblasts and Osteocytes

Osteoblasts are derived from mesenchymal tissue along a tightly regulated pathway. Mesenchymal cells can form connective tissue fibroblasts, adipocytes, and bone. Differentiation of mesenchymal cell into osteoblasts occurs along a pathway involving regulation by autocrine, paracrine, and endocrine factors. Endocrine factors including parathyroid hormone, growth hormone, and insulin-like growth factor stimulate proliferation and in certain instances differentiation for pre-osteoblastic cells.

Critically, RUNX2, a nuclear transcription factor, must be expressed for a mesenchymal cell to differentiate along an osteoblastic lineage. The mechanisms by which expression of RUNX2 lead eventually to an osteoblast phenotype are beyond the scope of this chapter. However, it should be noted that bone morphogenetic proteins (BMPs) are critical for the induction of RUNX2 expression. BMPs are a member of the transforming growth factor family of

*Practical Periodontal Diagnosis and Treatment Planning*, Second Edition. Edited by Serge Dibart and Thomas Dietrich.
© 2024 John Wiley & Sons, Inc. Published 2024 by John Wiley & Sons, Inc.

proteins, and to date 30 have been identified. BMPs are present in bone and become soluble following demineralization. At that point they are able to exert inductive effects on differentiating cells in the osteoblast lineage. Thus, bone formation, at least in adulthood, is critically dependent on bone destruction occurring first. Several existing and emerging therapeutic approaches in bone grafting are intended to introduce autogenous BMPs, allogenic BMPs, or more recently, recombinant BMPs to a surgical site.

Once fully differentiated, osteoblasts synthesize an extracellular matrix principally composed of type 1 collagen but also containing other molecules. This matrix eventually becomes calcified and the osteoblasts are encased within the mineralized tissue. At that point the osteoblast is called an osteocyte. Osteocytes communicate with one another via dendritic processes, and the function of viable osteocytes with bone appears to be one of mechanosensation. Thus, bone that is not being mechanically stimulated tends to atrophy, while the converse is true of bone stimulated by exercise.

### Osteoclasts

Osteoclasts are multinucleated cells of hematopoietic lineage, specifically of the monocyte/macrophage lineage. Differentiation of monocytes to osteoclasts requires physical contact with osteoblasts or stromal cells. Osteoblasts express receptor activator of nuclear factor $\kappa\beta$-ligand (RANKL) on their membrane surface, which binds to the RANK receptor on osteoclast precursor macrophages and induces them to differentiate and eventually fuse into multinuclear cells, called osteoclasts. Osteoblasts also produce monocyte colony stimulating factor (M-CSF), which stimulates proliferation of osteoclast precursors. Whereas RANKL binds to RANK and stimulates osteoclastogenesis, the soluble molecule and decoy receptor osteoprotegrin (OPG) competitively binds RANKL and inhibits osteoclastogenesis. The relative proportions of RANKL and OPG have been termed the RANKL/OPG axis and seem to be instrumental in inflammation-dependent bone loss. This is especially significant for maintaining long-term stability of bone levels around the osseointegrated implant. This will be discussed later in this chapter.

### BMUs

Osteoblasts, osteoclasts, and osteocytes are organized into BMUs. These units are organized as cutting cones, which are led by osteoclasts that resorb bone and are trailed by osteoblasts that lay down new bone and eventually become osteocytes. BMUs have a limited life span and new units are continually formed to replace old, inactive ones. In good health, about 3–5% of an individual's skeleton is being

replaced at any given time and there is a relative homeostasis between bone formation and resorption.

## Bone Healing Following Implant Placement

Osteotomy preparation for implant placement, and implant placement itself, results in the destruction of both trabecular and cortical bone. It should be noted that the proportion of each varies such that a much higher percentage of cortical bone is present in the anterior mandible vs. the posterior maxilla. Whenever an implant is placed, there will be regions where the implant is in direct contact with the bone and areas where there are gaps. The areas with gaps are initially filled with blood clot and bone debris, which eventually give way to bone formation. These gaps may be evident only at a microscopic level or, in the case of immediate implant placement, they may be 3 mm or more. It has been shown by Botticelli et al. (2004) and Paolantonio et al. (2001) that gaps of 2 mm and perhaps as large as 5 mm can be expected to heal with osseointegration, even in the absence of membranes or grafting materials.

The areas of bone implant contact provide initial primary stability. However, Roberts et al. (1988) have shown that there is at least 1 mm of necrotic bone adjacent to an osteotomy site, even with optimal surgical technique, and that bone initially in contact with the implant remodels before integrating. In humans, the remodeling cycle, or sigma, is about 4.5 months. In other words, 4.5 months are required for osseous resorption, osteogenesis, and subsequently resorption. Hoshaw et al. (1997) have shown that the rate of bone remodeling increases following implant site preparation. Initial implant loading protocols of four months in the mandible and six months in the maxilla were based on the concept of sigma (Branemark et al. 1977). However, the success of contemporary protocols that emphasize much shorter or even immediate loading suggests that complete remodeling is not a requirement for long-term implant success (Esposito et al. 2007).

Given that de novo bone formation is required along the length of the implant, Osborn and Newesely (1980) have described two ways in which this may occur. Contact osteogenesis describes the formation of bone in direct apposition to the dental implant, whereas distance osteogenesis describes formation of bone from the mineralized surface toward the implant surface (Davies 2003) (Figure 14.1). Davies has discussed extensively the benefits of contact osteogenesis vs. distance osteogenesis (Davies 2003). A series of papers from his group, as well as others, have shown that where gaps occur, fibrin adherence to the implant surface is critical for de novo bone formation on

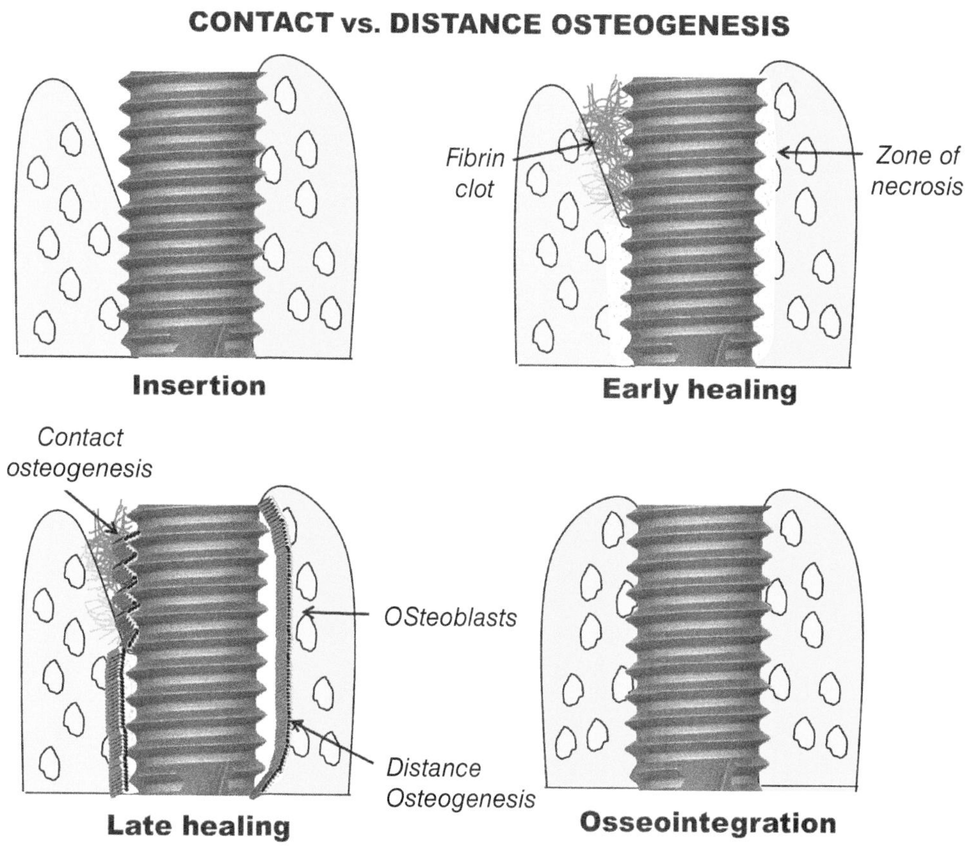

## CONTACT vs. DISTANCE OSTEOGENESIS

Figure 14.1   Contact vs. distance osteogenesis leading to osseointegration.

the implant surfaces—contact osteogenesis—and that this adherence is improved when the implant surface is textured as opposed to machined. Methods for texturing have included acid etching, sand blasting, electrolysis, plasma spray, and coating with hydroxyapatite. The relative advantages and disadvantages of each surface treatment are beyond the scope of this volume, but in terms of bone implant contact (BIC), all have been shown to be superior to machining (Cochran 1999).

A matrix is required for bone to form. In non-endochondral bone formation, this matrix is usually preexisting bone. In the case of implant placement, it has been shown that fibrin can be used as a matrix. Osteoblasts migrate through fibrin to the implant surface and first deposit a thin layer of glycoprotein similar to a cement line seen at the junction of old and newly formed bone. Bone is then deposited on the surface of the implant itself; this is contact osteogenesis.

Conversely, no blood clot is present in areas where bone is initially in contact with the implant. Rather, the necrotic bone that results for the osteotomy preparation serves as the substrate for new bone formation. As a result, bone forms from the surface of the bone toward the implant. Distance osteogenesis is expected to predominate in cortical bone, given its more dense nature, vs. trabecular bone.

## Inflammatory Bone Loss Around the Integrated Implant

Whether by contact or distance osteogenesis, osseointegration is normally expected to result. However, bone is a dynamic structure and maintenance of integration is an ongoing dynamic process. Homeostasis and stability of bone around an implant are characterized by an absence of inflammation.

The precipitating causes of peri-implant bone loss are not entirely clear. Known periodontal pathogens have been localized to peri-implant lesions associated with a progressive crestal bone loss similar to periodontal disease, peri-implantitis. Excessive force or stress has been implicated at least in animal models in the loss of peri-implant bone, but this evidence is equivocal (Heitz-Mayfield 2008a,b; Isidor 1996; Kozlovsky et al. 2007). Smoking and diabetes have been suggested as risk factors for peri-implantitis, as they are for periodontitis (Heitz-Mayfield 2008a,b). A very interesting study recently published by Heckmann et al. (2006) suggests that the presence of both stress and inflammation together induce peri-implant bone loss more than either factor on its own.

While periodontal bone loss and peri-implant bone loss are not the same disease, there are important similarities.

These include the presence of periodontal pathogens in both lesions, progressive bone loss over a long period of time and often in the absence of obvious local predisposing factors, and the presence of inflammation (Heitz-Mayfield 2008a,b; Van Dyke and Sheilesh 2005).

Periodontal bone resorption has been shown to be caused by inflammation as opposed to bacterial lytic enzymes. The OPG/RANKL/RANK axis has been suggested as a mechanism for understanding the dynamics of bone formation and resorption, particularly as it relates to loss of bone around teeth, and this may have important implications for the management of bone loss around implants (Cochran 2008). As discussed above, RANKL promotes the resorption of bone, whereas OPG interferes with this process by binding to RANKL and thus preventing the binding of RANKL to RANK (Figure 14.2). In the absence of RANKL-RANK binding, osteoclast differentiation does not occur and osteoclast apoptosis increases. Stability of the ratio of OPG/ RANKL is expected in homeostasis, where neither bone formation nor loss occurs. Increased bone formation is expected to be the result of an increase of OPG relative to RANKL, and an increase of RANKL relative to OPG is expected to result in an increase in bone loss. As was

discussed earlier, in classical models, RANKL is produced by osteoblasts, then binds to RANK on osteoclasts, induces osteoclast differentiation and bone resorption, and inhibits osteoclast apoptosis. OPG, which is also produced by osteoblast, binds to RANKL, and in so doing prevents it from binding to RANK. This provides the coupling mechanism between bone formation and resorption in homeostatic conditions.

There is an alternative pathway for production of RANKL that does not involve osteoblasts and results in the net loss of bone. It has been shown that T- and B-lymphocytes and fibroblasts also produce RANKL, and that this occurs in response to stimulation by pro-inflammatory molecules including IL-1, IL-6, $PGE_2$, and TNF-$\alpha$. Production of RANKL by inflammatory processes such as these results in increased RANKL relative to OPG; osteoclast-mediated bone loss is stimulated in the absence of bone formation and the result is the net loss of bone.

Ongoing loss of peri-implant bone (Figure 14.3) may similarly be characterized not only by a state of inflammation but also by a failure of inflammation to resolve (Van Dyke 2008). The most up-to-date research has begun to make it clear that the resolution of inflammation is an active process, just as is the development of inflammation,

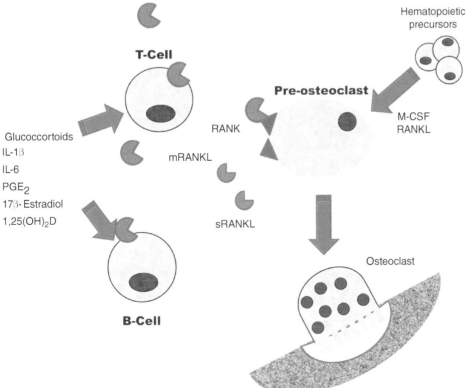

Figure 14.2   The inflammatory RANK-RANKL axis.

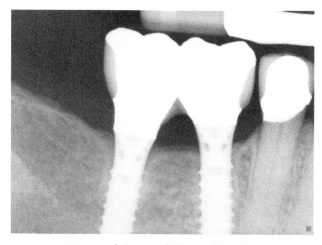 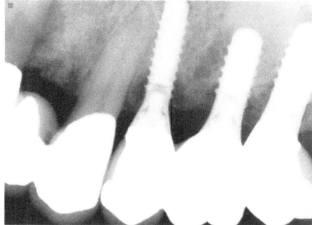

### Normal Crestal Bone Height          Peri-Implant Bone Loss

Figure 14.3   Radiographs showing normal bone height (left) and bone loss around implants (right).

and that specific molecules including IL-4, -10, -12, -13, and -18 as well as Interferon-β (IFNβ) and -γ (IFN-γ) all play an important role in promoting this process. In addition, a new class of polyunsaturated fatty acids (PUFA) present in fish oil has been implicated in the resolution of inflammation. These molecules have been termed lipoxins, protectins, and resolvins, and have been shown in in vitro and in in vivo animal studies to promote resolution of inflammation (Serhan et al. 2008).

Early studies showed that using nonsteroidal anti-inflammatories (NSAID) to interfere with the production of proinflammatory molecules such as $PGE_2$ mitigated periodontal bone loss in humans and animals (Jeffcoat et al. 1995). Unfortunately, undesirable side effects preclude the use of these medications over the long term. Lipoxins, protectins, and resolvins and our understanding of them have shed important new light on the dynamics of resolution of inflammation and hold special promise as the basis for a new class of therapeutic agents in the future. These may have a significant impact on the management of inflammatory bone loss in the oral cavity.

## References

Botticelli, D., Berglundh, T., and Lindhe, J. (2004). Hard-tissue alterations following immediate implant placement in extraction sites. *J. Clin. Periodontal*. 31 (10): 820–828.

Branemark, P.I., Hansson, B.O., Adell, R. et al. (1977). Osseointegrated implants in the treatment of the edentulous jaw. Experience from a 10-year period. *Scand. J. Plast. Reconstr. Surg. Suppl*. 16: 1–132.

Cochran, D.L. (1999). A comparison of endosseous dental implant surfaces. *J. Periodontal*. 70 (12): 1523–1539.

Cochran, D.L. (2008). Inflammation and bone loss in periodontal disease. *J. Periodontal*. 79 (8 Suppl): 1569–1576.

Davies, J.E. (2003). Understanding peri-implant endosseous healing. *J. Dent. Educ*. 67 (8): 932–949.

Esposito, M., Grusovin, M.G., Willings, M. et al. (2007). The effectiveness of immediate, early, and conventional loading of dental implants: a Cochrane systematic review of randomized controlled clinical trials. *Int. J. Oral Maxillofac. Implants*. 22 (6): 893–904.

Heckmann, S.M., Linke, J.J., Graefe, F. et al. (2006). Stress and inflammation as a detrimental combination for peri-implant bone loss. *J. Dent. Res*. 85 (8): 711–716.

Heitz-Mayfield, L.J. (2008a). Diagnosis and management of peri-implant diseases. *Aust. Dent. J*. 53 (Suppl 1): S43–S48.

Heitz-Mayfield, L.J. (2008b). Peri-implant diseases: diagnosis and risk indicators. *J. Clin. Periodontal*. 35 (8 Suppl): 292–304.

Hoshaw, S.J., Fyhrie, D.P., Takano, Y. et al. (1997 May). A method suitable for in vivo measurement of bone strain in humans. *J. Biomech*. 30 (5): 521–524.

Isidor, F. (1996). Loss of osseointegration caused by occlusal load of oral implants. A clinical and radiographic study in monkeys. *Clin. Oral Implants Res*. 7 (2): 143–152.

Jeffcoat, M.K., Reddy, M.S., Haigh, S. et al. (1995). A comparison of topical ketorolac, systemic flurbiprofen, and placebo for the inhibition of bone loss in adult periodontitis. *J. Periodontol*. 66 (5): 329–338.

Kozlovsky, A., Tal, H., Laufer, B.-Z. et al. (2007). Impact of implant overloading on the peri-implant bone in inflamed and non-inflamed peri-implant mucosa. *Clin. Oral Implants Res.* 18 (5): 601–610.

Osborn, J.F. and Newesely, H. (1980 April). The material science of calcium phosphate ceramics. *Biomaterials* 1 (2): 108–111.

Paolantonio, M., Dolci, M., Scarano, A. et al. (2001). Immediate implantation in fresh extraction sockets. A controlled clinical and histological study in man. *J. Periodontal.* 72 (11): 1560–1571.

Roberts, E.W. (1988). The oral surgeon-dental anesthesiologist team. *Anesth. Prog.* 35 (1): 18.

Serhan, C.N., Chiang, N., and Van Dyke, T.E. (2008). Resolving inflammation: dual anti-Inflammatory and pro-resolution lipid mediators. *Nat. Rev. Immunol.* 8 (5): 349–361.

Van Dyke, T.E. (2008). Inflammation and periodontal diseases: a reappraisal. *J. Periodontal.* 79 (8 Suppl): 1501–1502.

Van Dyke, T.E. and Sheilesh, D. (2005). Risk factors for periodontitis. *J. Int. Acad. Periodontal.* 7 (1): 3–7.

15

# How to Write and Read a Scientific Paper

*Cataldo W. Leone*

Dentistry is a healing art that is well founded in science. Demands from within and outside the profession require that standards of practice be increasingly based on scientific evidence. Such evidence is acquired largely through published peer-reviewed research reports, commonly referred to as "the literature." This chapter, which is adapted from the author's postdoctoral course in research writing, discusses how scientific papers are structured according to the principle components of the research process.

> The literature in a scientific field consists of various types of written communications, of which the primary sources of knowledge are peer-reviewed publications, called original reports.

One of the tenets of research is that the work be communicated publicly. A research report is the primary way to disseminate the findings of a study once it has been completed (after the fact). Similarly, a research proposal is written prior to beginning a study to obtain funding and/or permission to conduct the work (before the fact). Research reports and proposals have similar formats designed to explain to readers what the investigators did and found, or what the investigators will do and think that they will find, respectively.

Several types of research reports are found in the scientific literature. The predominant type is the original report, often referred to as a paper or article. Original reports typically are publications narrowly focused on a specific research question or idea that adds new knowledge, or confirms existing knowledge, in a particular scientific discipline. Most readers are familiar with the standard format used in original reports; namely, introduction, methods, results, and discussion, as described in detail below.

Another type of research report is the review, which summarizes sets of original reports in a scientific discipline. For the most part, reviews traditionally have been written by experts who often provide their own interpretation of the collected findings, and are therefore referred to as narrative reviews. Increasingly, however, a related type of review known as the structured review is being published, in part, to minimize the potential bias that may be associated with narrative reviews. Structured reviews follow stringent criteria regarding how articles are included and analyzed. These publications are particularly useful in documenting solid evidence in a field and also in identifying gaps or misperceptions that may exist.

Structured review articles can be both qualitative and quantitative in format. Qualitative structured reviews often use evidence tables to present summaries of articles that have been reviewed. Evidence tables are comprehensive listings of the salient aspects of each article that has been included in the review. These evidence tables allow the reader to judge the relative merit of the available evidence comprehensively and efficiently. Quantitative structured reviews additionally provide what is called a meta-analysis, which is a computational method for analyzing the data reported in a set of published papers. In essence, meta-analysis allows the reviewer to treat data compiled from individual studies as if such data were from one larger study. This is an extremely powerful technique to establish the strength of evidence, or lack thereof, in a scientific discipline.

Other examples of research reports include abstracts or proceedings of scientific conferences, which can be in the form of posters or oral presentations. A graduate dissertation or thesis is also a type of research report. Chapters in textbooks and monographs also can be categorized as research reports. Opinions of experts expressed in editorials or letters in journals can sometimes be considered as a type of scientific publication, although there are obvious limitations to how such information should be interpreted and used.

The predominant type of research proposal is the grant application. To be successful, grant applications must clearly describe the rationale, importance, and feasibility of a proposed research study. Grant applications also must clearly describe how the study will be performed, what results are anticipated, and how the results will be analyzed.

*Practical Periodontal Diagnosis and Treatment Planning*, Second Edition. Edited by Serge Dibart and Thomas Dietrich.
© 2024 John Wiley & Sons, Inc. Published 2024 by John Wiley & Sons, Inc.

Increasingly, research proposals in the biomedical sciences have multiple levels of investigation: human, animal, and in vitro. By using humans as research subjects, investigators can identify clinical evidence of a particular disease or condition and can test new interventions or treatments. Animal models allow specific ideas or interventions to be tested that would not be feasible to do in humans. This is especially true in research activities that have little or no known benefit and relatively high risk for subjects. In vitro cellular, molecular, genetic, biochemical, and biophysical analyses are useful in identifying or confirming biological mechanisms that explain a particular condition, risk factor, or treatment outcome. As part of the grant application process, investigators often must apply for institutional permission to use humans, animals, and certain hazardous materials such as radioisotopes, recombinant nucleic acids, or toxic chemicals. Such applications themselves are proposals that must justify the particular permission being sought.

## Original Reports Reflect the Basic Format of the Research Process

Research can be defined as any focused, systematic inquiry or activity designed to contribute to generalizable knowledge and enhanced understanding of a particular subject (Centers for Disease Control and Prevention 1999). It is critical that the activity be systematic; that is, it must follow set rules or patterns designed to produce valid conclusions and allow repetition and confirmation. Often called the scientific method, this approach ensures that the knowledge in a scientific discipline is based on objective facts rather than on unsupported opinions. The criterion of generalizability further ensures that such knowledge can be applied to populations or conditions outside the sample group or condition being studied within a particular research investigation. The research process follows a logical sequence. Typically, research begins with an idea or observation that forms the basis of a hypothesis that can be tested and subsequently evaluated. The process is cyclical in that subsequent systematic investigations modify the accumulated knowledge base as new evidence is obtained (Appendix Figure 15.1).

Research writing, like the research that it describes, also is a process having a logical structure. Scientific reports and proposals both follow a formulaic pattern designed to communicate the various components of a particular research endeavor. As indicated in Appendix Figure 15.2, research writing is designed to answer the following questions in original reports (or grant proposals).

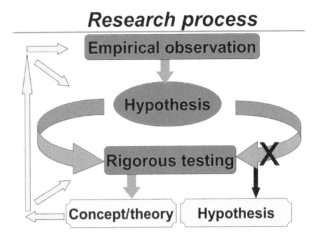

**Appendix Figure 15.1** Algorithm for the general sequence of events in the research process. Research typically begins with an interesting observation or idea that is then developed into a hypothesis that can be tested. If the results are consistent and repeatable, then the initial idea may become part of an accepted concept or theory, which is subsequently modified as new knowledge is gained in the future. Without rigorous testing of the hypothesis, the original interesting idea remains speculative.

## General Format of Reports/Proposals

| | Reports ("did") | Proposals ("will") |
|---|---|---|
| What ___ you do? | ⇔ Purpose | Specific Aims |
| Why ___ you do it? | ⇔ Introduction | Background |
| How ___ you do it? | ⇔ Methods | Experimental Design |
| What ___ you find? | ⇔ Results | Preliminary Data |
| What ___ it mean? | ⇔ Discussion | Relevance |
| What next? | ⇔ Future Directions | Contingency Plans |
| Who to thank/ask? | ⇔ Acknowledgments | Collaborators |

**Appendix Figure 15.2** Component questions addressed by research writing. Scientific papers attempt to convey to the reader the significance of the research, why and how it was conducted, and what the most likely interpretation and conclusion should be. Similarly, grant proposals seek to prove to the funding agency why the work should be done, provide the grant reviewers with some evidence that the proposed study can actually be done, and indicate what the investigators will do if unforeseen problems arise. In both published papers and grant applications, respectively, it is important to acknowledge those who have provided or will provide significant help with the project.

- What did (or will) you do?
- Why did (or will) you do it?
- How did (or will) you do it?
- What did (or will) you find?
- What does (or will) it mean?
- What might you do next (or do if you hit a roadblock)?
- Who helped (or will help) you, including paying for it?

These questions form the basis of the standard format used in original reports or grant proposals. The essential components of a scientific report or proposal often are presented as separate sections of the written work, but also can be collapsed and combined as deemed appropriate. The remainder of this appendix discusses these various components.

> The initial idea for an original report is developed into a justifiable and testable hypothesis through review of the existing literature (the "Introduction").

The introduction section of original reports generally states the purpose of the study, and also describes the background information that supports why the study was conducted. In performing the study, the researchers had to establish a balance between how interesting or important the research question was and how feasible it was to test, in terms of time, resources, and available methodologies. As suggested in Appendix Figure 15.3, a research question that is easily answered oftentimes may lack significance. On the other hand, an important research question may not be testable due to scientific or logistical constraints.

Any interesting research idea needs to be developed and refined so that it can be tested; otherwise, it remains merely an interesting idea with little practical merit. The process has analogy to the popular riddle: Which comes first, the chicken or the egg? In other words, one needs to know at least something about an area to come up with an interesting research question in the first place. The research question may be too broad or ill-defined at first, which then requires one to review the literature in the field to focus the question. This becomes a repetitive, iterative process until the nascent idea is transformed into a precise hypothesis worthy of investigation; that is:

> The research question is *developed* from a review of the available literature.
>
> ↑↓
>
> The review of the available literature is *focused* on the research question.

The key point to be made is that the steps taken to develop a research question into a testable hypothesis are the same as the steps taken to conduct a focused review of the existing knowledge base for that same research question (Appendix Figure 15.4).

## The Hypothesis

The hypothesis is a clear and concise statement of the research idea that is to be tested. Often, the hypothesis is presented as the purpose of a particular study with specific aims or objectives that list how the purpose was (or will be) achieved. Hypotheses are built according to relatively simple logical patterns: if/then, cause/effect, and intervention/outcome. In simplest terms, a hypothesis of any clinical study has the following structure:

## Research Question

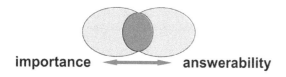

- Is it important ?
- Can it be answered ?
- What is the best approach/modality to answer the question ?
- How much $$ will it cost to do ?

Appendix Figure 15.3    Balance between the significance of a research study and the feasibility of realizing the study's objectives. A research question that is easily answered may not be deemed important by the scientific community, and likely would not advance knowledge in any meaningful way. On the other hand, potential scientific, logistical, or financial constraints may render a research study overly ambitious and practically impossible to conduct. Thus, investigators seek to find a middle ground that allows them to actually answer a research question of reasonably high importance.

## Steps for Developing the Hypothesis

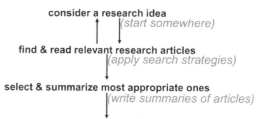

Appendix Figure 15.4    The generation and refinement of a research hypothesis is an iterative process. It begins with a nascent idea that is developed through a targeted search of the literature. Oftentimes, the question is modified based on evidence that may or may not be found in the literature. Articles are read and summarized in the context of the investigator's hypothesis. That is, articles are used strategically to produce "a story" that is rational, convincing, and scientifically exciting. The hypothesis then represents a reasoned justification for conducting the proposed study.

Such a structure points out four key factors to be considered in focusing the research question into a testable hypothesis: (1) **P**roblem and patients, (2) **I**ntervention, treatment, or risk factor, (3) **C**omparison intervention or group, and (4) **O**utcomes or effect. The acronym PICO describes this well-accepted format for framing hypotheses (Richards 2007). Each of these four factors addresses the following questions, respectively:

1) What is the problem of interest and the patients or subjects it concerns?
2) What is the main intervention, treatment, or risk factor being considered?
3) What is the main alternative to which the intervention, treatment, or risk factor will be compared? To what group will patients or subjects of interest be compared?
4) What do the researchers hope to accomplish? What do they realistically expect to see? To what will the risk or exposure lead? What outcome would be particularly worrisome?

Some examples of PICO-formatted research questions are listed in Appendix Table 15.1. It is important to note that by following this format each example makes clear not only what will be tested but also what general methods or measurements most likely will be used.

## Publication Databases and Search Strategies

There is little doubt that the biomedical literature has burgeoned during the past several decades. Increasing numbers of original reports are being published in increasing numbers of journals. This presents a considerable challenge for researchers interested in focusing a research question; that is, how to identify relevant publications efficiently and effectively without missing important ones and without obtaining ones that are not directly relevant. An important first step is to recognize that the literature is organized in several electronic databases that can be searched.

The most popular data base is MEDLINE, which is produced by the National Library of Medicine (NLM) in Bethesda, Maryland. MEDLINE is a comprehensive bibliographic database of citations to published journal articles in the biomedical sciences. It covers all aspects of healthcare: dentistry, medicine, nursing, allied health fields, biomedical and preclinical sciences, pharmacy, psychiatry, etc. MEDLINE indexes approximately 4,800 journals containing more than 15 million citations, dating from 1950 to the present. MEDLINE is free, open to the public, and available 24 hours/day, 7 days/week on the Web from any computer worldwide. This database is dynamic, with citations updated weekly. It can be readily accessed online through the PubMed portal (PubMed): http://www.ncbi.nlm.nih.gov/entrez.

MEDLINE is not the only database available to biomedical and social scientists. Others include Biosis; CINAHL (Cumulative Index to Nursing and Allied Health Literature); Cochrane Central Register of Controlled Trials; Cochrane Database of Systematic Reviews, Genetics, Genomics and Proteomics Databases; PsycINFO; TOXLINE; TOXNET; and the Web of Science databases known as Science Citation Index and Social Sciences Citation Index. These databases would also be searched depending upon the particular research question being asked.

After an appropriate database has been identified, it next becomes necessary to execute an effective strategy to search for relevant publications. In this regard, it is useful to

**Appendix Table 15.1** Examples of hypotheses formulated using the PICO format.

| | Problem/patients (P) | Intervention/treatment/ risk factor (I) | Comparisons (C) | Outcomes (O) |
|---|---|---|---|---|
| Example 1 | Among adults ... | ... does moderate-to-severe periodontal disease ... | ... compared to mild or no periodontal disease ... | ... lead to increased myocardial infarctions? |
| Example 2 | In patients with fixed orthodontic appliances ... | ... would use of an electric toothbrush ... | ... compared to a manual toothbrush ... | ... lead to improved plaque removal? |
| Example 3 | In patients with aggressive periodontitis ... | ... does flap surgery ... | ... compared with scaling and root planing ... | ... decrease the need for extraction during the maintenance phase? |
| Example 4 | Among adults with type 2 diabetes ... | ... is periodontal treatment ... | ... compared with no treatment ... | ... associated with improved glycemic control? |
| Example 5 | Among adults who smoke ... | ... do tapered implants ... | ... compared with cylindrical implants ... | ... demonstrate identical success rates? |

Given A, B, and C (the current state of knowledge), if subjects do or have X (an intervention, treatment, or a risk factor), then they are expected to demonstrate Y (an outcome or effect) in comparison with subjects without X.

recognize that databases are compiled by library science personnel who read and catalogue the articles according to set criteria. For MEDLINE, these criteria constitute a controlled vocabulary thesaurus known as medical subject headings (MeSH), which represent the subject content of each article. MEDLINE uses more than 50,000 MeSH terms (also referred to as subjects) with more than 30 subheadings that are attached to the MeSH to further describe a particular subject. MeSH subjects also are grouped in hierarchies called trees that organize the relationships among diverse subject headings. A tree progresses from the most general (broad) term to the most specific (narrow) term. The indexers at the National Library of Medicine assign 8–20 MeSH for each article, which can then be used by researchers in their literature searches.

The literature search process is generally organized into successive steps that result in the retrieval of a manageable number of relevant articles. The first step is to use various search terms (or fields) as needed. The MeSH terms are frequently used, as are specific text words from an article's title or abstract. The key words listed in articles are also useful terms. Searches can also be conducted according to the names of known authors or specific titles of journals. Once a first pass through the available literature is completed, the search is then either widened or narrowed, depending on the initial results. This is referred to as exploding or focusing, respectively. So-called limits can be applied to large sets of articles to reduce the number of articles identified and refine the search. These limits can be according to subject age or gender, type of publication, years of publication, language, dental specialty, or other criteria. The search results can be combined to include only articles that contain more than one of the search elements. Once these are done, the most efficient next step is to review the title and abstract of each individual article, without reading the entire article, to determine if the retrieved article is relevant to the topic. This entire process then repeats until the researcher is satisfied with the search results.

It should be noted that universities appoint professional searchers, typically library staff, to assist researchers in developing their research agenda. These individuals are experts in information recovery and generally provide ongoing training for researchers in need of assistance. Such training is very useful in improving the efficiency and effectiveness of one's literature searches.

## Summarizing the Literature

The net result of the literature search is to establish a set of articles with the most relevance to the intended research investigation. These articles must then be read and summarized so that they can form the basis for justifying why the intended investigation is necessary, and what is hoped to be accomplished. This constitutes the introduction section in an original report (or the background/significance section in grant proposals). How these articles are actually summarized is usually a matter of preference of the individual researcher. However, to be useful, each article retrieved from the search process should be summarized with the following questions in mind:

1) What was the authors' research question?
2) How did the authors attempt to answer that question (i.e., research design and methods)?
3) What were the results?
4) What is the article's relevance to my own research question or project?
   a) Does it help indicate the current state of knowledge?
   b) Does it help argue the case for my own research question?

Once reviewed and summarized, the information reported in selected literature is compiled into a narrative that provides general background information and the details of the current state of knowledge in the relevant area. Arguments are then presented defending the need to answer the specific research question, which is formulated as a testable hypothesis. As indicated in Appendix Figure 15.4, these summaries are organized into a hopefully convincing story that provides the rationale for the intended research investigation.

## Citations and Citation Management

The format of citations in original reports is specified by the scientific journal in which they are published. In the biomedical literature, these tend to follow the Uniform Requirements for Manuscripts Submitted to Biomedical Journals (International Committee of Medical Journal Editors 2007). Typically, one of two general formats is used: the numbering method for citing articles or the name and year method for citing articles. As the name implies, the numbering method cites references according to the order in which they appear in the publication. These are then listed in ascending numerical order at the end of the paper. In contrast, the name and year method cites references by indicating the name of the author(s) and the year in which the reference was published. These are then listed alphabetically at the end of the paper. Although each journal has its own rules, typically only up to three authors' names are listed in the body of the text, whereas all authors are listed at the end of the paper. An excellent resource that describes citation management can be found at The Writing Center, University of Wisconsin-Madison (The Writing Center).

It also should be noted that several software programs to facilitate the management of references are commercially available. These help organize one's personal electronic database of articles to which future articles can be added. These software programs allow citations to be easily inserted into the text of manuscripts that are being prepared for publication. A useful advantage is that the citations can then be listed at the end of the paper according to the varying formats specified by different journals; these formats come preset within the software program.

> The hypothesis is tested systematically using relevant protocols in established study designs (the "Methods").

In discussing the methods used in research studies, it is helpful to distinguish between the general design of a particular investigation and the specific protocols used to generate data.

## Study Designs

The design of a study refers to the general format of how the investigation is conducted. Several formats are commonly used in clinical studies, as reviewed in Callas (2008). These formats are based on several defining characteristics: the timing of data acquisition, the extent of influence or direct action by the researchers, and the amount of involvement and risk for the study subjects.

In the broadest sense, research study designs are either descriptive or explanatory. Descriptive studies are those that identify and report various characteristics of interest such as age, gender, race, geographic location, and incidence or prevalence of a particular disease, as examples, without testing a specific hypothesis. Descriptive studies are useful in generating information that can be subsequently used to develop hypotheses that can be tested. Clinical case reports, specifically those reported as case series, are examples of descriptive studies.

Explanatory studies (also referred to as analytical studies) are designed to answer and explain specific questions; that is, to actually test research hypotheses. These studies can be either prospective or retrospective: prospective studies collect and analyze data going forward from the start of an investigation, whereas retrospective studies collect data after an outcome has occurred or they analyze existing data that have been collected previously. Explanatory studies can be further classified as observational or experimental (also referred to as interventional). As the name implies, observational studies are those in which "natural" changes or differences in one characteristic

(variable) are studied in relation to changes or differences in another variable(s), without any direct intervention by the investigator. In contrast, experimental studies are those in which the investigator actively intervenes by changing a particular variable and then measures what happens to other variables.

Observational studies can be further classified as cohort studies (also referred to as longitudinal), case-control studies, and cross-sectional studies. In cohort studies, groups selected by the presence or absence of a risk factor or other characteristic suspected of being a precursor for an outcome of interest are followed prospectively over time and the outcome is subsequently measured. In case-control studies, two groups are analyzed retrospectively to determine possible causes or risk factors for a particular outcome of interest. The two groups are defined by the presence (case) or absence (control) of the relevant outcome. In cross-sectional studies, data are collected at one point in time and then analyzed for the concurrent presence or absence of a factor suspected to be associated with a particular outcome characteristic. If data are compared between groups of subjects with and without the outcome characteristic, then the cross-sectional study is considered to be explanatory. If data for only one group of subjects is reported, then the cross-sectional study is more aptly considered to be descriptive.

Experimental or interventional studies are collectively referred to as clinical trials, which are designed to produce cause-and-effect relationships among variables of interest. In clinical trials, subjects are assigned into either experimental (test) or control groups. The experimental group is actively subjected to a suspected causal variable or intervention, while the control group is not, and predetermined outcome variables are then measured prospectively. There are several types of clinical trials that are characterized according to how subjects are assigned into the study groups and the nature of the control group.

The randomized clinical trial (RCT) has long been considered the gold standard in clinical research design. In the RCT, subjects are randomly assigned into either the experimental or the control group. Randomization is very important from a design standpoint because the process ensures that the two comparison groups are as similar as possible in multiple characteristics (for example, age, gender, health status), except for the suspected causal variable or intervention.

Nonrandomized clinical trials also can be found in the literature, but these studies are not considered as strong as the RCTs. Studies that compare two different groups (i.e., experimental and control) within the same study are considered stronger than those in which each research subject serves as its own control (called self-controlled trials, in which subjects participate in both the experimental and control groups at different times during the study). Along the same lines of reasoning, studies that compare two different groups within the same study are considered much stronger than studies in which the experimental group is compared with an external control group, either the general population itself or different groups studied in previous research investigations (called historical controls).

As described above, a systematic review is a type of literature review that attempts to identify, pool, and interpret available evidence on a specific research question, usually from RCTs, so that the strengths and weaknesses of the evidence can be made clear.

The various study designs can be summarized as follows:

**Case Series Description: Did you see something interesting?** These are a grouping of anecdotal observations about a particular outcome that helps to generate initial research ideas.

**Case-Control Studies: What happened?** In this type of study design one group of subjects already has a particular outcome (cases), as compared to another group that does not (controls).

**Cross-Sectional Studies: What is happening?** Groups are examined at one point in time for the presence or absence of a particular outcome.

**Cohort (Longitudinal) Studies: What will happen "naturally"?** Groups are followed over time for the occurrence or non-occurrence of a particular outcome.

**Clinical Trials: What will happen "experimentally"?** One group (experimental) is subjected to a specific manipulation while another group (control) is not; both groups are examined at a future point in time for the presence or absence of a particular outcome.

**Systematic Reviews/Meta-Analyses: How can existing data in separate studies be critically summarized so that the "real" answer to a research question is identified?** A systematic review uses rigorous, objective criteria to retrieve, evaluate, and summarize published scientific papers that are relevant to a topic. A meta-analysis is a statistical method used in certain systematic reviews that allows quantitative data published in different scientific papers to be evaluated and combined as if they were all from one large study.

## Hierarchy of Evidence

One of the fundamental goals of biomedical research is to discover and advance knowledge for alleviating human abnormalities and diseases and improving overall quality of life. Thus, research study designs have been ranked according to how directly applicable their respective findings may be to the human population and how well potential sources of study bias or error have been reduced. This ranking is often referred to as the hierarchy of evidence and includes in vitro, animal, and human clinical studies. This hierarchy can be illustrated by an evidence pyramid, as shown in Appendix Figure 15.5. The figure is available from the online Evidence Based Medicine Course at the Medical Research Library of Brooklyn, State University of New York Downstate Medical Center. This is an excellent tutorial on evidence-based medicine that can be accessed freely (Markinson).

The different types of evidence are labeled in the figure, with the least clinically relevant at the bottom and the most clinically relevant at the top. The top five layers indicate evidence generally considered strong enough to be clinically relevant (i.e., directly influencing clinical decisions). The bottom layers have considerable merit in terms of providing scientific information, but do not provide sufficient strength of scientific evidence to warrant direct relevance to humans. As illustrated, systematic reviews and meta-analyses are considered to be the highest level of evidence in biomedical research. These serve to increase the credibility and power (discussed below) of individual studies, and are extremely useful in helping busy practitioners distinguish between reality and hype, so to speak, regarding diagnostic and treatment interventions.

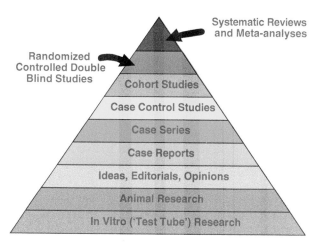

**Appendix Figure 15.5** The evidence pyramid. Available evidence can be ranked according to its relative strength in clinically relevant contexts. In general, this ranking reflects how directly applicable the evidence may be to the human population, and to how well potential sources of bias or error have been reduced. It is important to point out that all types of evidence have intrinsic value but that only the study designs listed in the upper levels of the pyramid provide evidence that may be of immediate use for the practicing clinician. (Reproduced with permission of Dr. Andrea Markinson, Evidence Based Medicine Course, State University of New York Downstate).

## Study-Specific Protocols

These are intuitively understood as constituting the methods of a study. In a periodontal clinical study, for example, measurements of attachment loss, probing pocket depth, recession depth, gingival index, plaque index, or bleeding on probing would each be done according to specific protocols. Researchers determine a priori what measurements would be made, how many teeth or sites would be evaluated (for example, Ramfjord teeth) (Fleiss et al. 1987), by which instruments (for example, manual vs. electronic periodontal probe), and how often (for example, number of posttreatment recall visits). Oftentimes, these protocols are well established and commonly used across many different studies. In such instances the protocol is merely indicated by a published citation without much description of the details of the technique. A classic example of this is the highly cited Gingival Index (GI) of Loe and Silness (1963). On the other hand, if a well-accepted protocol has been modified, or if a new method has been developed for the particular research study, then it is expected that a more detailed description will be provided. Thus, a balance is established between clarity and brevity in published reports. Appendix Figure 15.6 provides some examples of study-specific methods. The list is for illustrative purposes only and is not meant to be comprehensive. Moreover, many of these are applicable to human subjects and animal models, depending on the objectives of the research study.

### *Examples of Some Specific Protocols/Techniques*

| Clinical | Animal | Laboratory |
| --- | --- | --- |
| Plaque score | Birth weight | H & E stain |
| Gingival index | Food Intake | Cell counts |
| Caries | Caries | RNA expression |
| Pulp vitality | Pulp vitality | Protein Levels |
| Intercanine distance | Behavior | Bond strength |
| Fluorosis | Sedation | Leakage |
| Use of Services | Sacrifice | Moment of Inertia |
| Attitudes | Phlebotomy | Stress/Strain |

Appendix Figure 15.6   Some types of measurements or procedures that may be found in research studies. Each would be described in varying detail within scientific papers or grant proposals, depending on how well known and accepted the particular measurement or procedure may be to the scientific community. Intuitively, measurement protocols that are standardized and frequently used can be described by a simple citation, whereas novel techniques or common techniques that have been significantly modified should be described in detail. The important point to note is that the scientific community should be provided sufficient technical details to allow the study to be repeated. Such repetition by different groups of investigators is critical for confirming the validity of findings presented in the literature.

---

> There are a number of important scientific principles to be considered when designing and conducting a research investigation.

## Sampling, Sample Size, and Power

The concepts described in this section are shown in greater detail in the Research Methods Knowledge Base (Trochim 2006). Because it is highly impractical, if not impossible, to study all individuals in a population, researchers select a representative subset to study (i.e., the sample). This subset must be truly representative if valid conclusions are to be drawn from the research findings. Consequently, the methods section of a published scientific paper often describes how the research subjects were chosen and recruited. The reader should be confident that the subjects represent the full range of individuals who present with a particular condition, or who are exposed to a particular risk factor, or who require a particular intervention.

It is also important that inclusion and exclusion criteria are clearly identified. Inclusion criteria are those characteristics that subjects must demonstrate to be accepted into the study. In studies of periodontal disease, for example, subjects must often present with a minimum amount of attachment loss on a predetermined number of teeth prior to enrollment. Exclusion criteria are based on subject characteristics that, when present, would likely interfere with interpretation of the research data. In studies of periodontal disease, again for example, concurrent or recent use of systemic antibiotics due to a medical condition often would cause a prospective subject to be deemed ineligible.

Thus, appropriate sampling strategies for clinical studies are critical for ensuring that comparison groups are well-matched and that subjects do not present with characteristics that could diminish the strength of the research (Trochim 2006). Several sampling strategies are commonly used to recruit subjects in clinical trials. In random sampling, as the name implies, subjects are selected at random. In consecutive sampling, all potential subjects who meet the inclusion criteria over a specified period of time are recruited. In convenience sampling, subjects who are easily accessible are recruited. Stratified and cluster sampling strategies are similar in that a population is subdivided according to demographic or geographic characteristics, respectively, and then random samples are taken from the subgroups.

In addition to using appropriate sampling methodologies, it is important for researchers to determine how large of a sample must be studied (i.e., the sample size) (Whitley and

Ball 2002). If the sample is too small, there is uncertainty about how much the findings are due to random chance instead of the study design. If the sample is too large, extra effort and costs are incurred unnecessarily. In both instances the possible risks to human subjects are unacceptably increased. Researchers are therefore obligated to calculate the sample size that is appropriate for their study. Although formulae and tables for calculating sample size are readily available, these require several pieces of information that should be known or estimated before the study is conducted.

One important estimate is the variability (variance) of the measures to be made in the study. In simplest terms, this represents the "natural" measurement error of a particular technique. Such an estimate can be determined from the available literature or from general consensus from practitioners in the field. For example, measures of probing pocket depth using a manual probe in clinical periodontics are generally accepted as ±1 mm. If this variance is unacceptably high for a proposed study, the use of an electronic probe would be required to reduce this inherent variability in the measure of pocket depth.

Another important determination is how large or small a difference between sample groups will be considered to be real. Intuitively, if the difference to be found is small, then larger samples must be measured to find the difference. On the other hand, large or gross differences between sample groups may be detected with smaller sample sizes. In the example of probing pocket depth measured with a manual probe, a difference of ≥3 mm pocket depth between two sample groups would be much easier to detect than would a 1 mm difference.

A third important parameter in calculating sample size is power (Danya International Inc. 2005). Power refers to the ability of a research study to detect a difference between comparison groups when such a difference does, in fact, really exist. Power, variance, difference, and sample size are interrelated. A study that is underpowered would not be able to adequately test a hypothesis because (1) the variance is too large, given the sample size and difference to be detected, (2) the difference to be detected between the groups is too small, given the variance and sample size, or (3) the sample size is insufficient for detecting the specified difference, given the variance and difference to be detected. To adequately test a hypothesis, therefore, a study must be appropriately powered. Increasingly, journals are requiring investigators to provide justification for their sample size and/or a power calculation in the methods section. This assures the reader that the work was worth the effort and expenditure of resources, and also that the potential risks to research subjects were acceptable. Without adequate power, the findings of a particular study will not be generalizable, which is one of the main goals of research.

## Reliability and Validity

The terms reliability and validity describe different aspects of what may generically be called the credibility of a study and its results (Colorado State University). Reliability is concerned with accuracy and precision of the actual methods, procedures, tests, instruments, etc. in a particular study. Specifically, reliability is a function of how well the measures reflect relevant characteristics or variables of interest, and how consistent these measures are over time. Validity is concerned with the degree to which the research study itself accurately tests the hypothesis. Validity is a function of how well the study is designed to answer the research question; that is, that the study actually measures what it is supposed to measure. Therefore, for a study to be considered valid it must not only have reliability of its measures, but also these reliable measures must be appropriate for testing the stated hypothesis.

A simple example can be used to illustrate the relationship between reliability and validity. Let us suppose that a particular investigation is evaluating the hypothesis that susceptibility to periodontal disease is related to the degree of surface mineralization of teeth. In this imaginary example, clinical attachment is measured at six sites in all teeth and periodontal disease is defined as clinical attachment loss of more than 3 mm in at least four teeth per subject. To test the hypothesis, the investigators designed a cross-sectional study that uses standard shade guides to evaluate the color of natural crowns in subjects with periodontal disease. After all data have been collected, the investigators will look for any associations between tooth shade and periodontal disease. Here, both attachment levels and tooth shade are reliable measures because they can be obtained with high accuracy and repeatability, when necessary, by an experienced clinical investigator. However, the study probably would not be valid even if an association was found between tooth shade and periodontal disease because tooth color per se does not necessarily reflect the surface mineralization status of either the crown or root.

In this example the investigators could generate lots of accurate and consistent data, but those data would probably have little to do with testing the relationship between surface mineralization and periodontitis. Despite any statistically significant associations that may be found, this study would have failed to test its hypothesis. Instead, the study would actually have tested a different hypothesis than intended; that is, that periodontal disease is associated with the color of natural crowns.

Several types of reliability have been described (Colorado State University). Publications of clinical studies often provide information about interrater reliability. This is the extent with which two or more investigators demonstrate agreement when measuring a particular characteristic or variable. Interrater reliability defines how well calibrated the clinical examiners may be, and this is often reported in scientific papers as the Kappa statistic. Intrarater reliability describes how consistent one clinical examiner is with herself over time. Internal reliability describes the extent to which two or more measures assess the same outcome; that is, the consistency of the tools that are measured by reliability tests such as Cronbach's Alpha and Spearman-Brown Split Half Coefficient. Stability reliability describes the extent to which the same measures remain consistent over time and is measured by the test-retest method. Equivalency reliability is the extent to which two or more outcomes co-occur; that is, the consistency of finding an association between measures. Importantly, equivalency reliability does not describe causal relationships but instead describes coincidental associations or correlations that are reported as correlation coefficients (r).

Several types of validity have also been described, but these generally fall into two main categories: internal validity and external validity (Colorado State University). Internal validity is concerned with how good the results of a study actually are in testing the hypothesis and, consequently, relates to factors inside the experiment or study design. One group of factors constitutes what may be viewed as the "rigor" of the study. These involve critical elements such as the appropriateness of the study design, whether or not correct decisions were made about what or what not to measure, and whether or not the methods and technical aspects of the study were carefully applied. Internal validity also establishes whether or not any cause-effect relationships have been identified and explained correctly, and if alternative explanations exist.

In contrast to internal validity, external validity is concerned with how well the results of the study can be generalized or transferred to larger groups or different populations. Consequently, external validity defines the applicability of the results beyond or outside the particular research investigation (i.e., generalizability). In simplest terms, the various types of validities can be considered as components of a logical hierarchy. The validity of a study increases as it answers the following levels of questions:

1) Is there a relationship between characteristic or variable X and characteristic or variable Y?
2) If yes, is this relationship causal (i.e., "If X, then Y")?
3) If yes, can this causal relationship be generalizable?

## Chance, Bias, and Confounds

The validity of a study can be diminished by a number of factors. Again, these generally fall into two main categories: internal validity-related and external validity-related. Internal validity is decreased when the study is not sufficiently controlled to be internally consistent. The main factors are chance, bias, and confounds (Colorado State University). Chance can be considered to be random error or experimental "noise." Causal associations may be found, or not found, merely due to chance error that can be reduced but never completely eliminated in research studies. The often published significance level of <0.05 is commonly interpreted to mean that the reported findings have only at most a 5% probability that they are due to chance alone. In other words, there is at least a 95% probability that the findings are real. Typically, the effect of chance on diminishing validity is not overly important in well-designed and -controlled studies.

In contrast with chance, factors that introduce bias into research studies are important to identify and eliminate or minimize. These affect the rigor of the study and lead to conclusions that deviate from reality. Bias can involve any aspect of the research process. Hawthorne-type effects are the well-known biases related to performance of the research subject, wherein the subject responds in certain ways due to self-awareness of being in a research study (i.e., placebo effect). Subjects also can exhibit recall bias, which is a systematic error due to differences in accuracy or completeness of their memory of past experiences. Repeated-order effects are biases introduced when subjects learn a test that is repeated the same way over time, which produces data on how well subjects learn to take the test instead of the knowledge that the test is intended to identify. Investigator bias can also be introduced due to the selective gathering of data, either subconsciously or consciously on the part of the investigator. Loss to follow-up bias often occurs in long-term prospective studies when subjects drop out and do not complete participation in the study for whatever reason.

Confounding factors are those that negatively affect the cause-effect determination of the study. In the "If X, then Y" scenario, outcome Y depends on characteristic X. Confounding factors are additional variables that coexist coincidentally along with the independent variable X that is being studied. These extraneous factors are sometimes readily identifiable and controlled, but they can also be poorly known or measurable variables that may be unrelated or related to the independent variable. If, for example, smokers were on average younger than nonsmokers in a study examining the effect of smoking on the outcome of periodontal guided tissue regeneration, then age might confound the results. In other words, it might be possible that the younger age (and putatively better healing potential) could offset the factor of smoking, unless the analysis is adjusted for age. When confounding factors are not adequately accounted for, it becomes highly likely that something else caused the effect that the investigators measured so reliably.

External validity is decreased when the study is based on a sample of the population that is not sufficiently accurate to allow generalizability. This occurs due to sampling errors such as selection bias, or errors in the study due to systematic differences in characteristics between study participants and nonparticipants. Generalizability is also indirectly influenced by publication bias, which is the unwillingness of most journals to publish negative results.

Finally, it is important to point out that researchers use a number of methods to reduce bias and confounds in study designs. Many of these methods are commonly known, for example, the use of double-blinding in clinical trials to reduce both subject and investigator bias. The use of placebo groups helps facilitate the generalizability of a study. Dropouts in long-term prospective clinical trials can be handled by an intent-to-treat analysis, which is a statistical method that allows incomplete data on a subject to be retained and analyzed rather than being discarded (i.e., lost to follow-up).

One way to control extraneous factors is through random assignment of subjects/samples to the experimental and control groups. Randomization is arguably the most important method to reduce selection bias and mitigate the effects of confounding variables, because any factor that participants bring to the study that might influence the outcome are randomly distributed across the groups. Researchers, and particularly statisticians, use a number of different randomization schemes to control for nuisance variables and ensure that experimental and control groups are equally matched except for the variable, intervention, or treatment of interest.

> There are also a number of important regulatory considerations in designing and conducting a research investigation.

## Institutional Review Boards

The use of humans as research subjects in university and industry studies is highly regulated. Federal and state regulations mandate that institutional review boards (IRB) review and approve all research that involves human subjects. The regulations specify the composition of the IRB, which must include scientific/medical experts, nonscientists, and outside consultants as needed. The IRB is charged with protecting the rights and welfare of human research subjects.

Protocols submitted to the IRB are judged according to three ethical principles: beneficence, justice, and respect for persons (US States Department of Health and Human Services). Beneficence refers to activities or actions that maintain or improve the well-being of subjects. The principle of beneficence obligates researchers to prevent harm and promote good. The principle of justice obligates researchers to ensure that both the risks and benefits of

research are distributed fairly across different groups and are not disproportionately borne by any one particular group. Respect for persons obligates researchers to treat individual research subjects as autonomous agents allowed to make informed choices freely. The primary expectation is that subjects will be respected as fellow human beings and not be viewed merely as means to an end.

The IRB determines whether risks to subjects, be they physical, psychological, sociological, or economic, are reasonable and justified given the potential benefits of the study. These benefits may be applicable to the individual research subject, to others in the larger population, and/or to the advancement of general knowledge. The IRB ensures that the consent process is clear, fair, and free from coercion. It also ensures that consent forms are written so that a layperson with a 7th- or 8th-grade education can understand exactly what he will undergo as part of the study. In addition, the IRB makes a judgment on how well subject confidentiality will be maintained. Privacy is an important consideration mandated by the federal Health Insurance Portability and Accountability Act (HIPAA), which regulates research activities as well as clinical practice.

It is interesting to note that the use of placebos as a method to control for bias and confounding factors in clinical trials is being questioned for ethical reasons. Such questions arise when researchers and IRBs consider the ethics and fairness of withholding treatment to subjects in the placebo or sham group, or continuing treatment in the experimental group, solely for the sake of the study. In drug trials, for example, the research is often discontinued before the study is completed when a drug is found to be effective. In such instances all subjects, including those in the placebo group, are then offered the use of the drug. On the other hand, drug trials are also terminated prematurely when a particular drug is found to be grossly ineffective or unacceptably dangerous. These decisions are made by the IRB, study-specific independent entities known as data safety and monitoring boards (DSMB), or data safety committees (DSC) during interim analyses performed at various times during the study. This illustrates how the protection of human subjects is a dynamic, ongoing process.

Journals require scientific papers to indicate that IRB approval was obtained for any research involving humans. This information typically is provided in the methods section of original reports.

## Institutional Animal Care and Use Committee

Universities and industry are sensitive to the ethical issues involved in using animals as research subjects. Federal, state, and local regulations ensure the humane treatment of animals in research studies, in particular nonhuman primates and other vertebrate animals. All universities are mandated to have an institutional animal care and use committee (IACUC) charged with overseeing such research (Office of Animal Care and Use). Like the IRB, the IACUC is composed of individuals having mandated expertise and interest in animal welfare. Specifically, the IACUC must include at least one doctor of veterinary medicine with training or experience in laboratory animal science, one practicing scientist experienced in research involving animals, one nonscientist layperson, and one individual who is not affiliated with the institution in any way other than as a member of the IACUC. Protocols submitted to the IACUC are reviewed for scientific merit and clear justification for the number and species of animals for which authorization is being requested. The IACUC is the legal mechanism through which institutions give researchers permission to purchase, house, and use animals specifically for research purposes.

Investigators submitting applications to the IACUC are required to demonstrate compliance with the three R's of animal research: reduction, refinement, and replacement. Reduction refers to decreasing the number of animals actually used in the study. Investigators must provide sample size and power calculations that justify the number of animals to be used, and they should use the fewest number of animals possible without compromising the statistical power of the study. Refinement refers to modifications in the research plan that lower the incidence or severity of pain and distress in the animals. The IACUC is especially concerned with animal pain and distress for practical as well as ethical reasons; animals respond to pain and distress with changes in their normal physiology that may skew any data being collected. Replacement refers to the substitution of nonsentient material for animals, or to the substitution of a lower species that might be less sensitive to pain and distress than a higher species. The replacement strategy also has a practical aspect; lower species tend to be less expensive to purchase, house, and feed.

As with human subject research, journals require scientific papers to indicate that IACUC approval was obtained for any research involving animals. This information typically is provided in the methods section of original reports.

## Laboratory Safety

Universities and industry are required to follow established regulations and standards for laboratory safety. These are designed not only to protect the researchers but also to ancillary and noninvolved personnel. Radiation safety committees, for example, oversee the use of radioactive materials and modalities, including radiographs and CT scans when performed for research purposes rather than routine clinical care. Biological safety committees ensure that dangerous microbes and recombinant genetic material are handled safely in approved settings. Investigators are required to be up to date with chemical safety (including material safety data sheets, or MSDS), fire safety, and infection control protocols. Although not usually indicated in scientific papers, it is presumed that the study has followed all applicable regulations.

> Testing of the hypothesis generates findings that are compiled, analyzed, and presented systematically (the "Results").

## Data Compilation

The specific aims and design of a particular study dictate how data are acquired. In all research investigations, the results must be collected systematically to minimize bias and ensure consistency and integrity. The collection process often follows predetermined rules for recording the data and also for sorting or reducing the data so that they can be managed effectively. This is especially true for large clinical trials that may be conducted across multiple locations.

The standard instrument for data collection in clinical trials is the case report form (CRF). Typically, these are paper or electronic forms specifically designed so that an investigator can record necessary information in an organized format that has a logical flow related to a specific visit or procedure for the research subject. For example, an important use of CRFs is to verify and document the eligibility (inclusion criteria) or ineligibility (exclusion criteria) of research subjects during the recruitment and enrollment phase of a study. CRFs are also designed to facilitate data transfer into electronic databases or spreadsheets for subsequent analysis. A large clinical study may use several different CRFs, depending on the number of variables or study characteristics that need to be measured and recorded. Appendix Figure 15.7 lists some examples of CRFs that might be used in clinical trials. Additional information on CRFs can be found in Incorporating Cancer Clinical Trials into Your Practice (Module 3) (National Cancer Institute).

## *Examples of Case Report Forms*

| General CRFs | Study-specific CRFs |
|---|---|
| • P.I. Verification Form | • Biomarker Forms |
| • Subject Enrollment Form | • Apoptotic Index |
| • Eligibility Form | • Cell Differentiation |
| • Subject Randomization | Biomarkers |
| Form | • Inflammatory Cytokines |
| • Medical History | • DNA Ploidy Analysis |
| • Physical Examination | • Inflammatory Cell Infiltrate |
| • Clinical Laboratory Data | • Intracrypt Apoptotic Index |
| • Compliance | • Nucleolar Morphometry |
| • Concomitant Medication | • PGE2 Levels |
| • Adverse Events | • Proliferation Analysis |
| • Off Study | • Nuclear Morphometry |
| • Death | |

See also: http://cme.cancer.gov/c02/s02/c3_4b_01.htm

Appendix Figure 15.7 Some types of case report forms (CRFs) that may be found in research studies. CRFs provide research investigators with standardized formats with which to record relevant data. These can be paper or electronic forms specifically designed to have a logical flow related to a specific visit or procedure for a given research subject or a particular test or laboratory measurement. Large clinical studies often use several different CRFs, depending on the number of variables or study characteristics that need to be measured and recorded. (Adapted from the public access Web site/online tutorial Incorporating Cancer Clinical Trials into Your Practice, National Cancer Institute, National Institutes of Health).

## Data Analysis

Data analysis, like data collection, must also be done systematically to ensure consistency and integrity of the research study. Myriad statistical methodologies, ranging from simple to complex, are available for analyzing data. These are described in original reports under the standard heading of "statistical analysis." The plan for statistical analysis follows predetermined rules for accepting or rejecting the data, characterizing the data, and identifying which statistical methods will be used. The use of professional statisticians is usually highly recommended, if not required, in complicated or large-scale research investigations. It is also important to note that data may be both quantitative and qualitative. Quantitative data are represented by actual numbers and are, consequently, considered to be objective in nature. Qualitative data are considered subjective in nature and are represented by comments, opinions, or impressions that may be collected from study participants in focus groups or by surveys, for example. Although a comprehensive discussion of statistical methodologies is beyond the scope of this chapter, it is useful to review some fundamental knowledge regarding quantitative data.

Quantitative data are characterized by a hierarchy according to their properties (TheReasearchAssistant).

These properties constitute a commonly described four-level scale: nominal, ordinal, interval, and ratio. Nominal data have the property of identity; that is, each number has a meaning such as "1" for female and "2" for male. Numbers in the nominal scale have no inherent magnitude, order, or linear relationship to each other. In contrast, ordinal data have both identity and magnitude; that is, the numbers can be ordered by size such as "mild," "moderate," or "severe." Although numbers in the ordinal scale can be ranked relative to each other, they have no quantitative linear relationship to each other. Numbers in the interval scale have fixed equal differences between them, for example, height in inches or attachment loss in millimeters. The ratio scale is identical to the interval scale with the additional property of having an absolute or true zero within the scale. That is, the number zero represents the absence of the characteristic that is being measured.

The properties of numbers determine which statistical tests may be applicable. For purposes of conducting statistical analyses, the four scales just described are collapsed into two types of data: categorical and continuous. Categorical data comprise those measured in categories or classes, and include those numbers that are nominal and ordinal. Continuous data comprise those measured on a numeric scale, thus representing a true quantity. Continuous data include interval and ratio numbers and are further classified as having a normal (bell curve) distribution or a non-normal (skewed or multimodal) distribution.

Both categorical and continuous data can be described by two general statistical approaches: descriptive and inferential. As the name implies, descriptive statistics are those that use procedures for describing or summarizing data, and are also called summary statistics. Inferential statistics use procedures for actually making inferences or drawing conclusions about the data.

Inferential statistics allow analyses to be made according to three levels: comparisons, associations, or predictive relationships. Statistical tests of comparison evaluate the properties or characteristics of two or more groups of variables to determine if there is a difference between the groups. Tests of association identify the existence of a relationship between two or more variables. Tests of prediction determine if one or more variables can be predicted by one or more other variables. Tests of prediction are also used to quantify the association between two or more variables. Inferential statistics are further classified as parametric and nonparametric. Parametric statistical procedures are those used for continuous data and generally require that the data be normally distributed. Nonparametric statistical procedures are those used for categorical data or non-normally distributed continuous data.

Appendix Tables 15.2 and 15.3 list the common descriptive and inferential statistical tests, respectively, used in research studies (TheResearchAssistant).

## Data Presentation

The development of the personal computer and a large variety of graphics software has led to an unfortunate tendency to overcomplicate figures by emphasizing the visual display over the data per se, which many times are relatively simple sets of numbers. As a consequence, the use of many different graphic effects can give the appearance that the data convey more information than actually may exist. An example of this is the increasing use of 3D or "depth" effects in published figures. The author of this chapter believes that figures in scientific reports should display data simply and efficiently. The noted statistician and expert in informational graphics, Edward Tufte, has succinctly noted that "What is to be sought in designs for the display of information is the clear portrayal of complexity" (Tufte 1983). Thus, the graphics should be the means to clearly and simply point out to the reader what important relationships may exist in the data.

Appendix Figure 15.8 presents data from an imaginary study of periodontal disease progression, measured in both smokers and nonsmokers one year after completion of some new type of experimental procedure. The figure may be viewed as visually plain, but it is quite effective in conveying important findings. Even without a figure legend to provide details about the study, the reader can quickly and easily evaluate the results that are displayed. The title at the top of the figure indicates that the graph depicts disease progression measured at a specified time after treatment has been provided in a clinical study on humans. The label of the Y-axis at the left of the figure specifies how disease progression was defined in this study; that is, sites that exhibited more than 1 mm of additional attachment loss during the posttreatment follow-up period. The label also indicates that the data are being reported as the average number of sites per subject in each group with disease progression, plus or minus the standard deviation. The label of the X-axis indicates that the two groups have been differentiated on the basis of smoking status, and also indicates how many subjects are included in each group. Of course, the figure does not provide all relevant information, nor is it necessarily expected to do so. The reader would need to review the methods section of the scientific paper, or the

**Appendix Table 15.2**   Common types of descriptive statistics (used for data summarization).

| Type of data | Statistical measure | |
| --- | --- | --- |
| | Measures of central tendency | Measures of dispersion |
| Continuous—for normally distributed continuous data | Mean: the numerical average of the observations | Range: the difference between the largest and smallest observation (i.e., the spread) |
| | Mode: the value corresponding to the most frequently occurring observation | Standard deviation: measures the spread around the mean |
| Continuous—for non-normally distributed continuous data | Median: the numerical value at which half of the observations occur above and half of the observations occur below this value (i.e., the 50th percentile) | Interquartile range: the spread occurring around the middle 50% of the observations (i.e., between the 25th and 75th percentiles) |
| | Mode: may also be used to describe non-normally distributed continuous data | |
| Categorical—for ordinal data | **Statistical measure** | |
| | Mode: again, the most frequent observation | |
| | Median: again, the middle observation; half the observations are smaller and half are larger | |
| | Frequency: quantifies the various observations according to occurrence | |
| | * Frequency expressed as counts: summarize the number of observations in each category | |
| | * Frequency expressed as proportions: summarize the percentage of total observations for each category | |
| Categorical—for nominal data | Mode: as above | |
| | Frequency: as above (both counts and proportions) | |
| | (Note: the use of the median is not appropriate for nominal data) | |

Appendix Table 15.3  Common types of inferential statistics (used for data analysis).

| Type of data | Types of test | | |
| --- | --- | --- | --- |
| | Tests of comparison (reported as the particular test statistic, ex. t, $\chi^2$ [Chi-squared], or U) | Tests of association (reported as the correlation coefficient [r] or the ratio value) | Tests of prediction (reported as the regression value [$R^2$]) |
| Parametric—for normally distributed continuous data | t-test (Students): compares two means<br>*One-sample t-test: compares the mean from your observations to a standard or norm value<br>*Two-sample t-test: compares the means from your observations of two independent groups<br>*Paired t-test: compares the means from two Independent observations from one group<br>Analysis of variance (ANOVA): compares three or more means either between or within groups | Pearson correlation coefficient: measures the relationship between two variables or observations within one group | Linear regression: used when the outcome (i.e., dependent) variables are continuous (either normally or non-normally distributed) or ordinal |
| Nonparametric—for ordinal or non-normally distributed continuous data | Wilcoxon signed-ranks test: compares median from your observation to a standard or norm value | Spearman's rho: measures the relationship between the ranks of two variables or observations within one group | Linear regression: used when the outcome (i.e., dependent) variables are continuous (either normally or non-normally distributed) or ordinal |
| | Mann-Whitney U test: compares medians from two independent groups<br>Wilcoxon matched-pairs signed-ranks test: compares two Independent medians from one group<br>Kruskal-Wallis test: compares medians from three or more independent groups<br>Friedman test: compares medians for three or more observations from one group | Kendall's tau: similar to Spearman's correlation coefficient | |
| Nonparametric—for nominal data | Binomial sign test: compares counts or proportions for your observation with a population standard | Relative risk: the chance of an outcome occurring relative to the presence of a risk or predisposing factor; used with cohort or clinical trial studies in which patient is followed over time | Logistic regression: used when the outcome (i.e., dependent) variables are nominal; often used when outcome data are dichotomous (e.g., bleeding-on-probing positive and bleeding-on-probing negative) |
| | Chi-square test: compares counts or proportions for data from two or more independent groups (including a standard or norm value)<br>Fisher's exact test: compares counts or proportions for data from two or more independent groups (including a standard or norm value)<br>McNemar test: compares counts or proportions for two observations from one group<br>Cochran Q test: compares counts or proportions for three or more observations from one group | Odds ratio: the chance that a group with a particular outcome was exposed to a particular risk or predisposing factor; used with case-control or cross-sectional studies | |

figure legend that may accompany the illustration, to learn additional information such as the age, gender, or racial characteristics of the subjects, how the smoking status was defined, and what comprised the experimental treatment.

Nonetheless, the figure readily illustrates that the two groups of subjects, smokers and nonsmokers, had little difference in disease progression. The figure effectively communicates research findings without unnecessary fanfare.

**Appendix Figure 15.8** Presentation of findings from an imaginary study of periodontal disease progression measured in smokers and nonsmokers one year after completion of a new type of experimental procedure. Although the data can be presented by several different graphical formats, the graphic illustrated here effectively conveys the results. It should be noted that some investigators prefer graphics that show the actual range and scatter of data points, in addition to the mean score. Similarly, some investigators advocate the use of illustrations that minimize the "ink area" in the graphic. The graphic layout illustrated here is one type commonly seen in scientific papers.

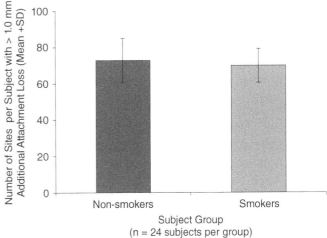

Disease Progression in Humans with Agrressive Periodontitis 12 Months after Experimental Treatment

---

> The results of a scientific investigation are explained according to the available literature and within the limitations of the study design (the "Discussion").

The discussion section of a scientific paper is often the most difficult section to write, especially for newer investigators. Whereas the introduction provides the background literature to justify the study, the discussion focuses primarily on the prior literature that supports and/or contradicts the findings of the present study. Thus, the discussion section serves to explain the results in the context of existing knowledge about the research topic.

Although scientific journals have varying guidelines governing the length, extent, and logical flow of discussion sections, most require that certain key components be presented. The majority of the discussion presents the authors' own interpretation of their results, including reasons for agreement or disagreement with the published findings of other investigators. Important relationships among the results are emphasized, as well as the perceived usefulness. The discussion describes how the present results confirm existing knowledge or, due to the use of newer or improved techniques, indicate that previously published findings need to be reinterpreted. Well-written discussion sections also discuss the critical factors that influenced the study's findings, specifically those variables that may have diminished reliability and validity.

The appropriateness of the study design in answering the research question is often described, as are potential limitations of the techniques and measurements performed in the study. Some investigators prefer to restate briefly the most significant findings of their study, usually in the opening paragraph of the discussion. This is not necessarily required but, when provided, does help focus the reader on data having the most relevancy or generalizability. This is especially true for high-impact studies that provide evidence for a novel concept or new scientific field. Alternatively, the authors may choose to present the most important findings as topic sentences in separate paragraphs throughout the discussion. Discussion sections typically end with concluding remarks that present the "take-home message" of the study, and that may identify additional work that should be performed in the future.

> The results often may have more than one interpretation, or lead to additional questions that might warrant further investigation.

If the study design and specific protocols are both appropriate and well executed, and if the data are appropriately evaluated, the results of any given study will be credible regardless of whether the results are expected, unexpected, or even disappointing to the researchers. That is to say, the data themselves "are what they are" and should be unequivocal. What may be equivocal, on the other hand, is how such data are interpreted. Caution is required in reading the discussion section of original reports because this is where the authors interpret their results according to their own professional opinions. Alternative viewpoints may be possible and equally viable, so that many times the research data may be interpreted in more than one way.

Let us return to Appendix Figure 15.8. Such graphics usually indicate if the measurements exhibit statistically significant differences, for example, by an asterisk drawn above the bars. Because no asterisk or other indication is shown, we can reasonably conclude that the two groups of subjects, smokers and nonsmokers, had no difference in disease progression. This would be the primary finding that the figure serves to illustrate. However, other information can also be gleaned from the figure. On closer inspection it appears that subjects in both groups continued to demonstrate aggressive disease, because some 60–70 sites per subject had disease progression measurable one year after treatment. Assuming that each tooth was measured at six sites in 28 teeth, then a range of about 10–28 teeth per subject had additional attachment loss.

The experienced reader would wonder why these subjects were so prone to continued disease. Was the experimental treatment grossly ineffective? Was there a control aggressive periodontitis group that received no treatment at all (and would withholding treatment be ethical)? Was there something particularly unique about the subjects in this study? Could the findings be explained by the presence of a very aggressive (i.e., extremely downhill) subset of subjects, who just happened to be recruited into the study by chance? If so, could this subgroup account for most of the continued disease progression measured in the study? Could the definition of disease progression be too stringent? Would a cut-off value of 2 mm or 3 mm possibly show a difference between smokers and nonsmokers? These are the types of questions that are intended to be asked when the reader is exhibiting the important, albeit overused, notion of critical thinking. Critical thinking is the hallmark of so-called evidence-based dentistry or medicine. Stated simply, critical thinking implies that the informed reader decides for herself how to interpret the data.

Let us consider another imaginary example. A study reports retrospective data on patient mortality rates following cardiac bypass surgery in three different hospitals, A, B, and C. The data is reported in terms of absolute numbers of deaths and show that hospital C has the highest number of patient deaths after the procedure.

Assuming that the study is appropriately designed, powered, and evaluated, what can be concluded about hospital C? It is tempting to conclude that hospital C is worse than hospitals A or B; specifically, that the surgeons and the postsurgical care are not as good as in the other two hospitals. But, do we have sufficient information to support this conclusion? Would our interpretation be different if we knew that hospital C performs many more procedures than hospitals A or B? That is, how do the numbers of deaths compare to the overall caseloads in the three different hospitals, when expressed as a percentage of total procedures? Would

our interpretation again be different if we knew that hospital C performs the procedure primarily on very sick patients not usually treated at hospitals A or B? That is, what would we conclude about hospital C if the data were normalized to the patient status and show that hospital C has markedly lower percent death rates for the sickest patients than do the other two hospitals? Perhaps our take-home message would be that the surgeons and the postsurgical care at hospital C are actually better than in the other two hospitals, especially when patients are severely compromised.

These examples point out the widely accepted view that a good study leaves one with more questions than answers, provided that the hypothesis, study design, and methodology have been appropriate.

---

Research requires intellectual, technical, and financial resources that must be planned for and acknowledged (the "Acknowledgements").

---

The cliché that nothing in life is free certainly is applicable to biomedical research. Research investigations have inherent costs that must be paid for somehow. Typically, funding for research in dental schools is derived from both intramural and extramural sources. Intramural funds are those provided to the researchers by the school or university to help establish a laboratory or clinical research center and to allow preliminary work that will allow the researchers to compete for extramural funding. Extramural sources are government, industry, and philanthropic organizations. It is widely appreciated that a good deal of researchers' time and energy are devoted to the arduous task of securing financial support for their research endeavors. As a consequence, these sources of support are gratefully acknowledged in published reports.

Extramural funding helps to defray both direct and indirect expenses of a study. As the name implies, direct costs are those incurred in the actual conduct of the study. These include a number of large- and small-scale expenses such as labor, materials, subject-related payments, consultant fees, statistical analyses, publication costs, travel to professional conferences, and even photocopying and mailing expenses. Indirect costs are those associated with overhead expenses incurred due to facilities-related costs, such as electricity, heating, and air conditioning, and to administrative costs such as grants management personnel, within the dental school and university. Not surprisingly, these indirect expenses are referred to as facilities and administration (F and A) costs and, although not directly related to a particular research question, must also be accounted for when conducting research. Thus, the total cost of a research study is the sum of direct and F and A costs.

Significant nonfinancial support is also acknowledged. This type of support may be quite varied, and could include collaborative arrangements with other investigators for the use of equipment, supplies, and technical help. Intellectual support, in the form of advice and technical training from colleagues, is also acknowledged. Many times, key administrative personnel on a research study are given a special "thank you" by the authors.

## Conclusion

The research process typically begins with a proposal to obtain funding for the work, and ends with a published report to communicate the findings of the work. Research writing is the modality by which the research process and outcomes are communicated to the profession. This chapter has described the key components involved both in the research process and in the writing and reading of a scientific paper. The underlying aim has been to point out the necessity of critical thinking in evaluating the scientific merits of any given research study.

In conclusion, it should be added that good studies are those worthy of being reported by the researchers and read by the practicing professionals. Good studies are those that have addressed an important question and have provided valuable insight into a particular area. In turn, a well-written paper offers the reader a sense of excitement and a desire for even more knowledge in the subject area.

## References

Callas, P.W. (2008). Searching the biomedical literature: research study designs and critical appraisal. *Clin. Lab. Sci.* 21 (1): 42–48.

Centers for Disease Control and Prevention (1999). Adapted from guidelines for defining public health research and public health non-research. United States Department of Health and Human Services. (revised 4 October 1999). http://www.cdc.gov/od/science/regs/hrpp/researchdefinition.htm (accessed 14 September 2008).

Colorado State University. Overview: reliability and validity, an online writing course. http://writing.colostate.edu/guides/research/relval (accessed 14 September 2008).

Danya International, Inc. (2005). Computing sample size for scientific studies: a non-technical overview. In: "TheResearchAssistant," a comprehensive web-based resource developed by Danya International, Inc., through the Small Business Innovation Research Program funded by the National Institute on Drug Abuse, National Institutes of Health (Contract No. N44DA-8–5060).

(revised 22 August 2005). http://www.theresearchassistant.com/tutorial/4-power.asp# (accessed 14 September 2008).

Fleiss, J.L., Park, M.H., Chilton, N.W. et al. (1987). Representativeness of the "Ramfjord teeth" for epidemiologic studies of gingivitis and periodontitis. *Community Dent. Oral. Epidemiol.* 15 (4): 221–224.

International Committee of Medical Journal Editors (2007). Uniform requirements for manuscripts submitted to biomedical journals: writing and editing for biomedical publication. (Revised October 2007). http://www.icmje.org (accessed 14 September 2008).

Loe. H. and Silness, J. (1963). Periodontal disease in pregnancy. I. Prevalence and severity. *Acta. Odontologica. Scand.* 21: 533–551.

Markinson. A. Evidence based medicine course. State University of New York Downstate. http://library.downstate.edu/EBM2/2100.htm (accessed 14 September 2008).

National Cancer Institute. Incorporating cancer clinical trials into your practice (Module 3). *National Institutes of Health.* http://cme.cancer.gov/c02/s02/c3_4b_01.htm (accessed 14 September 2008).

Office of Animal Care and Use. Animal care and use. US Department of Health and Human Services. http://oacu.od.nih.gov (accessed 14 September 2008).

PubMed. Home page. US national library of medicine and national institutes of health. http://www.pubmed.gov (accessed 14 September 2008).

Richards. D. (2007). Creating a DEBT. *Evid. Based Dent.* 8 (2): 35–36. Editorial in Evidence-Based Dentistry. 8, 2. doi: 10.1038/sj.ebd.6400484. http://www.nature.com/ebd/journal/v8/n2/full/6400484a.html.

TheResearchAssistant. Statistical support on the web. http://www.theresearchassistant.com/research/link.asp (accessed 14 September 2008).

The Writing Center. University of Wisconsin-Madison home page. http://www.wisc.edu/writing (accessed 14 September 2008).

Trochim, W.M. (2006). *The Research Methods Knowledge Base,* 2e. revised October 2, 2006. http://www.socialresearch-methods.net/kb. This is a comprehensive web-based textbook that covers the entire research process including formulating research questions, sampling, measurement, research design, data analysis, reliability of measures, study validity, ethics, and writing the research paper.

Tufte, E.R. (1983). *The Visual Display of Quantitative Information.* Graphics Press. 191.

US States Department of Health and Human Services. IRB Guidebook. Office for Human Research Protections. http://www.hhs.gov/ohrp/irb/irb_guidebook.htm (accessed 14 September 2008).

Whitley, E. and Ball, J. (2002). Statistics review 4: sample size calculations. *Crit. Care.* 6 (4): 335–341. Epub May 10, 2002.

# Index

Please note: Page numbers is *italics* refer to figures and those in **bold** refer to tables.

*Practical Periodontal Diagnosis and Treatment Planning,* Second Edition. Edited by Serge Dibart and Thomas Dietrich.
© 2024 John Wiley & Sons, Inc. Published 2024 by John Wiley & Sons, Inc.